500 of the most important WAYS TO STAY YOUNGER LONGER

500 of the most important WAYS TO
STAY
YOUNGER
LONGER

The Ultimate A–Z Guide
to Anti-Ageing

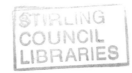
Daily Mail Columnist
Hazel Courteney
with Robert H Jacobs, Shane Heaton, Stephen Langley

CICO BOOKS

London

First published in Great Britain by
Cico Books
32 Great Sutton Street
London EC1V 0NB

Copyright © Cico Books 2003

Text copyright © Hazel Courteney 2003

10 9 8 7 6 5 4 3 2

A CIP catalogue record for this book is available from the British Library.

ISBN 1 903116 58 9

Front cover photograph copyright © Rex
Design by Paul Wood
Edited by Mary Lambert
Printed and bound in Singapore by Tien Wah Press

Hazel Courteney is an award winning journalist, author and broadcaster who has spent the past 10 years researching, documenting and lecturing on advances in alternative medicine. In 1997, she was voted Health Journalist of the Year for her alternative health columns in *The Sunday Times* and *The Daily Mail*. She is currently working on the sequel to **Divine Intervention**, which will be her seventh book. Her website is at: www.hazelcourteney.com

Other Books by Hazel Courteney include:
What's The Alternative ? – Boxtree MacMillan
Mind and Mood Foods – Reader's Digest
Body and Beauty Foods – Reader's Digest
Divine Intervention – Cico Books
500 of the Most Important Health Tips You'll Ever Need – Cico Books

Robert H. Jacobs NMD, PhD, HMD, DipHom (MED) is the medical director for the Society for Complementary Medicine. He practises naturopathy and is a member of the British Naturopathic Medical Association, The General Register of Naturopaths and the Homoeopathic Medical Association UK. He has been practising natural medicine since 1975 and specializes in immune system function, hormone balance, brain chemistry, metabolism, and nutrition. Tel: 0207 487 4334.

Shane Heaton Dip.ION is a clinical nutritionist trained at the Institute for Optimum Nutrition in London. He is the author of the much acclaimed Soil Association report *Organic Farming, Food quality and Human Health* published in May 2002. Up until June 2002, Shane ran a busy nutritional practice in London, but he has now returned to live and work in Australia where he continues to practise as a nutritionist. He specializes in research, but also gives lectures and writes health features for numerous publications including the ION magazine. He currently works in the USA and Australia. You can reach him via shane@dontjustsurvive.com

Stephen Langley ND, DipHom, DBM, DipAc, OMD is a Registered Naturopath, Homoeopath, Acupuncturist, Doctor of Chinese Medicine and Medical Herbalist. He lectures in Naturopathic Medicine at the College of Naturopathic Medicine (CNM) in London, Dublin, Galway and Belfast as well as running a busy health practice at The Hale Clinic in London and lecturing globally. Stephen has studied Holistic Medicine in China, India, America, Australia, Tibet and Japan. He can be reached via the Hale Clinic in London on 0870 167 6667.

For Stuart.
For being so very special.

ACKNOWLEDGMENTS

Within a month of beginning this book, I realized that the subject of "ageing" is more complex than even I had imagined. And so I enlisted the help of three wonderful men who have endured endless questions, phone calls and e-mails as well as helping with specific conditions in which they have clinical experience and encyclopedic knowledge.

Bob, I thank you and Peta with all my heart for your invaluable contribution to this book – and for being such wonderful, patient and dear friends.

To Steve, thank you for all those journeys from Surrey on the M25 in the rush hour, for the acupuncture to help me sleep, and for sharing so much of your knowledge and experience. You are a true friend.

To Shane, England is a sadder place now that you have left. You are a rising star in the alternative health field and Australia is lucky to have you. I thank you all for your commitment and professionalism, which I will never forget.

Enormous thanks also to my friend Dr Keith Scott-Mumby, a nutritional physician based in London and Manchester who gave me some great interviews, copy and advice which is featured throughout the book.

Thanks to nutritionist and founder of the Institute for Optimum Nutrition, Patrick Holford, for a great interview, for being a good friend and for allowing me to use his Anti-Cancer Diet.

Big hugs to nutritionist Kerrin Booth for checking seemingly endless subjects and for all her advice and kindness – I thank you.

Heartfelt thanks to my ex-secretary Lindsey Ross-Jarrett, for coming to my rescue yet again, by doing all the layouts and checking every phone number in her "spare" time. You are a star.

And a big thank-you to all the doctors, surgeons, scientists and experts named throughout the book who helped me with their speciality subjects.

To Debbie Heron, my true and dear friend, thank you for your back massages, your magical Reiki healing – and most of all – for listening.

To Said and Pat – thank you for coming back, and for all your healthy food.

Finally to my husband Stuart, for keeping your temper, and for your unflinching support during the last eight months. I could not have done it without you baba. You really are the best.

INTRODUCTION

A woman born today has a 40% chance of living to 150. Within 15 years, 1.2 billion people, that's 1 in 5 of us will be over 65 – and more than one million people will be aged 100 or more. And if you choose – with help from this book – to begin taking more care of yourself from today onwards, you will have a far greater chance to live a healthy, active and useful life until you are 100 or more.

You will discover how amino acids like carnosine have been proven to regenerate ageing cells, which in turn help to regenerate your skin, brain and muscles. You will discover the main causes of ageing, from free radicals and insulin resistance to Syndrome X, toxicity and pollution. Find out why sugar is one of the most ageing foods you can eat and what you can do to reverse the damage; also, how to use the proven power of your mind to slow and reverse many of the physical signs of ageing.

Find out the difference between stem cell therapy and live cell therapy – and discover how to rejuvenate yourself inside and out with the latest anti-ageing therapies such as chelation with added nutrients, which is now available.

In the West, the majority of women seem to think it's necessary to lie about their chronological age, but there are many parts of the world where old age is revered and inhabitants often add years to their true age, and consider someone aged 100 as being young. They are respected for their wisdom and common sense. On the island of Okinawa near Japan, at the time of going to press, there are 427 residents aged over 100 in a population of just 1.27 million. Of the Hunza people of Northern Pakistan, the Vilcambamba in Equador and the people of Georgia in Russia – almost all live, happy, useful and healthy lives. Externally these people may look weather-beaten and aged, but internally their cells stay far younger than those of people living in "modern" societies. These people hardly suffer age-related diseases. They experience 80% fewer heart attacks, and less than a quarter of Western levels of breast, ovarian and prostate cancer. In their women, the menopause usually arrives 10 years later than their Western counterparts – and the majority have never heard of HRT. They do not understand the concept of retirement, and remain active and involved in their local community all their lives.

But in so called "civilized" societies, youth and the pursuit of it, has for many people become an all-consuming obsession, which can reduce their quality of life. From the covers of practically every glossy magazine, stare the stunning, flawless, line-free faces of teenage models. Every TV station seems to cater for the under thirties – this is the age of youth.

When I was seventeen, I vividly remember admiring the skin of a girlfriend who was 25, and saying "I hope my skin looks that good when I get to your age!" It was pathetic, and yet I thought everyone over 25 was positively ancient. My views have changed somewhat over the years, but I remain fascinated as to why we age. Scientists are now on the verge of offering us ways to become ageless and, more than ever before in our history, we now have access to knowledge that can help us turn back the clock.

In this book, we have done our best to share with you hundreds of ways, that if you begin today, will enable you to stay younger for longer.

Above all, this book is all about choices, about living consciously at every level. You can choose what you eat to help yourself to live longer – but food is also meant to be fun. And so I invite you to eat and live more consciously. For instance, if you decide to live on croissants, cappucinos, fast food and vodka-martinis, have insufficient sleep, smoke and so on – and that is your conscious choice – then don't be surprised when your skin wrinkles prematurely and your bones begin to thin. It was your choice.

Living consciously, and making more right choices could save our ailing health service. Late-onset diabetes, which is totally preventable, costs the NHS £5.2 billion a year, smoking £1.5 billion, alcohol related illnesses £3 billion and obesity £500 million – all because we make too many wrong choices. We have forgotten the need for balance in all things.

Having said this, believe me I'm no saint, I love apple crumble with whipped cream and adore organic chocolate, but I eat my treats consciously. I also eat plenty of healthy organic foods, exercise, meditate and take anti-ageing supplements.

I want to have fun too. You do not have to become a slave to a regimen which restricts your life and makes you miserable, and so my conscious choice is to take a middle path. The calorie restricted diet of raw foods and sprouting grains, which has been proven to reverse many biological markers of ageing, is not for me – but if you choose to take that path – then I wish you a long and happy life. It's all about choice.

Currently, the longest-lived mammals appear to be whales and some species are known to survive over 2 centuries. If we lived in a perfect stress-free world, eating fresh, seasonal, organic food, taking regular exercise, breathing fresh air and so on, there would be no reason, logically, why one day we could not do the same.

Right now, we live in a less-than-perfect world, but if were all willing to live more consciously, be more adaptable, positive, and practise more prevention, then without doubt the world could become a far healthier place and we could all live and look younger – for longer.

From today you need to forget your chronological age, as you cannot change your birthday, but you can change the rate at which your cells age. Begin thinking young, don't become fanatical about ageing – as the worrying will age you even faster – and above all, enjoy your journey.

Hazel Courteney, November 2002.

IMPORTANT HINTS YOU NEED TO KNOW ABOUT TAKING SUPPLEMENTS

- If you are taking any prescription drugs – you should advise your doctor of any supplements or herbs you wish to take – in case of contraindications. For instance the drug Warfarin thins the blood – but so does vitamin E, garlic, fish oils and the herb ginkgo biloba. If you decide to begin taking supplements, you would need to have regular blood tests. In time, by eating a good diet, taking the right supplements, and with your doctor's permission, your drug intake can hopefully be reduced.

- Never use supplements as a substitute for a healthy, balanced diet. If you really want to stay younger longer, you need to do it all!

- When taking fat-soluble nutrients such as Vitamin E, Co Enzyme Q 10 and Vitamin K – take them with a little fatty food such as a salad with French dressing, a little avocado or a slice of buttered toast to aid absorption.

- Suppliers of portable toilets report that large numbers of vitamin/mineral pills (and prescription drugs) can pass through the body undigested, and that they can even read the manufacturer's name on the pills and capsules! Read the section on *Absorption* for more help.

- If you take vitamin E as part of your anti-ageing regimen – then ask for full-spectrum natural-source vitamin E that contains tocoperols and tocotrienols, which taken together have a greater anti-ageing effect.

- If you are on a detoxification programme, don't take too many supplements – as these for the most part need to be metabolized by the liver. Powdered green food supplements at this time would be most beneficial – see under *Detoxing*.

- Supplements taken regularly in the long-term almost always produce beneficial effects, but don't expect miracles overnight. Supplements are not magic bullets, but stimulate the body's natural healing processes to encourage the body to heal itself

- Never self-medicate with hormone supplements that are freely available over the counter in many countries and on the web – always find out if you need them first.

- In most cases, supplementation with nutrients produces improvements in health more slowly than prescription medications, which normally just suppress symptoms. If you start a course of vitamins, minerals or any supplements, take them regularly for at least two months in order to see the benefits. Any changes in your health may be very subtle.

- Many supplements currently on the market have less than optimum quantities of beneficial ingredients. In general, you get what you pay for. Some low-priced supplements contain relatively small amounts of nutrients or forms of nutrients. The better-quality, and usually more expensive, supplements generally provide better value for money in the long-term. All the companies I recommend on pages 13 and 14 are known to sell good-quality supplements. Remember that vitamins, minerals, essential fatty acids and essential sugars (see *Essential Sugars*) are nutrients essential to life, but herbs are powerful medicines. Many prescription drugs are based on herbs. nutrients essential to life, but herbs are powerful medicines. Many prescription drugs are based on herbs.

■ Herbs are not essential to life, but when taken in the appropriate amounts and for the appropriate time, have proven to be of benefit for many conditions. Generally, take herbs for no more than three months at a time, have a month or so without them and then if you feel the need, or under supervision, begin taking them again.

■ Do not take extra iron supplements if you are over 50, unless you have been diagnosed with a medical condition that requires extra supplementation, as iron accumulates in the body and is linked to heart problems. Always keep iron tablets away from children.

■ Keep all supplements away from young children. Any substance (including water) taken to excess can cause negative side effects. Follow the manufacturer's or your health professional's instructions.

■ Most vitamins have a good shelf life but cease to be effective if you keep them for too long. Be aware of sell-by dates and always keep your vitamins in a cool, dry place – don't expose them to direct sunlight.

■ Supplements should be taken with food unless otherwise stated on the label, as it aids absorption.

■ Amino acids such as Carnosine, L Glutamine and so on are best taken on an empty stomach about 30 minutes before food, or in-between meals. Follow the directions on the label.

■ Some people have reactions to certain supplements but this is quite rare. Reactions are usually caused not by the nutrients themselves but by a reaction to one or more of the other ingredients contained in the supplement. In general, better-quality supplements containing hypoallergenic ingredients are less likely to give rise to adverse reactions.

■ If you take Niacin, a B vitamin, unless directed to do otherwise **always ask for the no-flush variety**, or your skin will turn a bright lobster red for around 45 minutes!

■ B vitamins cause your urine to turn a deep yellow-orange colour which is perfectly normal.

■ If you suffer a negative reaction to any supplement or herb, stop taking it immediately, and consult a health professional. For example, most Glucosamine supplements are derived from crushed crab shells – so if you are highly sensitive to shellfish – avoid this supplement.

■ Vitamin C is more effective when taken in repeated small doses throughout the day. It should always be taken with food. Ask for a non-acidic ascorbate or esther form, which is less likely to upset the stomach in cases of sensitivity.

- The supplements suggested in this book can be taken by anyone over the age of 16. For children's dosages, or if pregnant, seek professional guidance.
- Probiotics (or friendly bacteria) more commonly known as acidophilus should also contain bifidus strain bacteria. All probiotic preparations keep better in glass bottles and should be kept either in a fridge or freezer. Take these with or after meals. You can now buy coated acidophilus capsules to use when travelling that don't need to be kept in the fridge.
- If you are pregnant, or planning a pregnancy, do not take any supplement containing more than 3000iu of vitamin A. Most manufacturers state whether supplements are unsuitable during pregnancy.
- If you have any problem taking pills, and cannot find liquid formulas at your health shop, use an inexpensive tablet crusher. To order call Health Plus on 01323 737374 www.healthplus.co.uk
- If you are suffering from any form of cancer, especially hormone related cancer, avoid soya based products. If in doubt, please consult a health professional.

If you are in any doubt about the amount of supplements you or your children should be taking – always consult a qualified health practitioner.

HOW TO USE THIS BOOK

Throughout this book we have suggested various remedies which are now widely available in health shops and many supermarkets worldwide. In case you cannot find certain new or more specialist supplements, I have given the name of the company that manufactures them or a retail outlet where they can be found – and all these contact details are on this and the following page.

There are hundreds of brands and if we had tried to name them all, this book would never have been completed. Therefore the companies listed here are those that I trust, and I have used many of their products for several years. I do not in any way wish to infer that other brands are inferior or less effective. All the companies mentioned, and all reputable vitamins companies, have their own in-house, trained nutritionist who can give you advice. Even if you don't want to buy their supplements, don't be afraid to ask for help. All these companies are happy to post their products worldwide.

BioCare Ltd
Lakeside, 180 Lifford Lane, Kings Norton, Birmingham B30 3NU
Tel: 0121 433 3727
Fax: 0121 433 3879
Sales Fax: 0121 433 8705
E-mail: biocare@biocare.co.uk
Website: www.biocare.co.uk

Blackmores UK
Willow Tree Marina, West Quay Drive, Reading, Middlesex UB4 9TA
Tel: 0870 7700976
Fax: 020 8841 7557
E-mail: sales@nhb-company.co.uk

The Health and Diet Company
GNC Direct, PO Box 5736 Freepost MID23007, Burton on Trent DE14 1BR
Mail Order: 0845 601 3248
E-mail: customerservices@gnc.co.uk
Website: www.gnc.co.uk

Higher Nature Ltd
The Nutrition Centre, Burwash Common, East Sussex TN19 7LX
Tel: 01435 884 668 (Sales Line)
E-mail: info@higher-nature.co.uk
Nutrition Department E-mail: nutrition@higher-nature.co.uk
Website: www.higher-nature.co.uk

Kudos Vitamins and Herbal

2nd Floor, Parkway House, Sheen Lane, East Sheen, London SW14 8LS
Freephone in the UK: 0800 3895476
Tel: 020 8392 6524
Fax: 020 8392 6540
E-mail: info@kudosvitamins.com
Website: www.kudosvitamins.com

The NutriCentre

The Hale Clinic, 7 Park Crescent, London W1N 3HE
The Hale Clinic's Main Number is: 0870 167 6667
For the NutriCentre, tel: 020 7436 5122
Fax: 020 7436 5171
Bookshop Tel: 020 7323 2382
E-mail: enq@nutricentre.com
Website: www.nutricentre.com

Pharm West Inc

4640 Admiralty Way, Suite 423, Marina Del Rey, California, USA 90292
Tel in UK: FREEPHONE 00 800 8923 8923
Tel in Ireland: 00 35 3469 437 317
E-mail: info@pharmwest.com

The Sloane Health Shop

27 King's Road, Chelsea, London SW3 4RT
Tel: 020 7730 7046

Solgar Vitamin and Herb Company (UK)

Aldbury, Tring, Hertfordshire HP23 5PT
Tel: 01442 890355
Fax: 01442 890366
E-mail: solgarinfo@solgar.com (for general/sales enquiries, not orders)
Website: www.solgar.com

Solgar Vitamin and Herb Company (USA)

500 Frank W. Burr Boulevard, Teaneck, Jersey, NJ07666,USA
Tel: +1 201 944 2311 or +1 201 944 7351

AUTHOR'S NOTE

Throughout this book Bob, Shane, Steve and myself have in many instances suggested specific amounts of certain nutrients. This is to ensure that sufficient amounts of these nutrients are taken to benefit a specific condition. In places where no specific amounts are recommended, take the supplements daily, according to the instructions on the label, or on the advice of your health professional.

We have mentioned numerous books that we have found useful, but whatever you are suffering from, believe us, there is a specialist book out there waiting to be read.

This book is not intended as a substitute for medical counselling. Never stop taking prescribed medicines without first consulting your doctor. It is wise to inform your doctor of any supplements or herbs you are taking in case they are contraindicated with any prescription drugs you may be taking.

During the past 15 or so years, Bob, Steve, Shane and I have read hundreds of books and research papers and we have retained many phrases and facts. Wherever possible, we have acknowledged the source of these phrases and facts. And to any whose names we have forgotten, our apologies for any unintentional oversight.

ABSORPTION

(See also *Diet, Digestion* and *Stomach*)

We are not only what we eat, but also what we can absorb and eliminate. In fact it's a false assumption to believe that whatever you swallow is automatically absorbed into your system: there is a vital intermediate stage. You swallow food, and if you chew it thoroughly, amylase, an enzyme in your saliva, begins breaking down your food. But as we age, levels of amylase fall. For instance, it is 30 times more abundant in the average 25 year-old than the average 80 year-old.

The chewing process also alerts the stomach that food is coming, which triggers stomach acid production, ready to begin the digestion process. Chewing is the first and very important stage of digestion. Your stomach does not have any teeth!

And with ageing, stomach acid production is also reduced. Without these natural digestive aids, absorption of nutrients through our gut walls and into the bloodstream is greatly diminished. Therefore valuable nutrients needed for tissue repair and cellular regeneration can in some instances pass through the body and out the other end undigested.

As the pace of modern life is increasing, more and more people, even young people, suffer varying degrees of absorption problems.

Stress also has a negative effect on the digestive process as it reduces absorption, and greatly increases the ageing process (see also *Stress*).

Symptoms of malabsorption include hair loss, low energy levels, chronic fatigue, weight loss or gain, poor bone density, dry and wrinkled skin, hair and nails. Naturopath, Steve Langley says:

"Almost all disease is linked to deficiency of nutrients and toxicity within the body, therefore if you get your digestive system in good working order, a huge amount of age-related diseases could be avoided."

Foods to Avoid

■ Reduce your intake of red meats and heavy, rich meals. Concentrated proteins and fats such as red meat and cheese are generally harder to digest as they require more oxygen to break them down completely. We need to maintain a high oxygen level in our tissues to slow the ageing process. And all junk foods reduce oxygen levels and accelerate loss of enzyme reserves in the body.

■ Avoid too much junk food especially croissants, burgers, fried foods, high-sugar foods and full-fat dairy produce. The more unnatural your diet the more the body has to produce enzymes to digest them, and over time symptoms emerge.

■ Cooked cheese is really hard on your digestive system.

■ Modern refined wheat and related products are often hard for us to digest as we lack the necessary enzymes.

■ Avoid drinking too much fluid with meals, which dilutes the stomach acid – the very substance you need for digesting your food.

Friendly Foods

■ Raw or lightly cooked foods contain enzymes, which aid digestion. Papaya is rich in papain, which aids in the breakdown of foods in the stomach and small intestine, and is best eaten before a main meal.

■ Pineapple is rich in the enzyme bromelain, which again aids digestion.

■ Generally increase your intake of fresh raw foods. Eat a salad at least once daily. Light stir-fries and steamed vegetables are also fine.

■ If you have a problem with wheat, try spelt, millet, buckwheat or quinoa-based breads, which are freely available in most supermarkets and health stores.

■ Try rice, corn or millet-based pastas, which are also easier to digest.

■ If you have a problem with cows' milk, try rice, oat or goats' milk, which are gentler on the stomach.

■ A glass of red wine can help to stimulate stomach acid production.

Useful Remedies

■ Take a digestive enzyme capsule (available from health stores) with all main meals.

■ You can also take an HCl with pepsin capsule with main meals, but only if you have been diagnosed as suffering from Low Stomach Acid (see also *Low Stomach Acid*).

■ Bitter herbs such as gentian, in tincture form can be taken 15 minutes before each meal to stimulate production of stomach acid and digestive enzymes.

Helpful Hints

■ Don't eat late at night as this places an extra burden on the digestive system.

■ Chew thoroughly and, as much as possible, eat sitting down in a relaxed frame of mind. Not always easy, but greatly aids digestion.

■ If you are going to take rigorous exercise, allow at least an hour after eating before exercising.

■ Don't eat large meals when you are under stress.

■ If your digestive system is playing up, try Food Combining. Basically this means separating concentrated proteins, such as meat, fish, eggs and cheese, from concentrated carbohydrates such as potatoes, rice, bread and pasta. So, if you want to eat fish for instance, eat it with vegetables rather than potatoes. And if you want to eat pasta, then also eat this with vegetables but not meat or fish. Eat fruit in-between or 15–20 minutes before a meal rather than after a main meal as fruit likes a quick passage through the gut and if it gets "stuck" behind a main meal, gas and bloating can result.

■ For the same reason, eat melon on its own as a starter, and don't combine with other fruits, as it has an even quicker transit time than other fruits, which again can trigger fermentation and bloating in the gut.

ACID–ALKALINE BALANCE

(See also *Digestion* and *Low Stomach Acid*)

For good health, the body needs to maintain a certain acid-alkaline balance, and keeping this balance is one of the most crucial keys to remaining healthy and slowing the ageing process. Every cell functions more efficiently when it is predominantly alkaline.

In general, the body needs to be around 70% alkaline and 30% acid. But in the West, the average person is 80% acid and 20% alkaline. Many people confuse the term "acid forming" with "acidic", but they are entirely different. Everything we swallow, once metabolized within the body, breaks down into either an alkaline or acid mineral-based ash or residue. Whether a substance is alkaline or acid is determined by its pH (potential Hydrogen).

Stomach acid can be as low as 1.5, very acid, whereas saliva after eating could be as high as 8, which is very alkaline.

Your blood has a pH which is slightly alkaline between 7.35 and 7.45 and this level has to be maintained at all costs. If it becomes too acid, the blood (via the kidneys) withdraws alkalizing minerals from anywhere it can find them; beginning with the hair, skin and nails and then moving on through the body until it begins drawing minerals from the bones.

Unfortunately, our Western lifestyle and diet is almost all acid forming and if the body remains in an acid state for too long, then acidosis triggers degenerative disease and early ageing. A high-acid-forming diet also has a negative effect on tooth enamel, especially pre-packaged concentrated fruit juices. Acid-forming foods deplete calcium from the body, while alkaline foods increase the body's ability to absorb calcium from the diet.

Emotions also affect this balance, for instance stress and anger cause more acidity in the body, whereas feelings of being in control, in love, and breathing deeply through the nose all re-alkalize the body. Basically, harmony alkalizes and disharmony acidifies.

And if you want to slow the ageing process, you need to maintain an alkaline reserve which buffers excess acidity, like having savings in the bank at times of crisis.

Practically every major degenerative disease, including some cancers, are triggered by an over-acid system. When the pH is out of balance, your skin and hair become dull, the nervous system is affected and you may suffer insomnia, arthritis, rheumatism, aching joints, skin conditions, candida, fungal infections, muscle pain and gout which are all common symptoms of an over-acid system.

Foods to Avoid

■ Just because a food is acid forming, this does not necessarily make it unhealthy. Proteins are acid forming, but they are also essential for good health. Therefore, if you eat two large meat-based meals daily, cut this down to two smaller portions.

■ Basically, all animal produce and egg yolks are acid forming. Duck, venison, grouse and pheasant, lamb, beef and pork are all acid forming.

■ Fish, turkey and chicken, are also acid forming, but do not contain such high levels of uric acid as red meat.

■ Milk and yoghurt are alkaline before digestion but become acid forming once digested. This is why milk products are calming to an over-acid oesophagus if you suffer from an acid type reflux after food. But in the long-term this would exacerbate arthritic-type conditions. It's just a case of getting a balance.

■ All nuts are acid forming except almonds, fresh coconut and chestnuts.

■ All grains are also acid forming with the exception of millet, amaranth and quinoa. Wholegrains are a healthy food and remember these foods are not to be eliminated per se, you just need to be aware of what is acid forming.

■ All refined sugars found in cakes, biscuits, pre-packaged desserts, whips and so on are acidic.

■ Wine, beer, spirits, coffee, tea, soft drinks and chocolate are all highly acidic.

■ All drugs, prescription and social, such as cannabis, are also acidic.

■ Cranberries, prunes and rhubarb are highly acid forming. But again I reiterate, these foods are healthy – in fact prunes (dried plums) are very anti-ageing. Everything in moderation

■ Mass-produced malt vinegar, a waste product of the brewing industry, is acid forming in the body.

Friendly Foods

■ Honey and brown rice syrup are alkalizing.

■ All vegetables are alkaline but the best are wheat grass, alfalfa, kelp, seaweed, parsley, watercress, carrots, endives, raw spinach, onions and celery.

■ Cabbage, kale, broccoli, spring greens, green beans and asparagus are all great alkaline foods.

■ All fruits are healthy, and should be eaten freely, but be aware that cranberries, prunes and rhubarb are highly acid forming and to a lesser degree so are blueberries, blackberries, raspberries and strawberries and plums.

■ The most alkalizing fruits are cantaloupe melons (and all melons), papaya, dates, especially dried dates, mangoes, lemons, limes and figs. In case you are wondering, it's the alkaline mineral content and not the sugar content that determines whether a food is acid or alkaline-forming in the body.

■ Oranges, grapefruit, pineapple, cherries, kiwi and tomatoes contain acids, but they make an alkaline ash within the body after they are digested. People who suffer indigestion immediately after a meal and may have an over-acid stomach, often say these types of foods make their problem worse. This is because they are acid on contact and until digested, but they make an alkaline residue once they reach the small intestine. This is why apple cider vinegar or lemon juice, with a little honey and warm water help to re-alkalize the body and reduce symptoms of arthritis and inflammatory conditions.

- Use a little organic sea salt, which is rich in alkalizing minerals.
- Drink more green tea, especially Bancha tea, with a little added honey.
- Apple cider vinegar, preferably organic, has an alkalizing effect within the body. It also helps increase stomach acid production as it is acid on contact – but alkalizing after digestion. Martlet's make a cider vinegar and honey formula already bottled and sold in most health stores.

Useful Remedies

- Ask at your health shop for powdered formulas that contain organic source wheat grass, spirulina, chlorella, alfalfa, broccoli and green foods.
- Dr Gillian McKeith makes a Living Food Energy Powder available from all health stores.
- Take a multimineral formula that contains 1000mg of calcium, 500–800mg of magnesium, 25mg of zinc, 200mg of potassium, in a colloidal or chelated form which are more easily absorbed.
- Sodiphos. Sodium phosphate helps to reduce lactic acid (and uric acid) build up and re-alkalizes an over-acid system. Take 600mg daily for three months (see Blackmores, page 13).

Helpful Hints

- Remember that stress, anger and smoking also contribute to acidosis.
- Breathing deeply and regularly helps to re-alkalize the body. This is because when you breathe in more oxygen into the body, it has an alkaline effect. When we are under stress, we tend to shallow breathe, which leaves more carbon dioxide, more acidity, in the tissues.
- If you ingest high-acid-forming foods and drinks, do not brush your teeth immediately afterwards as you can wear away the enamel. Simply drink a little water and swill it around the mouth to help neutralize the acids.
- Meditation also re-alkalizes the body (see also *Meditation p207*).
- When you first wake, the body is very acid, so having fruit for breakfast helps to re-alkalize the system. This is a great diet for summer breakfasts, but in winter you need to keep warmer and fruit won't do the job, so try porridge sweetened with a freshly grated apple or any chopped fruit. Breakfast is also a great time to drink freshly made juices. But too much orange juice can over-stimulate production of stomach acid, so try apple or pear as an alternative. Apple, carrot, celery with a little added fresh root ginger is also alkalizing.
- For more information on the subject read *Alkalize or Die* by Theodore A. Baroody, published by Holographic Health.

ACID INDIGESTION

(See also *Absorption, Acid-Alkaline Balance* and *Low Stomach Acid*)

Many people mistakenly believe they are suffering from an acid stomach, often presuming that they produce too much stomach acid – hydrochloric acid or HCl. In fact, sufferers regularly produce too much stomach acid at inappropriate times, such as when stressed or after ingesting too much caffeine, alcohol or sugar, which attack the stomach lining. This can trigger absorption problems in later life. And as the average person eats 100 tons of food in their lifetime, which requires 300 litres of digestive juices to break it down, it is no wonder we are suffering so many digestive disorders. Typical symptoms are feelings of heartburn, acid reflux, indigestion, bloating and general discomfort. Also when you are under prolonged stress or exhausted, your digestive system is impaired. Never underestimate how much stress and chronic exhaustion can affect the body.

Foods to Avoid

■ Reduce your intake of caffeinated coffee and tea, alcohol and sugar.

■ Reduce your intake of refined wheat-based foods, especially croissants, white bread and pre-packaged, mass-produced pies and cakes.

■ Avoid all full-fat cheeses and rich creamy foods.

■ Avoid heavy rich meals; especially avoid fried and fatty foods.

■ Don't drink concentrated fruit juices if you have an over-acid stomach. You can dilute them, but listen to your body and if they cause a reaction then avoid them.

■ Avoid fried and very fatty foods.

■ Avoid oily, spicy foods, such as an Indian take-away with lots of sauce, which are often packed with mass-produced refined vegetable oils.

■ Cut down on alcohol and smoking which both increase stomach acid production.

Friendly Foods

■ Eat more wholegrains, such as brown rice, buckwheat, quinoa, millet, kamut or amaranth and try rice, lentil, corn or spelt-based pastas, breads and cereals. Rice or oat cakes, amaranth and spelt crackers are often easier to digest than wheat.

■ If you adore bread, experiment with gluten-free breads.

■ Include plenty of lightly cooked vegetables and fruits in your diet, which are easier to digest.

■ Grilled pineapple with a little yoghurt and drizzled honey for dessert would aid digestion.

■ Choose low-fat meats such as venison, turkey, duck and chicken, without the skin, and include plenty of fresh fish in your diet.

■ Experiment with herbal teas such as fennel and liquorice, which are caffeine-free and reduce acidity. Camomile and meadowsweet teas also soothe the gut.

■ Fresh root ginger is very calming, as is lightly cooked cabbage or cabbage juice made from raw cabbage.

■ Eat more live, low-fat yoghurts, which aid digestion.

■ Choose decaffeinated coffees and teas that have been processed using water treatment, not chemicals as a solvent.

Useful Remedies

■ Deglycyrrhized liquorice helps to protect and heal the lining of the oesophagus and stomach. Chew one or two tablets 20 minutes before a meal. It can also be used as an alternative to antacids after meals. It is available from good health shops.

■ Herbcraft make a Peppermint Formula containing peppermint, gentian, fennel and camomile. Take either on the tongue or in water after meals. For stockists, call 01204 707420.

■ There are numerous formulas available to aid digestion. Look for ones containing slippery elm, aloe vera, marshmallow or meadowsweet, which all help to soothe the stomach lining.

Helpful Hints

■ Dr John Briffa suggests this home test for low stomach acid in his book *Body Wise*, Cima Books. Take a level teaspoon of bicarbonate of soda and dissolve in some water. Drink this mixture on an empty stomach. If sufficient quantities of acid are present in the stomach, the bicarb mixture is converted into gas, producing significant bloating and belching within 5 to 10 minutes of drinking the mix. Little or no belching denotes low stomach acid.

■ If you eat beetroot and your urine turns red, this can denote low stomach acid.

■ If you have pronounced longitudinal ridges in your nails, this is a common sign of low stomach acid.

■ Chew all foods thoroughly and avoid drinking too much with meals, as this dilutes stomach acid, which you need to digest your meal.

■ Eat little and often, avoiding large, heavy meals. The larger the meal, the greater the burden on your digestive system.

■ Small meals are especially important if you are stressed, as stress increases stomach acid production.

■ Take time out to eat your meals calmly and do not eat on the run. Never eat large meals when you are feeling upset.

■ If you are prone to nervous conditions, join a yoga or t'ai chi class and learn to relax. Get plenty of exercise but do not take strenuous exercise immediately after eating. But walking for 10–15 minutes will greatly aid digestion.

■ Drink fennel or camomile herbal teas after a meal to aid digestion.

- Food combining helps reduce an over-acid stomach: this means separating proteins and starches to aid digestion; basically if you are eating a protein such as meat or fish, eat this with salad or vegetables but not potatoes, pasta or bread; conversely when you eat bread, pasta or potatoes, eat them with vegetables or salad, not protein. Read *The Complete Book of Food Combining* by nutritionist Kathryn Marsden, Piatkus Books.

- Many people become addicted to antacids to control acid indigestion, but low stomach acid can also trigger similar symptoms, therefore check with your GP or health professional to ascertain the cause of your symptoms. Antacids can harm the body if used excessively and many contain aluminium, which has been implicated in Alzheimer's disease.

AGE SPOTS

(See also *Liver in Ageing* and *Skin*)

Melanocytes are your melanin, or colour producing cells, and as we age, and after years of exposure to the sun which triggers oxidative damage, these fatty pigments or lipids begin to "glue" together and age spots or uneven pigmentation of varying sizes and shapes begin to appear all over the body. They commonly appear on the backs of the hands, the face, the forearms and eventually anywhere that is exposed regularly to the sun. If you look at young skin, it's almost always clear with an even tone, and age spots don't normally appear until the early 40s and onwards. If you look at the buttocks of a 60-year-old woman (presuming she wears a bikini bottom that is) her buttocks will still look young and blemish-free.

The best ways to reduce and avoid age spots is to take less sun, look after your liver, and to ingest more antioxidants (see also *Antioxidants*).

Foods to Avoid
- Foods that rob your body of vital antioxidants will accelerate skin ageing. Avoid fried and barbecued foods, saturated fats found in full-fat dairy products, meat pies, cakes, fatty meats and chocolates.

- Alcohol and all fats place a strain on your liver (see *Liver*).

- Mass-produced refined foods and meals are often packed with hydrogenated and trans fats, plus sugar, which all age the skin (see *Fats for Anti-ageing*).

- Reduce non-organic foods that are often high in additives and pesticides.

Friendly Foods
- To help avoid age spots, it is important that the body is emulsifying and eliminating unwanted fatty deposits properly. This is best done with lecithin granules, which helps emulsify and break down fats. Take 1 tablespoon daily over cereals, fruits and yoghurts. Lecithin is available from all health stores. It is also found in soya products and eggs.

- Eat more antioxidant-rich foods, such as organic fruit and vegetables, especially red, orange or dark green fruits and vegetables such as carrots, apricots, pumpkin, broccoli, Chinese broccoli, pak choy, red peppers, red and purple berries and tomatoes.
- Use tahini or olive oil as a spread instead of hydrogenated margarines and spreads.

Useful Remedies

- Antioxidants help to mop up or neutralize the free radical reactions that are triggered when you over-expose your skin during sunbathing, therefore take a high-strength antioxidant formula (see details of Kudos 24, page 348).
- Beta-carotene helps to encourage melanin production. Make sure it's a natural source carotene complex that contains all the carotenoids.
- Potassium chloride is important also for removing congestion and fatty deposits in the tissues. Take 50mg potassium chloride three times a day (see Blackmores, page 13).
- Take active H (see *Antioxidants in Ageing*) – this is a very powerful antioxidant and many people taking this supplement have reported that after a few months of taking 2 x 250mg tablets daily, their age spots have disappeared.
- Take 1 gram of vitamin C daily.
- Essential fatty acids, known as EFAs, help to reduce the sun's negative effects. If taken regularly they help keep your skin looking younger for longer (see *Fats for Anti-ageing*).

Helpful Hints

- Begin at the age of 30 to use a factor 15 cream on the backs of your hands and on your face, and take more care in the sun, and you really will reap the benefits in later life.
- If you have young children, keep in mind that a huge amount of skin damage can be done before a child reaches 16. If children are allowed to burn, then they are more likely to suffer skin cancers in later life. A certain amount of sun is healthy, but all things in moderation.
- The secret is not to let the skin burn and turn bright red. We all know the sensible precautions – to cover up between 11am and 3pm and to always wear a hat in hot midday sun – but a huge majority are simply not doing it. Start protecting the skin from an early age. If you do want to tan, do it very slowly – don't burn (see also *Sunshine and Ageing*).
- Ask at your health store for an antioxidant-rich cream, there are now dozens of creams containing grape seed extract, vitamins C, E and so on. Use this on the age spots daily.
- Cigarettes will age your skin. If you seriously want to slow the ageing process inside and out – stop smoking.
- If you already have age spots, most pharmacies sell topical lightening preparations and if you keep them covered from the sun they may eventually fade.
- Modern lasers are highly successful at burning off age spots, but make sure you see a dermatologist or doctor who has experience of this work. I had mine done at a Lasercare

Clinic, 144 Harley Street by Dr Thomas Bozek (tel: 0207 224 0988). Lasercare have 12 clinics around the UK with qualified personnel. For further details and to find your nearest clinic call 0800 028 7222 or log on to: www.lasercare-clinics.co.uk

■ Read *Solve Your Skin Problems* by Natalie Savona and Patrick Holford, Piatkus Books.

AGEING

(See also *Antioxidants in Ageing, Cells and Ageing, Rejuvenation Therapies* and *Skin*)

Today, there are approximately 390 million people aged over 65 in the world – by 2030 over 20% of the world's 6 billion people will be over 65.

Governments worry about the health cost burden of the so called "pensioners" and yet if you begin taking more responsibility for your health from *today* – then you could have the capability to live a healthy, productive life until at least 100 years old.

An example of good nutrition and its effects on health and ageing can be seen in the Hunza population of northern Pakistan. The Hunzas are renowned for their average lifespan, between 100 and 120 years, which has been well documented. These simple people live a long life with virtually no illness. Dr Jay F. Hoffman was sent to study the Hunzas by the American Geriatrics Society. He wrote: "Here is a land where people do not have our common diseases, such as heart ailments, cancer, arthritis, high blood pressure, diabetes, tuberculosis, hay fever, asthma, liver and gall bladder trouble, constipation or many other ailments that plague the rest of the world"– in other words virtually all the modern-day Western illnesses that tend to accompany the process of ageing. And there is now no doubt that we can, in the majority of cases, greatly reverse this process as most people don't die from old age per se, but from the degenerative diseases that accompany old age, the majority of which can often be avoided.

As we age, biological changes take place throughout our bodies. Our heart muscle becomes thinner, the capacity of our kidneys reduces and all of our organs go through some physiological change. However, these changes are not necessarily associated with illness or disease. And none of these changes cause ill health or disease on their own. The process of ageing is the breakdown of key biological functions of our mind and body and is directly related to our environment, diet, lifestyle and outlook on life.

The single most common result of the process of ageing and the leading cause of death worldwide is cardiovascular disease. Dr Michael Colgan, an internationally renowned nutritional research scientist with his own research institute in America, says that if people could eat more of the right foods and change their lifestyles, then 98% of cardiovascular disease cases and 80% of cancers would be preventable. Also that diabetes, which is reaching epidemic proportions in Western countries, is a direct consequence of over consumption of sugar, plus stress and overuse of stimulants. It is both avoidable and manageable by healthier nutrition.

And if you eat the right foods, take the right supplements and hormones, then a 60 year-old can have the biological ageing markers, such as blood pressure, cholesterol count, lean body mass, bone density, skin thickness and so on, of a 40 year-old.

So, what causes the deterioration of our body that we call ageing?

It is now accepted by a huge number of scientists such as Professor Denham Harman from the University of Nebraska Medical School, that the ageing process and virtually all disease is the result of free radical damage to the cells in one form or another. Hence why antioxidant power holds one of the major keys to slowing the ageing process (see *Antioxidants p. 38*).

Free radicals are chemicals produced by our body when oxygen is used to create energy and during everyday processes such as breathing and eating. Our body is designed to cope with this production of free radicals (also known as oxidants), however, an excess of free radicals is produced within the body when we eat burned or smoked foods, are exposed to air pollution, pesticides, overuse of mobile phones, excessive sunbathing, additives and stress. These unstable molecules break down our DNA, trigger deterioration in our blood vessels and brain, and cause damage to virtually every cell of our body. And free radical damage accumulates with age.

While our body's natural antioxidant defence system is designed to successfully cope with a certain amount of free radicals, we are daily exposed to higher levels than our bodies can handle.

Inflammation is another major contributor to ageing. Degenerative diseases that are associated with inflammation in the tissues are arteriosclerosis, Alzheimer's, Parkinson's, diabetes, arthritis, ME, cancer and allergies. Sources of inflammation are chronic low-level infections, toxicity from ingesting too many foods packed with additives, deficiency of essential nutrients, foods to which we have an intolerance and heavy metals such as mercury and aluminium (see *Toxic Metal Overload*).

Physical activity is vital to prevent ageing but severe exertion generates large amounts of free radicals and can trigger inflammation in the body. This may explain a paradox: why people who spend so much time in the gym do not always survive longer and why some marathon runners and aerobics instructors age more quickly. As always, we need everything in a balance and this is the secret to anti-ageing (see *Exercise*).

Also, how often do you hear people say, "It's all in my genes" and if their parents died young, many people presume they have inherited the likelihood that they might do the same. Yes, our genes do play a huge part in the dice of life and how well or otherwise we age, but if our genes stay healthy then our bodies stay healthy. If you live a healthy lifestyle, you can change which genes are expressed. In other words if your parents and grandparents died of heart attacks you may well have a pre-disposition for heart problems at some point. But if you live a different lifestyle and eat healthier foods, you can change the chemistry within the body, and tip the scales in your favour. Genes are repairable and alterable, they adjust to our environment and state of mind. Scientists predict that within 10 years you may be able to have an anti-ageing gene chip inserted under your skin that can "switch off many of the processes of ageing" and until these become commonly available, there are a host of ways to stay younger longer (see also *Genes in Ageing p.151*).

Foods to Avoid

■ Sugar triggers an inflammatory response in the body, lowers immune function, and ages the skin faster than smoking or sunbathing. And if you don't use up sugar during exercise, it turns to fat in the body (see *Sugar in Ageing*). Therefore you need to cut down drastically on foods with a high sugar content such as refined carbohydrates: breads, cakes, biscuits, pastries, pasta, sweets and concentrated fruit juice. A diet of more than 40% carbohydrate intake can cause insulin resistance (see *Insulin Resistance*). Also, the body has a limited capacity to store carbohydrate in the liver and muscles and will turn excess carbohydrate into fat tissue.

■ Artificial sweeteners including Aspartame (NutraSweet and Canderel), saccharin, and Sucralose place a burden on the liver which accelerates ageing.

■ Avoid fried foods and all refined hydrogenated/trans fats (see *Fats for Anti-Ageing*).

■ Avoid artificial preservatives and chemicals, including monosodium glutamate (MSG).

■ Cut down on stimulants such as caffeine, fizzy drinks and alcohol.

■ Reduce your intake of full-fat dairy products.

■ Avoid shellfish which tend to feed in polluted coastal waters.

■ Preserved, smoked and cured meats (delicatessen-type meats and bacon, as the chemicals used are carcinogenic).

■ Avoid tinned, microwaved and pre-packaged foods.

■ Avoid mass-produced battery eggs and chickens.

■ Cut down on non-organic red meats.

■ Cut down on sodium-based table salts. Use mineral-rich sea salts in moderation.

Friendly Foods

■ Oily fish, linseeds, fresh fruit, vegetables, salads, nuts and oatmeal will all help to reduce inflammation in the body. As much as possible eat locally grown fresh foods.

■ Sip water throughout the day, the body can process and use about one glass of water an hour.

■ Eat organic when you can as it contains far lower levels of potentially dangerous pesticides and chemicals. Also, organic veggies have up to twice as many nutrients as non-organic ones.

■ A good anti-ageing diet will be composed of 50% vegetables, 20% protein, 20% fruits, and 10% grains. The vegetables should be raw or lightly cooked to preserve the nutrient content, the protein should include vegetable proteins as well as some animal protein and the fruits should be uncooked and whole as opposed to juiced. The grains are best as whole grains such as brown rice rather than flour-based foods.

- For a full list of anti-ageing foods see the *Diet – The Stay Younger Longer Diet (see page 114)*.

Anti-ageing Nutrients

- KUDOS 24 Multi-Active Age Management Complex is a multinutrient, up-to-the-minute highly absorbable formula containing food state, GM-free, vitamins, minerals, antioxidants, amino acids, brain nutrients, essential fats, isoflavones, green foods and specific anti-ageing `nutrients such as carnosine (see below) that both men and women of all ages can take daily. For full details and a list of the ingredients see page 348.

- If you prefer your own supplements, then take a good-quality multivitamin/mineral plus an antioxidant formula (see *Antioxidants in Ageing*). Always include an extra gram of vitamin C.

Below are listed the most up-to-date anti-ageing nutrients currently known:

- ALPHA-LIPOIC ACID is one of the most important antioxidants known and has the unique ability to pass into the brain, where it helps recycling of other antioxidants, such as vitamin C and E, plus glutathione. It is also removes heavy metals like aluminium, mercury and lead from the brain, which helps protect against Alzheimer's, Parkinson's and senile dementia. Because it is both water-and-fat soluble, it is easily absorbed in the gut. ALA also helps prevent and treat some of the complications of diabetes. Take 100mg daily with food.

- ACETYL L-CARNITINE (ALC) is a natural substance present in the human body, especially the muscles and brain. It helps to combat two major factors involved with brain ageing, diminished brain cell metabolism and reduced circulation in the brain. ALC easily crosses the blood-brain barrier and its role in protecting neurological function has been well established. The use of acetyl L-carnitine with alpha-lipoic acid is now being considered a major breakthrough for preventing the process of ageing. Take 1000mg daily on an empty stomach. Most companies now sell ALC and ALA in a combination formula (call Higher Nature for details, see page 13).

- CARNOSINE is a naturally occurring antioxidant made within the body and as we age the levels fall. High concentrations of carnosine are present in long-lived cells such as in nerve tissues and people who live longer have higher levels of this nutrient. Carnosine has been shown to help reverse age-related damage especially in the skin. It also blocks amyloid production, the substance found in the brains of Alzheimer's patients. Other emerging benefits are its apparent anti-cancer effects, its ability to remove toxic metals from the body and to boost the immune system. Food sources are lean red meat and chicken. For optimum anti-ageing results take 100–200mg daily. Take on an empty stomach in-between meals. It is best taken with natural source vitamin E x 200iu daily.

- ESSENTIAL FATS keep the skin hydrated and supple, are essential for hormone production, weight loss, the brain, the nervous system and controlling blood pressure. They are found in fish oils, flaxseed (linseeds), walnuts, hemp and pumpkin seeds and to a lesser extent soybeans. Include these seeds and unrefined oils in your diet and for more information see *Fats for Anti-ageing p.139*.

- Omega-6 essential fats are found in sunflower, sesame and pumpkin seeds, linseeds and their unrefined oils, and evening primrose oil. Most people have plenty of omega-6 EFA's in their diet from vegetable spreads and oils.

- S-ADENOSYL METHIONINE (SAMe) is an antioxidant which is naturally produced in the body. It helps protect brain cells against ageing, protects and improves joints function and mobility and fights depression. SAMe also helps the body generate more energy, helps prevent or reverse liver damage that has been caused by alcohol, viruses and chemical pollution and reduces chronic fatigue. SAMe is not available through the diet but can be supplemented. Take 200–800mg daily. It is best taken on an empty stomach in-between meals, with water.

Helpful Hints

- People who are adaptable and have a positive outlook on life tend to live the longest. Jeanne Calment, a French lady who lived to 122, gave up smoking at 120 in 1995 saying "it had become a habit" and died two years later. She had a great sense of humour, was adaptable and hard working – three vital characteristics of people who live a long life.

- Never underestimate just how much your thoughts and stress levels can affect not only your health but also the speed at which you age. If you keep saying over and over "it's to be expected at my age" – do not be surprised if you become sicker and age faster (see *Mind Power*).

- Learn to say YES to what you do want in your life and NO to what you don't.

- Have fun and laugh a lot. No one ever had engraved on their tombstone "I wish I had spent more time at the office". Find a balance.

- Stop worrying – as Dale Carnegie once said, "85 per cent of things you worry about never happen" so stop worrying about the things you cannot change – concentrate on what you can change. And if you really want to change things in your own life and environment then take the steps necessary to begin the changes that you require. Be willing to act positively for the good of all, rather than just talking about it.

- Stop smoking. Every cigarette you smoke takes 15 minutes off your life, ages your skin and depletes vital nutrients, such as vitamin C, which are needed for healthy skin and bones, energy production, and an active immune system.

- Take regular exercise, but not to excess (see *Exercise*).

- Being overweight can shorten your life by up to 10 years (see *Weight Problems in Ageing*).

- Supplementing the hormone DHEA (see *Other Vital Hormones p.237*) can help reduce inflammation and ageing in the body. Have your hormones checked.

- Reduce your exposure to mobile phones and excessive electrical equipment (see *Radiation in Ageing*).

- Reduce exposure to pesticides, herbicides and toxic chemicals. Eat organic foods/drinks as much as possible.

- Calorie restriction has been proven to reverse many of the biological markers for ageing but should only be attempted under medical guidance (see *Calorie Restriction in Ageing*). Otherwise, eat what you need – and don't overeat. Remember: "Eat to live – don't live to eat"!

■ Get sufficient sleep – it's the easiest way to look younger for longer.

■ Cut down your stress load as prolonged stress ages you (see also *Stress in Ageing*)

■ If you want to know how well or otherwise you are ageing, have your BioMarkers (this is your lean body mass, muscle strength, cholesetrol, blood pressure, bone density, basal metabolic rate etc) analysed at an anti-ageing clinic. One of the best anti-ageing clinics I have found is HB Health at 59 Beauchamp Place London SW3 1NZ. They have state-of-the-art equipment and a panel of longevity experts and doctors who can test your biological markers and offer you a complete and individual prescription (including chelation, hormones, supplements and therapies) for a longer life. For details call 0207 838 0765 or visit www.hbHealthOnline.com.

■ Under *Chelation in Ageing*, you will find a list of doctors who offer chelation and who would also be able to help with a longevity programme. Otherwise see *Useful Information and Addresses* on page 338 and find your nearest nutritional physician.

■ A great anti-ageing website is run by David and Kat Kekich in America – they have formed a non-profit organization called Maximum Life Foundation: www.maxlife.org

■ Another great website for anti-ageing research is the Life Extension Foundation on www.lef.org They run a very efficient postal service from the States and sell supplements that can be difficult to source in the UK. You can also order hormones like DHEA and melatonin from the Foundation.

■ Dr Nick Delgardo is a member of the American Academy of Anti-Ageing and his website www.growyoungandslim.com is well worth a look.

■ Dr David Wikenheiser, a US-based nutritional physician, has formulated an excellent questionnaire that will help you to discover your true biological age, a great way to find out how well, or otherwise you are ageing. For a free copy send an SAE requesting Dr Wikenheiser's Biological Age Questionnaire from Savant Distribution Ltd, Quarry House, Clayton Wood Close, Leeds LS16 6QE or call 08450 60 60 70.

■ There are hundreds of other anti-ageing hints throughout the book, otherwise see *General Anti-Ageing Health Hints*.

■ For further reading on Ageing see *Age Power* by Leslie Kenton, Vermilion, or *Longevity* by W. Lee Cowden MD, from www.alternativemedicine.com

ALCOHOL

(See also *Liver in Ageing*)

Every time you drink alcohol, which acts as a diuretic, the body excretes vital anti-ageing minerals and vitamins, especially the B-group vitamins which help keep your nervous system, hormone production and hair in good shape. Alcohol extracts water from cells which dehydrates every cell in the body, thus accelerating the ageing process. You also excrete vitamin C and the mineral zinc which help to keep your skin young and healthy. Alcohol is also acid forming within the body which contributes to osteoporosis (see *Acid–Alkaline Balance*).

Alcohol contains around 70 calories an ounce and so the body thinks it is being well fed, but in fact it is being slowly starved of essential nutrients.

The liver breaks down alcohol into sugar and over time this weakens the liver, which in the long-term can trigger cirrhosis. Also, alcohol generates huge amounts of free radicals that increase ageing at every level.

Moderate consumption, meaning a single unit (one shot of spirits, one glass of wine or half a pint of beer) of alcohol a day, has been shown to be slightly protective against heart disease. Enjoy an occasional drink, the ideal being a glass of aged red wine.

The nutrient content of alcohol is very low, but many people drink wine and spirits believing they are protecting their heart and tend to forget they are increasing their risk of hormonal cancers, particularly breast cancer. Alcohol also places an enormous strain on the liver, which reduces its ability to detoxify the body and contributes to ageing skin. Fatigue, dehydration, disrupted sleep patterns, weight gain, late-onset diabetes, mood swings, depression, dry skin and hair, plus poor eye sight and many other health problems can result from over consumption. Pregnant women risk foetal abnormalities if they consume more than one unit of alcohol a day during pregnancy and alcohol should be avoided if you are trying to become pregnant. During pregnancy give it up.

One in every 13 people now have a problem with alcohol and many young people in their 20s have liver damage that would normally only be seen in people over 40.

Foods to Avoid
- Certain foods can increase cravings for alcohol, these include milk, wheat, chocolate, meat and sugar – and the more sugary snacks you eat along with any alcohol the more likely you are to suffer from low blood sugar (see also *Low Blood Sugar p194*).

- Avoid eating fresh, tinned grapefruit or juice when drinking alcohol, as they increase the toxicity of the alcohol.

- Saturated fats also place a great strain on the liver, therefore reduce your intake of fatty meals, especially sausages, burgers, full-fat cheese, cream, chocolates, pre-packaged meat pies etc.

- Never ply anyone who is drunk with coffee, as coffee is a diuretic and as you urinate, the alcohol then becomes more concentrated in the body.

- Cut down on caffeine-rich foods and drinks plus sugar, which also place a strain on the liver.

Friendly Foods
- Any foods that help cleanse and support the liver should be eaten regularly if you like a drink.

Try eating broccoli, globe artichokes, fennel, cauliflower, beetroot, celeriac and radishes.

■ Onions and garlic are rich in the amino acid methionine, which helps support the liver.

■ All fruits and vegetables contain magnesium which is usually lacking in people who drink a lot.

■ Eat plenty of soluble fibres such as linseeds (flax), oat bran, psyllium husks and low sugar cereals or porridge.

■ Wheatgrass juice helps detoxify the liver, but needs to be used as part of a detox programme as it is very powerful and can trigger nausea if taken when the body is toxic (see *Detoxing*).

■ Avocado and raw wheatgerm are rich in vitamin E which helps to protect the cells against the damaging effects of alcohol.

■ Drink at least eight glasses of water daily.

■ If you wake up with a hangover – do not go out and have more alcohol. To help balance your blood sugar blend a banana, a cup of blueberries, a chopped apple, a pear (or any fruit you have to hand), a tablespoon of sunflower seeds, a teaspoon of any green powder from your health store and half a cup of organic aloe vera juice and drink.

■ Dandelion root tea is excellent for cleansing the liver.

■ See also *General Anti-ageing Health Hints p.147*.

Useful Remedies

■ Take a good quality multivitamin/mineral *and* an antioxidant formula daily such as Kudos 24 (see page 348).

■ Chronic consumption can constrict arteries in the brain, so also take an additional 500mg of magnesium daily to help keep blood vessels flowing more freely.

■ The herb milk thistle, a spiky-leafed plant contains the bioflavonoid silymarin, which promotes cell regeneration in the liver and it has been shown to help repair liver damage from alcohol. Take 600mg of standardized extract up to three times daily with meals for one month and then cut down to a maintenance dose of 600mg of standardized extract daily. Kudos Vitamins make a high potency capsule. For details call 0800 389 5476.

■ Obviously during this time you need to cut down your intake of alcohol to give the liver time to repair or it's like trying to put out the flames while you remain standing in the fire!

■ Take kelp – one tablet daily to support thyroid function.

■ The herb Chinese Kudzu contains diadzin, which has been known to be beneficial for treating alcoholism. Not only does Kudzu extract help reduce the craving for alcohol, but also acts as a muscle relaxant which helps to overcome some of the withdrawal symptoms. Take 10–20 drops of the tincture or two tablets before you intend to take a drink. For details call 01204 707420 or log on to www.gnc.co.uk

■ To avoid hangovers take 500mg of GLA (gamma linolenic acid) which is the main ingredient in evening primrose oil, one gram of vitamin C, a B complex, plus 500mg of milk thistle with a full glass of water before going out.

- Ask at your health store for an amino acid formula that contains methionine, cysteine and choline which help promote good liver function.

- The amino acid L-glutamine helps reduce the cravings for alcohol and helps heal the gut lining – take 500mg twice daily on an empty stomach.

Helpful Hints

- According to Chinese medicine, the body tends to detox the liver between 1am and 3am and the body detoxes more efficiently when you are lying down. So, if you are out late drinking, you place a severe strain on the body's natural repair processes.

- For every alcoholic drink make sure you have a non-alcoholic one in-between. Generally, drink more water as alcohol severely dehydrates the body.

- Alcohol causes less damage if taken with food. Never go drinking on an empty stomach.

- Avoid alcohol when flying because the pressurized cabins cause considerable dehydration.

- Take homeopathic Nux Vomica 30c – one before bed and one on waking to reduce a hangover.

- Bingeing on alcohol is extremely dangerous – it creates too much shock to the liver. If you begin to vomit, this is an indication that the body has reached a danger level and you must stop drinking. Unfortunately 37% of young men and 23 % of young women binge-drink regularly.

- If you must drink, have a couple of drinks daily. Better-quality red wine is the safest bet (unless you suffer migraines), due to antioxidant substances called polyphenols, present in the skin of red grapes. The skin of white grapes is discarded during the processing of white wine.

- Remember, it takes 20 minutes for alcohol to have an effect and over one hour for the body to process each unit (one unit = half a pint of beer, a small glass of wine or a single measure of spirits). If you are concerned about the amount that you (or a member of your family) are drinking, call Drinkline on 0800 917 8282 for advice and information. The line is open from 9am–11pm (Monday to Friday) and 6pm–11pm (weekends). All calls are treated in the strictest confidence and Drinkline provides a full support service for people with drink problems as well as their families.

ALZHEIMER'S DISEASE

(See also *Brain* and *Memory*)

What's the point of a long life if you can't remember it?

Alzheimer's affects half a million people in Britain with 60,000 new cases every year and these figures are expected to rise as the population ages. Experts estimate that within 30 years more than half the population over 85 will suffer with Alzheimer's Disease (AD). Alzheimer's has a huge economic impact on the Health Service and already costs the NHS £2billion every year.

Alzheimer's is a progressive, degenerative disease which attacks the brain, triggering symptoms such as memory loss, especially short-term memory, and a decrease in intellectual functioning. It is the loss of memory of how to do every day tasks that tends to make a familiar life almost impossible.

In the early stages, AD sufferers have symptoms of absent-mindedness and an inability to learn new things. Judgement and intellectual and social functioning begin to go awry. Later there is loss of logic, memory and poor coordination. Speech deteriorates and symptoms of paranoia may appear. In the final stages, the Alzheimer's sufferer completely loses touch with their surroundings and becomes unresponsive.

Needless to say this is very traumatic, not only for the sufferer but also their family. The tragedy is that Alzheimer's is a preventable disease and can even be reversed to a degree, sometimes remarkably so. If we could all eat a healthier diet, reduce our exposure to pollution, take the right supplements and so on, much heartache and billions of pounds could be saved. The key to prevention is to understand the numerous contributing factors. Many people state that "they can do nothing" thinking that AD is mostly inherited. Of course you can inherit a tendency for a particular ailment, but if you change your lifestyle and diet then you can stack the odds in your favour. But if you eat the wrong foods, are stressed etc, and there is some genetic influence, then the accumulation of factors may eventually overwhelm your body's ability to cope, resulting in AD.

One of the commonest theories for a cause of AD, is aluminium toxicity. A 1980 study of 647 Canadian gold miners who had routinely inhaled aluminium since the 1940s (a common practice thought to prevent silica poisoning) all tested in the "impaired" range for cognitive function, suggesting a clear link between aluminium and memory loss. And while aluminium is certainly harmful to the brain, there are other key factors that can lead to degeneration of the brain.

Researchers have found a significant imbalance of metals in Alzheimer's patients, especially mercury, mainly deposited in areas of the brain related to memory. Mercury is known to cause the type of damage to nerves that is characteristic of AD, and researchers have found that early-onset Alzheimer's patients having the highest mercury levels of all. (See also *Toxic Metal Overload*.)

Another factor is homocysteine, a toxic compound produced during the metabolism of proteins, and an increased homocysteine level is a strong, independent risk factor for the development of dementia and Alzheimer's disease. The higher the homocysteine level, the greater the damage to the brain. Homocysteine is readily recycled or broken down within the body by vitamins B6, B12 and folic acid. Therefore, by taking a B complex daily, homocysteine levels can be kept in check.

Cortisol, the stress hormone, can also harm the delicate balance of your brain, as cortisol causes the connections between brain cells to shrivel up which contributes to AD (see also *Stress in Ageing*).

Free radicals and an excessive intake of refined, processed foods, low in antioxidant vitamins such as A, C and E are also contributing factors (see *Antioxidants in Ageing*).

Basically, the more pollutants and refined foods we are exposed to, the more vital minerals and vitamins are excreted from the body and brain function deteriorates. Eating the right foods, taking supplements that nourish the brain and taking more exercise, increases circulation to the brain and memory can often be improved.

Foods to Avoid

■ Avoid refined grains in products such as white bread, rice and pasta. These grains have had most of their nutrients, including B vitamins, removed in the refining process, and remember that elevated homocysteine levels can be controlled by taking more B vitamins.

■ Avoid foods containing traces of aluminium such as commercial chocolate, desserts, baking powder, processed cheeses, chewing gum and pickles.

■ Eliminate any food containing the food additives aspartame (an artificial sweetener) and monosodium glutamate (MSG), which are suspected neuro-toxins.

■ Avoid ready-made meat pies, cakes, and pre-packaged meals that are not only cooked in aluminium containers but also packed with saturated fat, sugar and salt.

■ Reduce your intake of saturated fats found in fatty meats and full-fat dairy produce.

■ Reduce your intake of caffeine, sugar and alcohol, which can all deplete vital nutrients and interfere with brain function. Sugar is particularly deadly for brain function and contributes to beta amyloid deposits, which are now thought to be the main problem for Alzheimer's patients. Ronald Reagan's notorious sweet tooth may have led to his Alzheimer's.

Friendly Foods

■ Alzheimer's patients are often lacking in the vital brain nutrient acetylcholine, which is manufactured by the body, found in organ meats, such as liver or kidneys, oats, soya beans, cabbage and cauliflower.

■ Sprinkle a tablespoon of soya lecithin granules over breakfast cereals, into yoghurt or over fresh fruit. Lecithin is rich in acetylcholine but make sure the brand you choose contains at least 30% of this nutrient. Other foods containing this vital brain nutrient are egg yolks and fish, especially sardines.

■ Essential fats are vital for proper brain functioning and reducing inflammation within the brain (and body), as brain inflammation is also linked to AD. Include wild salmon, herrings, mackerel and tuna in your diet, which are rich in omega-3 essential fats. Include plenty of organic linseeds, sunflower and pumpkin seeds which are all rich in healthy fats. Sprinkle them into breakfast cereals, and these seeds are delicious, toasted or raw with salads and vegetables (see also *Fats for Anti-ageing*).

■ Include antioxidant-rich foods such as berries, dark green leafy vegetables, and any other brightly coloured fruits and vegetables. (See *General Anti-ageing Health Hints* and *Diet – The Stay Younger Longer Diet* on page 114).

■ Garden sage has been found to prolong and improve memory functioning, due to its powerful anti-inflammatory and antioxidant effects. Sage also inhibits the enzyme that breaks down acetylcholine. Use fresh sage over cooked foods or make sage teas. But don't use sage if you are pregnant as it stimulates the uterus.

■ Use fresh coriander over salads and sprinkle over cooked dishes, as coriander helps to remove toxic metals from the body.

Useful Remedies

■ Take a multivitamin/mineral/essential fats/antioxidant formula daily that also contains brain nutrients. Try Kudos 24 (see page 348).

■ Magnesium, 300mg daily, and potassium phosphate, 75mg daily, are important for nerve connections in the brain. They are available from Blackmores (see page 13).

■ Silica helps to eliminate aluminium from the body. Take 75mg per day.

■ Taking 600 iu of natural source, full spectrum vitamin E and 1gram of vitamin C three times a day with meals has been shown to slow the progress of Alzheimer's and to help prevent onset of dementia. Studies have shown that vitamin E is more effective than drugs in reducing the symptoms of Alzheimer's. However if you're on blood thinning drugs, check with your doctor before taking the vitamin E, as it thins the blood naturally.

■ Ginkgo biloba is a herb from leaves of what the Chinese call the memory tree. Try 120–240mg of standardized extract daily, which helps to increase circulation to the brain. In rare cases ginkgo can cause a rash in which case you should stop taking it. A study published in 1997 by the *Journal of the American Medical Association*, said ginkgo biloba was shown not only to prevent Alzheimer's degeneration but actually improved many cases.

■ Phosphatidylserine (PS) is another vital brain nutrient. The body can manufacture PS but only if you tend to eat offal. If like most people you avoid organ meats, which are often high in antibiotic residues, then take 100mg of PS twice daily.

■ B vitamins are destroyed by stress and alcohol, but are needed for the formation of acetylcholine and for the manufacture of other neuro-transmitters within the brain and nervous system, so take a high strength B complex daily, especially if you're stressed.

■ AGEBlock – containing aminoguanadine – has been shown to prevent destructive cross-linking of proteins with sugars in the brains of Alzheimer's patients. (It is available from the NutriCentre, see page 14 for details).

■ Curcumin, a substance found in the spice turmeric (widely used in curries), may be part of the reason Alzheimer's is uncommon in India compared to Western countries. Studies in India found a less than 1% incidence of Alzheimer's in the over-65s. Rat studies undertaken in California are reported to show that curcumin reduces brain amyloid (the protein deposit found in Alzheimer's) and also reduces the degenerative, inflammatory responses to amyloid. Try one or two curcumin standardized extract capsules daily.

■ See also *Essential Sugars*, as glyconutrients are having a profound and well documented healing effect on reducing Alzheimer's and dementia-type conditions.

Helpful Hints

- Avoid stress. Stress stimulates the adrenal glands to produce a hormone called cortisol, which can damage your brain. Learn to relax regularly, and walk regularly which is very relaxing, or try yoga, t'ai chi, massage or meditation.

- Stop smoking – research from Holland indicates that smokers are twice as likely to develop dementia in later life. Avoid drugs such as cannabis and Ecstasy, which are associated with memory loss if used in the long-term.

- Regular exercise has helped many sufferers restore some functions especially memory.

- If you have mercury fillings you are advised to have them removed. It is imperative this is done by a dentist who specializes in this procedure, as increased mercury poisoning can result if the proper precautions are not taken to protect you during the filling removal (see *Toxic Metal Overload*).

- Because of the link between aluminium and Alzheimer's, avoid aluminium cooking utensils and pans, and food stored in aluminium containers. Use stainless steel or glass cookware. Many antiperspirants contain aluminium, so use natural deodorants such as PitRok, or Tea Tree-based products, available from all chemists and health stores.

- Simple antacids are often based on aluminium salts and should also be avoided. Aluminium is also found in toothpastes, some cosmetics, processed cheeses, baking powder and buffered aspirin, and table salts often contain aluminium, which is used as a pouring agent. If our mineral levels are low, then the body tends to absorb more aluminium, so this is another reason to include a multimineral in your everyday health regimen.

- Chelation therapy helps to remove metal toxins from the body (see *Chelation in Ageing*).

- Use it or lose it. Keep the brain working with simple exercises like doing crosswords and force your brain to work by counting down from 500 each day in multiples of various numbers – such as 500 less 7 = 493, less 7 = 486 etc. Try writing and regularly using the opposite hand to the one you normally use. Extend your arms out at shoulder level, rotate one hand clockwise and the other anti-clockwise and then change over – make your brain work. Buy a dictionary and learn to use and spell at least one new word every day.

- Eat organically and drink filtered or bottled water. Many pesticides have been linked to neurological problems and these chemicals along with aluminium are finding their way into our drinking water. So use a good water filter that removes most of these residues. Contact the Fresh Water Filter Company Ltd. Tel: 0870 442 3633 or visit their website at www.freshwaterfilter.com.

- Minimize your exposure to mobile phones and computers. Certain studies have shown that exposure to electromagnetic radiation significantly increases the risk of Alzheimer's, or makes it rapidly worse. So working with or near computers, VDUs and similar equipment, may harm your brain and evidence of how mobile phones affect the brain is continuing to mount (see *Radiation in Ageing*).

- Maintaining circulation to the brain is essential, as poor blood supply to the brain will starve it of oxygen and nutrients. Hence why regular exercise is vital.

- Certain prescription drugs are known to cause side effects, which appear similar to symptoms of senile dementia. Anyone who feels that they may have the onset of dementia should immediately consult a qualified doctor, who is also a nutritionist (See *Useful Information and Addresses p.338* for details).

ANDROPAUSE
(See *Men's Hormones* and *Mid-Life Crisis in Ageing*)

ANGINA
(*See Heart*)

ANTIOXIDANTS IN AGEING

Antioxidants are major anti-agers, they help neutralize the excess build up of toxic free radicals in our body.

We breathe in oxygen, which is vital to life, and it is utilized or "burned" by every cell in the body to function properly, but during normal biochemical reactions such as in breathing and eating, oxygen and other molecules are altered and become unstable free radicals, also known as Free Oxidizing Radicals, or oxidants which attack our cells 100,000 times a second. When iron is exposed to air, it rusts and turns brown – it oxidises – so does an apple when it's peeled – and this is basically what happens to our cells as we age.

And yet certain free radicals are also vital to life, they are created by the billions daily, and no chemical reaction can occur in the body without free radicals. They help neutralize viruses and bacteria, they help to kill cancer cells, so there are positive purposes for a certain amount of free radicals in the body. For instance, part of the process of oxygen absorption into the blood is carried out by free radicals.

But once you begin to accumulate excess free radicals, from additional sources such as barbecued food, smoking, car exhausts, radiation and frying and as a by-product of our own body's cellular metabolism, then they begin to break down our blood vessels and brain and damage virtually every cell in our body, including our DNA. And as we age, free radical damage to our cells accumulates which causes 99% of the ageing processes.

The substances that help to neutralize free radicals are called antioxidants, which in simple terms mop up excess free radicals in the body. For the most part, if your immune system is in good shape, the body produces natural antioxidants, such as glutathione (young people usually make lots of this antioxidant), that can repair most of the damage triggered by excess free radicals or even stop it before it happens. When you are young and healthy, internal metabolic combustion processes can be managed, but become harder to keep in check as we age.

Virtually all degenerative disease is the result of accumulative free radical damage to your cells in one form or another. Hence why antioxidant nutrients are the most potent anti-ageing tools you can take to stay younger longer.

But as all the major antioxidants work together in the body, we need to take a formula that contains a broad spectrum – not just one in isolation. Most people are aware that vitamins A, C and E and the trace mineral selenium are powerful antioxidants, but new antioxidants are being discovered all the time. For instance research has shown that alpha-lipoic acid (similar in function to a vitamin found in red meat and potatoes) and acetyl-L-carnitine can help reverse some of the processes that are associated with ageing. Herbs also have powerful antioxidant properties. Dr John Wilkinson, head of the Phyto Chemistry Discovery Group at Middlesex University in the UK, which studies natural plant remedies, has found that garden sage is a powerful antioxidant which helps maintain neuro-transmitter levels in the brain. It improves memory functioning, but is not to be taken when pregnant. And grape seeds, green tea, pine bark and a myriad of other foods and plants are proving to be powerhouses of antioxidants.

Foods to Avoid

■ Microwaving food depletes vital nutrients from your food, and negatively affects blood chemistry, immune and endocrine systems and brain function. The cancer causing food contaminant acrylamide is generated by microwaving (and frying).

■ Avoid food additives; pesticides; and processed oils such as commercial, mass-produced vegetable oils and margarines (see *Fats for Anti-ageing*).

■ Avoid barbecued and fried foods, burnt or smoked foods.

■ Avoid excessive intake of red meat rich in iron, especially after the age of 50, as iron can accumulate in the body and generates more free radicals and excessive iron is linked to heart disease. (Obviously if you have a medical condition that requires iron, this would not apply to you.)

■ Cut down on refined sugar which also generates free radicals.

■ Many of the chemicals that generate free radicals are found in municipal water supplies. It is good to drink a lot of water, but avoid tap water as much as possible. Use a reverse osmosis or solid-carbon-block filter or drink spring water. For details contact The Pure H2O company on 01784 221180, or log on to www.purewater.co.uk. This company have offices in 40 countries (see also *Water in Ageing*).

Friendly Foods

■ Research from Tuft's University in Boston, USA has shown a new way to rate food's overall antioxidant power. Each food is assigned a certain number of ORAC (oxygen radical absorbance capacity), which means they are great foods for countering free radical damage.

- The top scorers are prunes (dried plums), raisins, blueberries and blackberries. Kale, spinach, strawberries, raspberries, plums, broccoli, avocado and alfalfa sprouts come a close second. A full list of ORAC ratings in food can be found on www.patrickholford.com.

- Eat organic unsalted and unrefined nuts, seeds and their unrefined oils such as pumpkin, linseed, sunflower and sesame seed, plus fish oils, whole grains (especially wheatgerm), fortified cereals, peas and apricots which are all great sources for vitamin E.

- Citrus fruits and fresh juices, green peppers, cabbage, spinach, broccoli, kale, cantaloupe melons, kiwi, and strawberries are all rich in vitamin C.

- Find natural source beta-carotene (which coverts to vitamin A in the body) in liver, oily fish, egg yolks, butter, spinach, sweet potatoes, watercress, peas, carrots, squash, broccoli, yams, tomatoes, cantaloupe melons and peaches.

- Garlic, onions, broccoli, cabbage, brown rice, eggs, shrimps, sunflower seeds, tuna, chicken, Brazil nuts and unrefined wheat provide selenium.

- Organic food contains more nutrients and fewer toxins, so as much as possible eat fresh, locally grown organic foods. The less you cook your food, the more antioxidants it will contain. Obviously raw foods have the highest antioxidant potential.

- Oregano, dill, sage, thyme, rosemary and peppermint rank even higher in antioxidant activity than fruits and vegetables (fresh herbs contain more antioxidants than dried ones).

- Drink green tea, which contains polyphenols and bioflavonoids, which act as super antioxidants that help to neutralize harmful fats, lower cholesterol and blood pressure.

- Co-EnzymeQ10 is found in beef heart, pork, chicken liver, salmon, mackerel and sardines.

Useful Remedies

- Vitamin E is the most abundant fat-soluble antioxidant in the body. It consists of eight compounds: four tocopherols and four tocotrienols. Many vitamin E supplements only contain alpha tocopherol, but most companies are now offering a full spectrum vitamin E capsule that contains natural source d-alpha tocopherols with tocotrienols. Take 100–400iu a day. For more details see the Life Extension Foundation website at www.lef.org

- Vitamin C is the most abundant water-soluble antioxidant in the body. It is particularly helpful in combating free-radical formation caused by pollution and cigarette smoke and is absolutely vital for healthy skin, collagen production and healthy cartilage, bones and eyes. Take between 50mg to 3grams daily in an ascorbate form, which is gentler on the stomach.

- Beta-carotene is an antioxidant, which is converted to vitamin A in the body. For anti-ageing take between 2500iu to 10,000iu a day.

- Selenium is an essential mineral that helps you to avoid cancer in later life, and which works with a zinc supplement. Take 200mcg of selenium and 25mg of zinc.

- Co-EnzymeQ10 is a fat-soluble vitamin-like substance produced naturally within the body and is found in all cells, where it is critical for the manufacture of energy molecules. CoQ10 is a powerful antioxidant that helps protect against the accumulation and deposit of oxidized fats in blood vessels, which can lead to atherosclerosis. Take 30–60mg a day. But any woman with a high risk for breast cancer should take 100mg per day.

- Grape Seed Extract and Pine Bark (known as pycnogenol) are also powerful antioxidants and both have been found to help maintain healthy skin.

- All the above (and a lot more) can be found in Kudos 24 – Multiactive Age Management Complex. For full details see page 348.

- Alpha-Lipoic Acid (ALA) is a co-enzyme (similar in function to a vitamin) which is made naturally within the body. ALA increases levels of the star brain antioxidant glutathione. Alpha-lipoic acid has the ability to pass into the brain, where is helps regeneration of other antioxidants, such as vitamin C and E plus glutathione. It is also helps remove heavy metals like aluminium, mercury and lead from the brain, which helps protect against Alzheimer's and Parkinson's disease and senile dementia. ALA also helps to prevent complications associated with diabetes, plus macular degeneration and cataracts. It is both fat and water soluble, which means it is easily absorbed within the gut. Take 100mg daily with food.

- Acetyl-L-carnitine acts as a powerful antioxidant needed for optimum brain functioning. It works well with alpha-lipoic acid. Some supplement companies are combining the two for optimum results. For details call Higher Nature on 01435 882880.

- Active–H is an antioxidant formula well worth a mention. The American physicist, Dr Patrick Flanagan, has shown that one tablet of Active H contains the same antioxidant, and anti-ageing abilities as 10,000 glasses of freshly squeezed organic orange juice.

I was extremely sceptical of this claim, until I read the large body of scientific research, and then tried it myself. Flanagan has spent 30 years trying to discover why certain people in remote areas of Pakistan, Russia and South America tend to live healthy lives often until well over 100. He eventually isolated the anti-ageing properties in their glacial waters, which are similar to distilled water in that they do not contain mineral salts, but microscopic colloidal – meaning insoluble in water – minerals, especially silica, an essential mineral which is found in every living tissue. Flanagan also found large quantities of negatively ionized hydrogen atoms, not found in other waters, which act as free radical scavengers. It took Flanagan another 10 years to re-create, stabilize and amplify the antioxidant properties of these waters, and the resulting supplement called Active-H, has been shown to be several hundred times more powerful than vitamin C. Raw, organic foods and drinks are also packed with large amounts of negatively charged hydrogen, or what Flanagan terms life force energy, which is destroyed during cooking. For more details see his website on www.flantech.com or to order call The NutriCentre on 0207 436 5122, www.nutricentre.com.

Helpful Hints

■ Pesticides, smoking, drugs or alcohol, all cause free radical damage.

■ Invest in an air filter in your bedroom to help clean polluted air which also triggers free radical reactions, avoid smoking and smoky environments.

■ Too much sun will trigger free radical reactions and accelerate skin ageing (see also *Sunshine in Ageing p305)*.

■ Regular exercise increases the body's production of SOD, superoxide dismutase, an anti-ageing enzyme that fights free radicals. However excessive exercise increases cellular metabolism and therefore free radical production, so if you exercise a lot, make sure you take extra antioxidants.

■ Stress reduction or relaxation has been shown to decrease the body's production of free radicals (see also *Stress in Ageing p293*).

ARTERIES IN AGEING

(See also *Circulation* and *High Blood Pressure*)

ARTHRITIS – OSTEO AND RHEUMATOID

(See also *Bones* and *Joints in Ageing*)

OSTEOARTHRITIS

Primary osteoarthritis develops when our natural cartilage repair process can no longer keep pace with the degenerative wear and tear we can suffer with age. Secondary arthritis is usually triggered by a trauma, such as a broken joint or a fall, or any underlying joint disease. Arthritis has now reached monumental proportions. In the UK, 54% of people over 65 suffer arthritis or joint pain. In America, a third of adults show X-ray evidence of arthritis in their hands, feet, knee or hips. By the age of 65, as many as 75% of the Western population are arthritic.

Over time the cartilage, which cushions and surrounds the joints, breaks down and the bones can become thickened and distorted restricting joint movement. In most cases it affects the load bearing joints – hips, knees, spine and hands. Some people believe that exercise makes you more prone to developing osteoarthritis. In reality, exercise helps to keep your bones healthy and joints supple.

Weight bearing exercise such as walking, weight lifting and so on help prevent bone loss (see *Exercise*). Yoga keeps you supple, but if you play contact sports like rugby, football or hockey, then the joints are more likely to be damaged.

The majority of people who suffer osteoarthritis eat too many acid-forming foods (see *Acid–Alkaline Balance*). Basically proteins such as meat and dairy produce from cows, plus refined carbohydrates like white bread and pizzas are acid forming, whereas fresh vegetables and most fruits plus millet are alkalizing. And if we could all eat less acid forming food, many illnesses could be eradicated. Arthritis can also be triggered by overuse of laxatives. People who develop osteoarthritis are often told to avoid the nightshade family, which includes tomatoes, potatoes, peppers and aubergines. Out of these tomatoes seem to be the worst offender, as tomatoes contain an alkaloid which can trigger inflammation in the joints. It has been shown that 60–70% of people who avoid these foods for at least 6 months or more see benefits. Being overweight places more stress on joints, which will add to the problem in later life.

In cultures where people eat a mainly wholefood, wholegrain, vegetarian diet, arthritis is virtually unknown.

Foods to Avoid

- Reduce your intake of black tea, coffee, alcohol, fizzy drinks, shop-bought cakes, pies, pastries, bread and pasta that are made with refined white flour and white sugar as these are are all acid forming.

- Avoid known triggers such as tomatoes, potatoes, aubergines and peppers.

- Oranges and orange juice can make symptoms worse in some individuals.

- Greatly reduce cows' milk, red meat, high-fat cheeses (especially Stilton), fried foods, sausages, meat pies and chocolate.

- Avoid all white and malt vinegars, which are highly acid forming.

- For anyone suffering gout-type problems, also eliminate foods containing large amounts of purines, which break down into uric acid in the body, as excess uric acid can trigger severe inflammation in small joints especially the toes. High purine foods are red meats, alcohol, shellfish, anchovies, mackerel, herrings, sardines and organ meats.

Friendly Foods

- Cherries, plums and blackberries are acid forming, *but* they help to move uric acid out of the joints, so that it is excreted in our urine. Cherries and cherry juice are best for gout.

- Pineapple contains bromelain which is highly anti-inflammatory.

- If you do not suffer gout then eat fresh oily fish such as mackerel, tuna, salmon or sardines at least 3 times a week.

- Sweet potatoes are rich in vitamin A, fibre and are a good alternative to ordinary potatoes.

- Grains such as millet, brown rice, amaranth, spelt, barley, quinoa etc are all preferable to refined wheat products. Choose wholemeal bread and try pastas made from corn, buckwheat, rice and lentil flours. Try 100% organic rye crisp bread, sugar-free oatcakes and low-sugar muesli or porridge

- Eat far more fresh green vegetables to re-alkalize your system. One of the quickest ways to do this is to buy a juicer and blend raw cabbage, watercress, celery, parsley, a little root ginger and drink immediately. You can also make delicious fruit blends (remember we are blending here, not juicing, so you get the peel which contains all the fibre). My favourite is half a cup of fresh blueberries, a chopped pear, apple and banana, a heaped teaspoon of any "green"-based powder from your health store, a tablespoon of linseeds and aloe vera juice all blended with a cup of organic rice or soya milk...Fabulous!

■ Fresh root ginger can be made into a wonderful pain relieving tea. Add a small cube of fresh root ginger to a mug of boiling water, add half a teaspoon of honey and apple cider vinegar and sip when warm.

■ Blackstrap molasses is rich in calcium, potassium and magnesium, which all help the joints. Try adding a teaspoon of the molasses to a tablespoon of organic apple cider vinegar or a little lemon juice into a cup of warm water, which helps you to absorb more minerals from your diet and helps to re-alkalize your system. For those who prefer honey, buy organic, preferably locally produced and, if at all possible, unrefined, which contains more natural minerals. If your symptoms are severe, drink this cocktail up to three times daily.

■ Use organic, unrefined olive, sunflower, walnut or sesame oils for your salad dressings.

■ Eat at least one tablespoon of linseeds, sunflower, pumpkin or sesame seeds daily, as they are rich in essential fats that are vital for healthy joints. Hazelnuts, cashew, almonds and walnuts are all rich in essential fats to nourish the joints. An easy way to eat more of them is to place 2 tablespoons of each in a blender, whizz for 10 seconds and store in an airtight jar in the fridge. Sprinkle over breakfast cereal, fruit salads or into low-fat, bio yoghurts daily.

■ Try herbal teas such as devil's claw and nettle and use dandelion coffee.

■ Add more turmeric and cayenne pepper to foods as they help to reduce inflammation.

Useful Remedies

■ One of the best nutritional supplements known to help this condition is the amino sugar glucosamine sulphate. A number of studies have found that 500mg taken three times a day taken for three months or more can substantially reduce pain and improve mobility. Initially take 500mg of glucosamine three times a day until symptoms improve and then lower dose to 500mg daily. Glucosamine is usually derived from crab shells, so if you have a severe intolerance to shellfish avoid this supplement.

■ Niacinamide (no-flush vitamin B3) – 500mg three times a day is a great alternative to glucosamine, which helps to reduce joint pain. Some people reap the benefits in as little as four to five weeks, but ideally three months to a year is a good time scale to take this vitamin. Incidentally, it has been noted that people who take niacinamide over a sustained period of time also have an improved sense of humour. Be sure to ask for the **no-flush variety**, as common niacin can cause a flushing effect that can be quite shocking if you are unprepared.

■ As all the B-group vitamins work together, add a B complex to your daily regimen.

- MSM (methylsulfonylmethane) is a form of organic sulphur which is involved with many key functions in the body. Extraordinary results are being reported in terms of pain relief from taking around 2–3 grams daily. It is also available in creams. For details call Higher Nature (page 13) or ask at your local health store.

- Nutricol Powder has been developed by Brian Welsby who designed the health programmes for most of the UK Olympic athletes. It contains glucosamine, MSM and hydrolysed collagen. For details call Be-Well Products on 01778 560868, fax 01778 560872 or website www.be-well.co.uk

- Take a couple of teaspoons of cod liver oil daily to help reduce the pain. The vitamin D in cod liver oil or capsules also helps to reduce pain. Or take three capsules daily. Many fish oils are now high in toxins that have been pumped into the world's oceans, most notably dioxins, deadly chemicals formed during incineration of plastic and PCBs, persistent industrial chemicals used in electrical equipment and many fish oils contain far too many toxins that can adversely affect hormones. Three of the safest found after extensive testing are BioCare's DriCelle Cod Liver Oil powder, Higher Nature's Omega-3 Fish Oil and Seven Seas One a Day pure cod liver oil. The Seven Seas is available at all health stores and for details of the others, see page 13.

- Natural source full spectrum (with 4 tocopherols and 4 tocotrienols) vitamin E 400–800iu daily helps reduce pain (but not if you take prescription blood thinning drugs, as vitamin E naturally thins the blood).

- Take 1–3grams of vitamin C daily in an ascorbate form with meals, which does not irritate the gut and has anti-inflammatory properties. Vitamin C is vital for healthy synovial fluid that surrounds the joints.

- Ginger, curcumin and boswelia are herbs with highly anti-inflammatory properties, take 3–4 tablets a day.

- The formula Ligazyme Plus made by BioCare (see page 13) contains vital minerals such as calcium, boron, magnesium, rutin, silica plus vitamins A and D and digestive enzymes, which all support connective tissue and encourage healthier bones.

- Sodiphos is a mineral (sodium phosphate) that helps to break down uric acid deposits in joints. It is especially useful for gout if you take 600mg daily. Available from Blackmores (see page 13 for details).

- Include a good-quality antioxidant formula in your regimen.

- Homeopathic Rhus Tox 6x helps to relieve stiffness when you first move around. It is especially good for people whose symptoms are worse when it's cold and wet.

- Homeopathic Ruta Graveoleans 30c often helps if tendons are sore and if spine and joints feel tender or worse when it's cold and wet.

RHEUMATOID ARTHRITIS (RA)

Rheumatoid arthritis is primarily an inflammatory disease of the smaller joints such as wrists, ankles, fingers and knees. It is an auto-immune disorder whereby the body's own immune system starts attacking joint tissue. It is a chronic disease and tends to progress with time but many people find the pain and stiffness comes and goes for varying periods of time. RA affects three times as many women as men and most often occurs between the ages of 25 to 50. Over acidity in the body and uric acid deposits in the joints is a contributing factor (see also *Acid–Alkaline Balance*).

The pain and stiffness are usually worse upon rising, and tends to wear off as the day progresses. The joints can become warm, tender and swollen. Fatigue, low-grade fever, loss of appetite and vague muscular pains can all accompany RA.

Researchers have found that at least one-third of people can completely control their rheumatoid arthritis by eliminating foods to which they have an intolerance. The most common culprits are any foods and drinks from cows, plus the nightshade group (see also *Osteoarthritis*).

Other triggers are a leaky gut, which is when food molecules pass through the gut wall thus triggering an allergic response. Many RA sufferers also have parasites and candida, a yeast fungal overgrowth. There can also be a genetic susceptibility (see also *Leaky Gut in Ageing p187*).

Heavy exercise may cause RA to progress faster, but gentle exercise such as swimming, t'ai chi, yoga, stretching and walking are more helpful. Researchers have found that many rheumatoid arthritis sufferers are deficient in the major antioxidant nutrients, vitamins A, C and E plus the mineral selenium, but particularly vitamin E. The majority of RA sufferers also appear to be low in stomach acid and supplementing with betaine hydrochloride (stomach acid) can help. (See also *Low Stomach Acid*.) Betaine helps to digest the proteins and most people who have allergies have a problem digesting certain proteins. If you have active stomach ulcers do not take the betaine and use a papaya or pineapple-based digestive enzyme capsule instead.

RA is virtually unknown in primitive cultures where the diet is mainly alkaline forming foods, nor do these people have antibiotics or refined foods, which also contribute to RA.

Foods to Avoid

- Animal fats eaten to excess tend to aggravate rheumatoid arthritis. Avoiding all dairy produce from cows, plus meat, sugar and eggs helps some people.
- Avoid known triggers such as tomatoes, potatoes, aubergines and peppers.
- Oranges and orange juice can be a problem for some people.
- Black tea, coffee, chocolate, peanuts, spinach, rhubarb and beetroot are all high in oxalic acid, which seems to further aggravate RA in some people.
- Greatly reduce your intake of refined sugary foods and drinks.
- Avoid wheat, citrus especially oranges and grapefruit, corn, food additives, colourings and flavourings. Keep a food diary and note when symptoms are more acute. Eliminate these

foods for a month and see if this helps.

Friendly Foods

- Eat more pineapple, which is a rich source of bromelain.
- Eat oily fish at least 3 times a week such as wild salmon or mackerel or take a couple of teaspoons of fish oil daily. These omega-3 essential fats reduce uric acid levels.
- Use organic linseed oil plus unrefined olive oil in salad dressings (see *Fats for Anti-ageing*) .
- A strict vegetarian, i.e. vegan diet, has been shown to help some individuals.
- Root ginger plus the spices turmeric and boswelia have anti-inflammatory properties that can substantially reduce the pain and give people more mobility.
- Make a tea using fresh ginger and lemon juice, and drink organic aloe vera.
- Eat plenty of cherries, garlic and use rice, oat or organic soya milks as alternatives to dairy produce from cows.
- Avocado and raw wheat germ is rich in vitamin E and essential fats.
- Eat lots more green vegetables especially raw green cabbage, spring greens, watercress, parsley, celery and endives or add a green food powder based on wheat grass, spirulina, alfalfa, chlorella and green foods, such as Dr Gillian McKeith's Living Food Energy, to cereals, juices and desserts. Available from health stores.
- Under professional guidance, juice fasts can greatly reduce symptoms (see *Detoxing*).

Useful Remedies

- For those who don't like fresh pineapple, bromelain is available as a supplement. Take one capsule of bromelain on an empty stomach to increase its effectiveness.
- I strongly recommend you read the section *Essential Sugars*, as this new food group is having profound beneficial effects with inflammatory and auto-immune conditions.
- Evening primrose oil can help, but you would need very high amounts and the reason people take EPO is for the GLA (gamma linolenic acid content). GLA is highly anti-inflammatory and is available as a supplement. Take 1– 2 grams daily.
- Vitamin C, 1–3grams daily, plus 400–800iu of natural source, full spectrum vitamin E.
- A multimineral formula containing 30mg of zinc, 70mcg of selenium plus traces of copper in either a food state or colloidal form taken daily helps to re-alkalize the body.
- EPA-DHA fish oil, take 1–2grams daily.
- Many sufferers of RA benefit from taking vitamin B5 pantothenic acid and 500mg can be taken four times a day. Pure Royal Jelly has a high B5 content.
- As B vitamins work together include a B complex.
- The herbs curcumin, turmeric and boswelia are also available in tablet and capsule formulas. Take 1200–1600mg daily of any one.

- Take 300mg celery seed extract daily to reduce uric acid levels

- L-glutamine 500mg taken three times daily, can help heal a leaky gut. Take between meals.

- Sufferers of RA are often lacking in healthy bacteria within their guts, therefore a daily acidophilus/bifidus capsule after meals can help increase assimilation of nutrients from food and supplements.

Helpful Hints For All Types Of Arthritis

- If you are overweight, this places more strain on the load bearing joints, so lose weight.

- Hot and cold compresses applied alternately will help reduce swelling and pain for 20 minutes at a time. Cold compresses are especially good if the affected joints feel hot to the touch. Moist hot packs help reduce pain and stiffness.

- Joint cartilage needs plenty of fluid, so drink at least 8 glasses of water daily, which also helps eliminate uric acid. Hard water can sometimes exacerbate arthritic type symptoms, as it is packed with minerals, but in an inorganic form which are hard to absorb. However, fruits and vegetables are able to absorb the inorganic minerals and aided by sunlight converts them to an organic form, and when minerals are in an organic or colloidal form, they become more bio-available to us (see also *Water in Ageing*).

- To ingest the 21 minerals that are essential for life, it makes sense to eat far more fresh fruits and vegetables. But unfortunately thanks to pollution, over farming and acid rain, most soils (especially in the UK) no longer contain sufficient minerals needed for good health. And if the minerals are not in the soil, they are never going to make it into our vegetables, however organic foods generally contain more minerals. This is why we all need to begin taking a daily multimineral.

- The purest forms of water are either distilled water or reverse osmosis (RO) waters, which are extremely pure and free of minerals. These types of waters re-hydrate your cells more easily. Really pure waters are filtered in such a way that gives you 99.999% pure H2O, like the rainwater that fell through an unpolluted atmosphere aeons ago. For further details of Reverse Osmosis Water call The Pure H2O Company on 01784 221188, or log on to www.purewater.co.uk. See under *Water* on p.325.

- To re-alkalize your system, take a good quality green powder such as Alkalife daily. The same company also make Alkabath salts which are more powerful than Epsom salts and help to eliminate toxins from the joints. For your nearest stockists call Best Care Products on 01342 410 303, fax 01342 410909 or www.bestcare-uk.com.

- Topically applied oil of wintergreen can help ease the pain and inflammation.

- Homeopathic Apis 30c helps in RA when there is swelling and rheumatic pains which are worse for heat.

- If the RA is in the small joints, ask at your homeopathic pharmacy for Actea Spicata-3c, which, taken three times daily between meals, helps reduce the pain.

- Wearing magnets has given pain relief to many people. There is now a new super magnet available that is 8000 times more powerful than the earth's magnetic field. Magnets placed on the painful area increase blood flow, bringing more oxygen to an injury or area of pain, which helps to reduce swelling and inflammation. For details of Super Magnets call Coghill Laboratories on 01495 752 122, or log on to www.cogreslab.co.uk

- The Chinese exercise regimes of t'ai chi or qigong have helped many sufferers, as they are easy to practise, even with severely impaired mobility. Rheumatoid seems to be affected by stress, so make sure you stay as calm as possible (see also *Stress in Ageing*).

- For help, ideas and counselling on arthritis call the Arthritis Care Helpline between 12pm–4pm, Monday to Friday, 0808 800 4050; website: www.arthritiscare.org.uk.

- Call the Arthritic Association on 020 7491 0233 between 10am–4pm weekdays or log on to their website www.arthriticassociation.org.uk. This charity provides very good dietary advice.

ATHEROSCLEROSIS
(*See High Blood Pressure*)

BLADDER PROBLEMS IN AGEING – FOR WOMEN
(*For Men* – See *Prostate*)

Incontinence, Prolapse and Urgency

As we age the muscles and ligaments that hold the bladder in place in the pelvic floor weaken. But gravity alone over time can lead to leakage and poor bladder control. Also a prolapsed or constipated bowel will push down onto the bladder. Following the menopause, the uterus can also begin pressing onto the bladder.

Varying degrees of incontinence can cause urine to leak out when the bladder is put under pressure when you laugh, cough, sneeze or exert yourself. It can also occur when you have eaten to excess and the bowel puts pressure on the bladder. This type of problem is referred to as stress incontinence. Exercise can help keep the pelvic floor strong and childbirth tends to weaken it, hence why it is a good idea to practise plenty of pelvic exercises after giving birth.

I suffered this problem during my 20s after giving birth to my daughter and it became so embarrassing that in my early 30s I found a gynaecologist who specialized in bladder repair and had surgery. It has made a huge difference to my quality of life and for over 20 years I have been free to exercise without embarrassment.

Urinary incontinence, or an urgency to urinate, is also associated with candida (thrush) and cystitis. Also when you become totally physically exhausted, especially from stress, then your adrenal glands also become exhausted and this can also cause you to urinate regularly. If you are exhausted, Siberian ginseng and esther vitamin C (a low acid formula) help support the adrenal glands.

If the pelvis is out of alignment or you suffer lower back problems, then the nerves to the bladder, if pinched, may be telling the bladder that it is full when it's not. If you have lower back problems, it's well worth consulting an osteopath or chiropractor who can check the pelvic area for misalignments.

Foods to Avoid

- Any food to which you have an allergy or intolerance can aggravate incontinence – caffeine being the most common culprit.

- Avoid fluoridated water, toothpastes and mouthwashes. I have received many letters from people who say that when fluoride is eliminated the problem stops, it also seems to help with children who wet the bed.

- The biggest culprits are usually yeast, wheat, dairy, alcohol and sugar.

- Food colourings, additives and preservatives can all irritate the bladder lining.

Friendly Foods

- Cranberry juice and fresh cranberries contain hippuric acid and if there are any bacteria clinging to your bladder walls, the cranberry will help remove them. Make sure any juices are low in sugar and free from aspartame and other sugar substitutes.

- Many bacteria in the bladder thrive in an acid environment, while others thrive in an alkaline environment. Therefore you need to keep the pH properly balanced (for foods see *Acid–Alkaline Balance*).

- Eat live, low-fat yoghurt, which helps to reduce problems like thrush and cystitis. These yoghurts contain friendly bacteria called acidophilus/bifidus, which are especially needed if you have taken antibiotics.

- Always drink six glasses of water daily, vital for healthy kidneys (see also *Kidneys in Ageing*).

Useful Remedies

- A multivitamin/mineral for women to help support surrounding ligaments and tissues, which contains no more than 50mg of B vitamins, as higher doses may irritate the bladder.

- 500mg of calcium with 250mg of magnesium to help muscle control. Take for six weeks before you will see the benefits.

- Inurin made by Bional is a formula containing horsetail and sweet sumach, herbs which are helpful if you find yourself having to go to the loo during the night. For your nearest stockists call 0800 328 4244. As I started popping to the loo in the night, which disturbed my sleep patterns, I started to take Inurin, it took two or three nights to click in, but I can now sleep through. Well worth trying.

- The mineral silica 75mg and the herb aquisetum (horsetail). 5mls of each tincture a day will help to strengthen the bladder.

- During the menopause, low oestrogen levels can trigger this problem, therefore if you are going through the menopause include soy extract (soya isoflavones), dong quai or black cohosh in your regimen (see also *Menopause p212*).

Helpful Hints

- Strengthening the pelvic floor muscles can reduce or eliminate stress incontinence. These muscles contract when you try to stop your urine flow. Squeeze this area and hold for at least four seconds, repeat regularly throughout the day, even if sitting at a desk.

- Try using a pelvic toner that used regularly helps to strengthen the muscles. For details call 0117 968 7744, or log on to www.naturalwoman.co.uk

- Aquaflex make weighted vaginal cones in various sizes, which also help strengthen the muscles. Tel 0808 100 2890 or log on to www.aquaflexcones.com

- Don't wait until you are absolutely "bursting" before you go to the loo, as in the long run you could end up with a very irritable bladder. Listen to your body.

- Women can empty their bladder more efficiently if they squat rather than sit on the loo.

- An osteopath or chiropractor can check the alignment of bones in the pubic area, because if the bones are out of balance urine flow in both men and women can be affected. Acupuncture has proven helpful to some people. (See *Useful Information and Addresses*).

- Contact the Continence Foundation, 307 Hatton Square, 16 Baldwins Gardens, London EC1N 7RJ, enclosing an SAE, or telephone their helpline on 020 7831 9831 (9.30am–4.30pm weekdays); website: www.continence-foundation.org.uk e-mail: continence-foundation@dial.pipex.com.

BLOOD TYPE IN AGEING

Eating the right foods for your blood type helps to slow ageing, encourages weight loss and increases absorption of nutrients from you diet.

Our blood type is our evolution, the genetic memory passed down from our ancestors. It is the key to our immune system and controls the influences of bacteria, viruses, chemicals and stress. For instance Type-0 is the oldest blood type (around 40,000 BC), whereas Type-AB is the more recent blood type (only 1,000 years old).

The immune system has a very sophisticated method to determine whether a food, additive or pollutant is foreign or not. The cells of our body have chemical markers called antigens, which determine your blood type.

We are not only what we eat, but also what we absorb and assimilate and the old saying "one man's meat is another man's poison" is certainly true and your blood type is a major factor in deciding which foods suit your body.

American, Dr Peter D'Adamo, has worked on the link between diet, disease and blood groups for more than 15 years. His father, Dr James D'Adamo, was credited with the discovery of these links when he observed differing responses to treatments offered to heart and diabetic patients based on their blood type. Treatments were better controlled in accordance with a diet based on their blood type, as foods were either compatible or incompatible to their blood.

In 1960, a Massachusetts study examined connections between blood types and heart disease and found a strong link between blood type and who survives heart disease. For instance Type-0s (aged between 39 and 72) had a higher survival rate than Type-As.

The four blood types are O, A, B and AB. Dr D'Adamo's theory revolves around certain toxic proteins in our food called lectins.

When you eat a food that contains these lectins such as cows' milk, pork or even chicken, if they are incompatible with your blood type, the lectins target an organ or bodily system (kidneys, brain, stomach etc) and blood cells start to clump together in that area. This reduces the blood's oxygen and nutrient capacity as well as placing huge demands on the liver and kidneys to excrete these "natural" toxins from the body. It is like running your car on poor fuel: it will still go but the life of the engine will be greatly reduced. In a similar way this is what is happening within our body, and over a lifetime it will have marked effects.

Lectins will interfere with digestion, slow down the rate of food metabolism, compromise the production of insulin and upset hormonal balance.

Examples of some of the differences in the blood types are:

- Type-0s (about 47% of the population) have hardy digestive tracts, do better on high-protein foods, combat their stress through vigorous exercise such as aerobics, are more prone to osteoarthritis, allergies, asthma and duodenal ulcers and tend to have higher instances of type 2 late-onset diabetes. They also tend to produce more stomach acid, are worse off in epidemics, for example the flu, and have thinner blood.

- Type-As (about 42% of the population) should be predominantly vegetarian and have sensitive digestive tracts. They combat their stress through quieter techniques such as yoga or meditation, have thicker blood, are prone to cardiovascular disease and high blood pressure, produce lower stomach acid and do better in epidemics. They also tend to produce a lot of mucus.

- Type-Bs (about 8% of the population) have strong immune systems, tend to combat their stress through moderate exercises such as t'ai chi, golf and cycling. They are not generally prone to allergies but are more likely to suffer from autoimmune disorders such as rheumatoid arthritis. In general, however, they have a much more balanced system.

- Type-ABs (about 3% of the population) are a modern merging of Type-A and Type-B. They have sensitive digestive tracts, can be prone to more parasites and may have difficulty eradicating candida (a fungal overgrowth). They have the least problems with allergies and are more like Type-A than Type-B, hence they tend to have thicker blood and high cholesterol levels. They also combat their stress in similar ways to Type-As, through meditation and yoga.

Foods to Avoid

These foods are not necessarily unhealthy, it's just that *if* you have the blood type these foods are harder to assimilate. If you want to eat these foods, don't eat them every day, once a week is fine.

- Type-O should avoid all cows' milk products including cheese, chocolate and ice cream, wheat and corn (Os tend to have an intolerance to gluten) pork, ham and bacon, oranges, avocado and peanuts.
- Type-A should avoid all meats and meat products, cows' milk, cheese and ice cream, tomatoes, oranges and bananas, chickpeas and vinegars.
- Type-B should avoid chicken, ham, pork and bacon, all shellfish and crustaceans, nuts and seeds, tomatoes, sweetcorn, wheat and rye.
- Type-AB should avoid cows' milk products including cheese and ice cream, beef, pork and chicken, most shellfish and crustaceans, buckwheat, sweetcorn, oranges and bananas.

Friendly Foods

- Type-O – organic beef, lamb, chicken or turkey, fish (especially cod, mackerel and salmon), goats' milk, oat milk or rice milk, goats' cheese, feta or mozzarella, oats, rice, barley and gluten-free breads and pastas (e.g. millet and rice noodle pasta), walnuts, broccoli, spinach, leeks, pumpkin, turnips, parsnips and onions, figs, plums, and pineapple, Rooibos tea.
- Type-A – fish (except sole, plaice and haddock), soya milk, rice, goats' and oat milk, goats' cheese, lentils, almonds and peanuts, tofu and all soya products, carrots, broccoli, onions and pumpkin, apricots, figs and pineapple, green tea.
- Type-B – lamb, fish (especially cod, mackerel and salmon), dairy foods (except blue cheese), millet, oats, rice and spelt, beetroots, Brussels sprouts and green leafy vegetables, bananas, grapes and papaya, peppermint and green tea.
- Type-AB – lamb, turkey and fish (especially trout, salmon, mackerel and sardines), goats' milk and goats' cheese, peanuts, lentils and walnuts, millet, oats, rice and spelt, cauliflower, celery, sweet potato and beetroots, and femented soya products, figs, cranberries, grapes and plums, green tea.
- Please note that if you would like a full list of foods to avoid and friendly foods for your blood type (see the suggested book at the end of *Helpful Hints*, page 56).

Useful Remedies

- Type-O – their diet is rich in all the most common vitamins and minerals, especially iron and vitamin C. They do however, tend to have sluggish metabolisms and would benefit from taking a good B-complex supplement daily.

■ It is also difficult for the Os to get adequate amounts of manganese in their diet as this mineral is primarily found in wholegrains and pulses, so a daily multimineral, which includes manganese, would be beneficial.

■ Because Os should not include dairy foods in their diet (apart from goats' milk and cheese), a multimineral that contains calcium, magnesium and boron is beneficial. Other good sources of calcium are sardines, canned salmon (unboned), and green-leafy vegetables especially broccoli.

■ Kelp is an excellent supplement for this blood type and can help with the sluggish metabolism. As Os tend to have high stomach acid, liquorice (deglycyrrhizinated liquorice) may be helpful.

■ If you are a Type-O but not used to a high-protein diet, taking a pancreatic digestive enzyme before a large meal may be necessary for a while until your system adjusts. BioCare make Polyzyme Forte (see page 13 for details).

■ Dandelion tea and coffee, peppermint, fenugreek and rose hip teas, ginger and parsley are also good for type O.

■ Type-A – they can be deficient in vitamin B12 because they should not eat animal proteins and may have a problem absorbing it due to a lack of intrinsic factor in their stomachs (intrinsic factor is a substance produced by the stomach which helps absorption of B12 in the body). This problem becomes more common in the elderly where it can be associated with neurological problems and dementia.

■ Soya foods such as organic tofu, tempeh and miso, contain B12 and can be eaten regularly but not if you have hormone related cancer.

■ A daily supplement of vitamin C (500mg twice daily) can help protect the stomach lining.

■ Iron may be lacking for the vegetarian, a teaspoon of blackstrap molasses in warm water each day, or a daily supplement of Floradix or Spatone can help. Molasses are also rich in calcium.

■ Goats' milk and cheese, broccoli, spinach, soya milk and sardines are also rich in calcium.

■ Zinc is another mineral often lacking in the vegetarian diet though this is generally because of eating processed food. Supplementing daily with 25–30mg of zinc picolinate on an empty stomach will help overcome this deficiency.

■ Beneficial herbs for Type-A are: camomile, fenugreek and rose hip teas, ginger, ginseng, alfalfa and aloe vera.

■ Type-B – their diet is rich in vitamins A, B, C and E as well as the minerals calcium and iron. Bs are very efficient in absorbing calcium, so much so that they run the risk of creating an imbalance between calcium and magnesium and consequent deficiency of magnesium. A daily supplement of magnesium (600–800mg daily) would be of benefit. Leafy green vegetables, wholegrains, pulses and beans are rich in magnesium.

■ If you are not used to eating meats and dairy foods, it may take a while to adapt to the diet and so taking a digestive enzyme such as bromelain (from pineapple) before each meal helps reduce any bloating.

■ Beneficial herbs for the Bs are, sage, peppermint and rose hip teas, parsley, liquorice, ginseng and ginger.

■ Type-AB – this blood type get plenty of vitamins A, B12, E and niacin from their recommended diets but would benefit from taking extra vitamin C (500mg twice daily with food), to help protect the stomach from nitrates (possible cancer-causing chemicals), due to having less protection because of low stomach acid. Their sensitive stomachs should also benefit from taking a bromelain- (pineapple) based enzyme before meals, especially if they suffer from bloating.

■ Taking the immune-boosting herbs echinacea or astragalus when a virus threatens can help boost the more vulnerable immune system of AB.

■ Other immune boosting herbs for this blood type are burdock root and rose hip teas, ginger, ginseng, alfalfa and liquorice.

Helpful Hints

■ Weight loss can be very difficult for some people and eating right for your blood type can be the answer. This way of eating has been the key to weight loss for thousands of people who have tried many different diets. Your system will become more efficient, and Steve Langley suggests eating this way for at least 3 months for best results. A gradual loss of weight, around one pound per week, is to be expected. People who follow the blood type diet (which is more a healthy eating plan than a diet) will find that their energy levels increase as they slowly shed the pounds. The following are some tips to lose weight for each of the blood types.

For Weight Loss

■ Type-O should avoid wheat (try gluten-free products), sweetcorn, lentils, kidney beans, cabbage, Brussels sprouts and cauliflower.

■ They should eat more seafoods, seaweeds such as kelp (sprinkle on your food instead of salt), kale, spinach and broccoli.

■ Type-A should avoid meat, all cows' milk products (milk, cheese and ice-cream) kidney beans and lima beans.

■ They should eat more flaxseeds (linseeds), fermented soya foods, vegetables (try and eat a wide variety) and pineapple.

■ Type-B should avoid wheat, buckwheat, sweetcorn, lentils, peanuts and sesame seeds.

■ They should eat more meat (lamb, venison, rabbit or beef), eggs, and green vegetables.

■ Type-AB should avoid red meat, wheat and buckwheat, kidney beans, lima beans, seeds (especially sesame) and sweetcorn.

- They should eat more fermented soya products, seafoods, seaweeds such as kelp, green vegetables, pineapple and alkaline fruits such as apples and pears.
- Read, *Eat Right For Your Type – Complete Blood Type Encyclopaedia*, by Dr Peter D'Adamo, Riverhead Books. Available from The NutriCentre Bookshop, tel: 0207 323 2382.

BONES

(See also *Exercise, Joints in Ageing* and *Osteoporosis*)

BOWELS

(See also *Elimination*)

In an ideal world, we should have a bowel movement after every meal, but most people in the West are lucky if they have one a day. Having clean bowels is one of the best ways to stay younger longer. Even if you have a daily bowel movement – you can still be constipated. As we age, we experience a gradual build up of mucoid plaque, a rubbery like substance, which adheres to the walls of the intestines. This plaque is caused by insufficient fibre and too many refined foods, and over time it inhibits proper assimilation of anti-ageing nutrients from the diet and supplements. It also adds to the weight of the colon, therefore placing more stress on the lower organs like the uterus and bladder.

Millions of men and women have large, protruding abdomens. This means that all the major organs in that area, such as the liver, heart and bowels are surrounded by a layer of deadly fat deposits. They are also likely to be carrying a lot of waste matter. Henry VIII had over 84 pounds of faeces in his bowel after his death and he had a very big stomach indeed.

When food leaves the small intestine, which is over 20 feet long, it passes into the large intestine or colon where it is gradually compacted into semi-solid faeces. The bowel is a term for the large intestines. Most of the absorption of nutrients from our diet and supplements happens in the small intestine. The large intestine (colon) is primarily involved with the breaking down of foods for elimination.

The more faeces in your bowel the more toxic your entire system becomes. If you are not eliminating properly these toxins are re-absorbed into the bloodstream and can be eventually dumped into the skin resulting in conditions such as acne. People from primitive cultures tend to evacuate twice the amount of faeces than their Western counterparts due to their higher intake of fibre and raw foods.

Peristalsis is the rhythmic movement of the colon, which helps to move the waste material out of the body. If you tend to eat a poor diet, low in fibre then the muscles in the colon can become lazy which over time can lead to chronic constipation. Also if you over-eat, food putrefies in the bowel, triggering symptoms such as bloating, gas, constipation/and or diarrhoea, irritable bowel, poor skin, dull hair and so on.

Haemorrhoids or piles (varicose veins of the anus) are the result of years of straining to go to the loo and straining also contributes to varicose veins in the legs. If ever you experience blood in your faeces, it is vital that you see a doctor immediately.

Foods to Avoid

- All animal products, especially red meats, have a long transit time through the bowel and should be eaten only in moderation.

- Many people do not have the enzyme needed to break down lactose, the sugar in milk, which can also lead to putrefaction in the bowel. This is especially common in African and Caribbean people.

- If you tend to be a big dairy fan, try cutting back on all dairy-based foods, as they are mucus forming, which adds to the plaque in the intestines. However, organic rice, oat or goats' milk are generally better tolerated.

- Refined sugars found in cakes, biscuits, desserts and highly processed foods ferment in the gut causing gas and bloating as healthy bacteria are destroyed. These bacteria help break down digested foods and aid in the manufacture of certain B-group vitamins. If these healthy bacteria are missing, your digestion and elimination are impaired.

- When you mix flour and water it makes a gooey paste, it does the same in the bowel, therefore cut down on pastries and flour-based foods.

- Low-fibre foods such as jelly, ice cream and soft desserts, all white flour products and refined breakfast cereals, which contain virtually no fibre and lots of sugar.

- Also avoid foods to which you have an intolerance, for instance cows' milk has been found to be responsible for a lot of infant constipation.

- Cut down on full-fat cheeses and don't eat melted cheese over food – it sets like plastic in the bowel.

Friendly Foods

- Eat more insoluble bran fibres derived from rice, or oats. The insoluble fibre is needed for stimulating the bowel to work properly. Wheat bran is fine so long as you don't have an intolerance to wheat, otherwise this can aggravate the problem.

- Try eating more brown rice (or rice bran) plus black-eyed beans, kidney, haricot, butter and cannelloni beans.

- Linseeds are a blend of insoluble and soluble fibres, which bulk the stool, encouraging it to move gently through the bowel. Linusit Gold are ready cracked.

- Wholewheat rye bread, Ryvita-type crispbreads, rough oatcakes, or amaranth crackers can be eaten as an alternative to wheat bread.

- Other high-fibre foods are fresh and dried figs, blackcurrants, ready-to-eat dried apricots and prunes, almonds, hazelnuts, fresh coconut and all mixed nuts.

- All lightly cooked or raw vegetables and salads will add more fibre to your diet.

- Eat more, live, low-fat yoghurts, which contain healthy bacteria – a lack of which can exacerbate constipation.
- Drink at least six glasses of water daily.
- Psyllium husks are a great way to add bulk to the stools. Take a tablespoon of psyllium husks in water before breakfast to help keep things moving.

Useful Remedies

- Dr Gillian McKeith's Living Food Energy Powder, take 1–2 teaspoons a day. This blend of fibres and nutrients helps improve bowel function and digestion. Available from all health shops.
- Acidophilus, bifidus are healthy bacteria, which can be taken after a meal, particularly if constipation has started after antibiotics.
- Taking 1 level teaspoon two to three times a day of Vitamin C powder with added calcium and magnesium, for a few days, can help soften the stool and increase the frequency of bowel movement. Magnesium also helps to tone the bowel muscles.
- One of the best ways I have found to eliminate constipation is to replace one meal a day with a fruit and vegetable blend whilst eliminating all flour from any source for at least two days. I put half a cup of aloe vera juice, a banana, an apple, blueberries and any fruit I have to hand, plus a teaspoon of any good green food mix, a teaspoon of sunflower seeds, a dessertspoon of linseeds and a teaspoon of olive oil into my blender. To this I add half a cup of organic rice milk and blend. It's delicious and packed with fibre. On alternate days I make a vegetable juice to which I still add the aloe vera juice but not the rice milk.
- Arabinogalactan (AG), a fibre from the larch tree, is very useful in the treatment of constipation. It acts as a normal stool softener, which helps to normalize bowel movements. Also when AG enters the colon, it reacts with existing bacteria to produce short chain fatty acids (SCFAs). These are a good food source of friendly bacteria in the gut and promote a lower pH in the colon, which in turn promotes peristaltic movement. Try one capsule twice daily. For details call The NutriCentre on 0207 436 5122 or log on to www.nutricentre.com

Helpful Hints

- Squatting to pass faeces helps to encourage elimination of waste products, as it is a more natural position for the colon.
- Over-use of laxatives makes the bowel lazy.
- It is very important that you eliminate any underlying causes for your constipation. Visit your GP and make sure there is nothing more serious going on.
- Do not bear down too much when you have a bowel movement as this places a strain on the vascular system and can, over time, lead to varicose veins, haemorrhoids or piles. Remember, rather than fall asleep after every meal, go for a leisurely walk. This will make you feel less bloated, aid digestion and encourage healthier bowels.

- In Chinese medicine the best time to walk is between 5am and 7am, which encourages the colon to work more efficiently – I think I'll pass on this one!!

- When you feel the need to pass a motion, be sure not to ignore the signal.

- For healthy bowel movements you need about a pint of fluid in-between each meal to get waste moving through successfully.

- Stress is a major factor for constipation as it slows down the peristalsis movements.

- When you add more fibre to your diet and you're not used to it, it is essential that you drink more water. Adding fibre without more fluid can actually aggravate the problem.

- In the elderly, a lack of folic acid has sometimes been found to be the cause of constipation, therefore, supplementing with folic acid in the form of a good-quality multivitamin/mineral should help.

- For severe constipation especially after surgery, and with your doctor's permission, try colonic irrigation. I have a colonic two or three times a year as a thorough cleanse, especially if I have taken antibiotics, which cause me real problems!

- You can also use a lukewarm-water enema at home. Available from Best Care Products on 01342 410303 or www.info@bestcare-uk.com.

BRAIN IN AGEING

(See also *Alzheimer's Disease, Memory* and *Mind Power*)

At the age of 75, you still have 85% of the brain cells that you were born with, and while previously it was always thought that loss of brain cells was permanent, we now know that brain cells can replace themselves. Researchers at the Salk Institute in California have now proven that we do have the potential to regenerate and revitalize our brains. This is great news.

If you don't use your brain and stay alert, with ageing gradual shrinkage can occur. How many people do you know in their 40s who are already showing signs of forgetfulness? You meet someone, you know their face, but cannot remember their name. Then you forget where you left the car keys. These types of symptoms do not always herald the onset of dementia, they can be a sign of low blood sugar (see also *Carbohydrate Control* and *Low Blood Sugar*).

As the years pass, you tend to think more slowly, it takes you longer to recall simple words and phrases, you may feel less motivated, have less mental energy, a lower sex drive and so on. But brain degeneration is not inevitable.

There are approximately 100 billion brain cells (neurons), each making between 5,000 and 50,000 hard-wired connections (known as "synapses") with other brain cells, totalling around 4 quadrillion connections. To help you understand the enormity of this, consider the Amazon rainforest. There are as many cells in your brain as trees in the Amazon, and as many connections as leaves!

This awesome power needs a great deal of energy. In fact our brain, which is only 2% of our body weight, uses 25% of the energy provided by the food we eat. And a combination of lack of oxygen, poor food, toxic overload and chemical deposits, including drugs, over time makes the brain vulnerable to damage and degeneration. So the more we look after our diet, avoid pollutants, take the right nutrients and keep our minds active – the better and longer our brains will work.

Foods to Avoid

■ Sugar ages your brain. Because the brain requires a lot of energy, we often crave "fast" sugar boosts to lift our mood or concentration. But the rapid rise of sugar in your system leads to a rapid fall, and you'll soon find that sweet foods no longer give you an energy boost, but instead make you feel tired. This includes all sugars: maltose, dextrose, white and brown sugar. Another way we seek a quick sugar rush is with refined carbohydrates: white bread, pasta and rice, cakes, biscuits, pancakes etc. (See also *Sugar in Ageing*).

■ Avoid artificial sweeteners such as aspartame (marketed as Nutrasweet, Equal and Spoonful), which is found in thousands of foods and drinks including diet foods, chewing gum, fizzy drinks, sweets, breakfast cereals, frozen desserts and yoghurt. Despite assurances from the US Food and Drug Administration that it is safe, a significant number of people have reported suffering from neuro-toxic ill-effects as a result of aspartame consumption, such as headaches, mood swings, hyperactivity in children, changes in vision, nausea and diarrhoea, sleep disorders, memory loss and confusion, convulsions and seizures. Aspartame also places a strain on the liver, which can exacerbate weight gain in the long-term.

■ For a healthy brain you need to reduce your caffeine intake. Found not only in coffee but also in tea, chocolate and cola drinks, caffeine is a powerful stimulant and brain toxin. Excess amounts can lead to headaches, insomnia, trembling hands, palpitations and in extreme cases convulsions. Adults should take no more than 3–4 cups of coffee a day, though less is better so as not to disrupt your blood sugar levels. A cup of coffee contains around 100mg of caffeine, cola 50mg, tea 60mg, green tea 25mg, chocolate cake 25mg per slice and dark chocolate 30mg per ounce.

■ Reduce your alcohol intake. Enjoy a drink but keep in mind that excess alcohol will have a negative effect on your brain.

■ Greatly reduce your intake of full-fat animal products, cheeses, red and fatty meats, full-fat chocolates, pre-packaged meat and sausage pies. Most mass-produced ready-meals contain considerable amounts of saturated or trans fats. Avoid hamburgers and fried foods.

Friendly Foods

■ Two-thirds of the dry-weight of your brain is made up from fat, and conclusive research shows that the amount and type of fat consumed throughout your life has a profound effect on how you think and feel. The brain and nervous system is highly dependent on healthy, essential fats (EFAs) for both its structure and function (see *Fats for Anti-ageing*).

■ Try to eat oily fish such as salmon, sardines, mackerel, herring and fresh tuna (not tinned as the omega-3 fats have been removed) at least twice a week as they are rich in omega-3 fats which nourish nerve fibres.

■ Seeds are also a good source of EFAs – sprinkle either whole or freshly ground flax (linseeds), pumpkin, sunflower, sesame and hemp seeds over cereals, fruit salads, salads, into desserts or blend with fresh juices. A convenient way to take more seeds is to buy a packet of each of these unrefined, organic seeds and pop them into a food mixer or coffee grinder with a few walnuts and Brazil nuts. Pulse for two to three seconds. Keep them in an air-tight jar in the fridge and sprinkle over salads, rice dishes and desserts.

■ For the brain to work properly we also need phospholipids, which make up the insulating layer or myelin sheath which protects most of our nerves. There are two types of phospholipids: phosphatidyl choline and phosphatidyl serine. Egg yolk is the richest source of phospholipids–look for eggs such as Columbus, now sold in most supermarkets, as their chickens are fed on an omega-3 rich diet. Otherwise buy free-range organic eggs. Avoid fried eggs – boiling and poaching is fine.

■ Lecithin is derived from soya beans and is rich in phosphatidylcholine. Take at least a heaped teaspoon of the granules daily. Make sure the granules contain at least 30% of the PC which not only helps increase memory but also reduces LDL, the "bad" cholesterol. I use Cytoplan High-Potency Lecithin Granules which are available from most health stores, or call 01684 310099.

■ Eat plenty of fresh fruits and vegetables, which are high in antioxidants that protect the brain from degeneration, the more colourful the better. Dark green leafy vegetables such as spring greens, sprouting broccoli, cabbage, beetroots, carrots, watercress, alfalfa sprouts, sweet potato and peas are also good choices.

■ Berries – dark blue, red or purple foods, such as blackberries, blueberries and bilberries, are rich in particularly powerful antioxidants called anthocyanins. Scientists at Tufts University in Boston have found that eating a half a cup of fresh blueberries daily helps to reverse brain ageing thanks to their high antioxidant activity.

■ Green Tea is high in antioxidants. Researchers at the National Institute of Nutrition in Rome have recently found that green tea and black tea have similar antioxidant power. Unfortunately, the antioxidant effect of both was neutralized by the addition of milk. Green tea also contains less caffeine and is normally consumed without milk.

■ Glutathione is a key amino-acid (part of protein) that works as an antioxidant in the body. It's made into the antioxidant enzyme glutathioneperoxidase (also dependent on selenium) that detoxifies car exhaust, carcinogens, infections, too much alcohol and toxic metals. As we age, glutathione levels in the body fall, so getting more from your diet or supplementing is important. Glutathione is found in white meat, tuna, lentils, beans, nuts and seeds, while selenium is high in Brazil nuts, sesame seeds and seafood.

- Replace refined wheat and rice with wholemeal bread and brown rice and pasta. Generally eat more grains.
- Almost half of your brain is made up of water, therefore, to help slow brain ageing, drink at least six glasses of water daily.

Useful Remedies

- A high-strength antioxidant formula is a great place to start to protect the brain. This should contain a range of antioxidants that protect your body and brain from deterioration. Try Kudos 24 (see page 348 for details).
- The star brain nutrient is glutathione, a naturally occurring amino acid, which aids brain function and also detoxifies the liver. As we age, levels fall and toxins such as heavy metals, pollution and pesticides reduce levels, in some cases dramatically. Glutathione is manufactured in our cells from precursors such as alpha-lipoic acid (ALA) and acetyl-L-carnitine. A well-publicized study involving rats fed on extra ALA and acetyl-L-carnitine lived 50% longer than normal rats and enjoyed greatly improved overall health. The animals were so vigorous that media headlines referred to the "dancing rats". After the age of 50, try 200mg of ALA, and 500mg of acetyl-L-carnitine on a daily basis. Many companies now produce these two supplements in one formula (see details of Higher Nature Ltd. on page 14).
- Phosphatidyl serine (PS) and phosphatidyl choline help to protect nerve fibres. Take a minimum of 50mg daily of either, or both.
- Lecithin – derived from soya beans is rich in phosphatidyl serine and choline (see *Friendly Foods* on page 61 for further details).
- Ginkgo biloba is sometimes referred to as the "memory tree" and is proven to increase circulation and act as a brain stimulant. Take 500mg of standardized extract daily. Remember that herbs are potent natural medicines, so take for 6 weeks, then stop for a month and then begin again.
- Vinpocetine – an extract of the wonder plant periwinkle; has been shown to dilate brain arteries which helps bring more nutrients into the brain; reduce the tendency of blood to clot (thus helping to protect against heart disease and stroke); speed up brain metabolism act as an antioxidant; and aid recovery after stroke (for details call The NutriCentre on 0207 436 5122).
- Take an extra 1gram of vitamin C a day.
- Also take 300mg of magnesium, which is known as nature's tranquilliser. A deficiency of magnesium has a detrimental effect on a huge array of enzyme reactions which take place in our bodies, and the brain is one of the first organs to feel the lack.
- Most health companies now make a "Brain Formula" such as Patrick Holford's Advanced Brain Food. Available from good health stores, or call Higher Nature Ltd (see page 14 for details).

Helpful Hints

- Dr Keith Scott-Mumby, a nutritional physician who specializes in allergies, says, "Many people who begin suffering 'woolly brain syndrome', a mixture of fatigue and slow cloudy thinking, often believe they are experiencing the early stages of dementia, but for the most part they are simply suffering food intolerances, and sometimes chemical sensitivities. Many patients also react badly to strong cleaning agents, paints, some cosmetics, prescription drugs and so on. The most likely food culprits are wheat and cows' milk and a detox usually helps reverse this trend. For 10 days eat only fruit, vegetables, fish, meat, herbal teas and spring water. Completely avoid bread, cakes, biscuits, pastries, pasta and anything containing flour. Eliminate all dairy products for the 10 days. No tea, coffee, alcohol or manufactured food of any kind. Absolutely avoid sugar. After 10 days your brain should feel altogether sharper, then start re-introducing the other foods gradually. For instance if patients eat some wheat and then their brain begins to feel 'foggy' again, they will begin to realize which foods are the culprits." For further details on Dr Scott-Mumby, log on to www.alternative-doctor.com.

- Chelation has also been found very useful for improving brain function and removing toxic metals. (See also *Chelation in Ageing* and *Toxic Metal Overload*.)

- I'm sure you will have heard the phrase "Use it or lose it" and this truly applies to the brain which thrives on activity. Science has shown that the number of connections in the brain can be increased, by simply making demands of the mind. More connections mean more brain power. Begin doing more crosswords, buy a dictionary and learn one new word every day. Begin making a mental note of telephone numbers until you know them by heart. Enjoy stimulating conversation with friends, join local educational classes, or take up a new sport.

- Daily exercise is also important. It stimulates and tones up both body and mind. Exercise releases endorphins, increases circulation and therefore oxygen supply to the brain. Endorphins are natural feel-good substances in our bodies.

- Laugh a lot which makes you feel more positive.

- Balancing your hormones can return brain function to more youthful levels (see also *Other Vital Hormones p237).*

- Essential oils such as cinnamon, lemon and rosemary help to stimulate the brain and aid mental alertness.

- Stress greatly affects the brain, it stimulates the adrenal glands to produce the hormone cortisol – which can damage the connections between brain cells (see also *Stress in Ageing p293*).

- Dr David Perlmutter, a neurologist in Naples, Florida has pioneered the use of intravenous glutiathione, which has helped many patients with brain related problems, such as Alzheimer's and Parkinson's disease and his book *BrainRecovery.com* makes fascinating reading. Published by the Purlmutter Health Centre. Available from the NutriCentre Book Shop on 0207 323 2382 or log on to his website: www.BrainRecovery.com.

- For more help read *Optimum Nutrition For The Mind*, by Patrick Holford, Piatkus or read *Brain Longevity* by Dr Dharma Singh Khalsa, Warner Books.

BREAST CANCER

(See also *Cancer*)

By 2015, as many as 1 in 8 women will have had a diagnosis of breast cancer at some point in their lives and it remains the most common cause of death in women aged between 35 and 54. It is not the death sentence that it used to be; today there is a lot we can do to help prevent and heal breast cancer.

A few women are so frightened of contracting breast cancer, as their mother, sometimes their grandmother and other relatives died of this disease, that they have their breasts removed as a precaution. My mother died from breast cancer, but I would never undergo such radical surgery unless I actually had cancer.

Our inherited genes control the structure and function of our body but if our genes stay healthy then our body stays healthy. If you live a healthy lifestyle you can change which genes are expressed. In other words if your parents and grandparents died of heart attacks, or cancers, you may well have a pre-disposition for heart problems and cancer. But if you live a different lifestyle and eat healthier foods, you can change the chemistry within the body and stack the odds more in your favour. Genes are repairable and alterable, they adjust to our environment and state of mind (see also *Genes in Ageing*).

Meanwhile, risk factors for breast cancer are using orthodox HRT, the contraceptive pill, excessive intake of saturated animal fats, dairy products, alcohol, pesticides, herbicides, and a poor intake of protective fruit and vegetables that are rich in antioxidants.

Many young women overproduce oestrogen and this is one of the reasons they suffer with symptoms of the pre-menstrual syndrome. If you eat a healthy diet, the body excretes these hormones via the liver. However, if the diet is high in saturated and animal fats or alcohol, not only is it harder for the body to excrete these oestrogens, it tends to recycle them into an aggressive form, which begin attacking tissue.

Residues of pesticides and herbicides known to cause cancer are now in our food chain and drinking water and these toxins live in fatty tissue within the body, so the more you avoid contact with such substances the more you reduce your chance of contracting cancer.

Foods to Avoid

- Reduce your intake of alcohol to no more than one unit a day.

- Animal fats should be kept to a minimum, eat only very lean organic meats.

- Reduce your intake of dairy, especially from cows, sheep and goats and if you do eat diary make sure it's low fat.

- Pesticides and plastics in the body act like strong oestrogens hence why you need to eat organic food as much as possible. Never re-heat a pre-packaged meal in its plastic container as the chemicals leach into your food. Transfer them to glass or stainless steel cookware before heating.

- There has been much misinformation in the media about fermented soya, saying that it causes hormone activity which is non-beneficial to health. In fact, fermented soya acts like a weak oestrogen, that blocks the stronger, negative oestrogens in our environment and in the body from binding to the breast cells, and it can really be beneficial in small amounts. If you already have breast, prostate or any hormonal type of cancer, then you must try to avoid all soya based products.

Friendly Foods

- Chickpeas, lentils, beans (dried beans are best) and fermented soya products like miso, tempeh and tamari. Japanese and Thai women have a much lower incidence of breast cancer and this appears to be due to their regular consumption of fermented soya-based foods rich in phyto-oestrogens and isoflavones, which contain genistein. And genistein inhibits the growth of cancer cells. As much as possible, only eat organic and/or GM-free soya in its traditional form: miso, soya sauce and tempeh, but cook it first.

- Broccoli, cabbage, Brussels sprouts and alfalfa sprouts all contain substances which are protective against breast cancer.

- Raw cracked linseeds sprinkled regularly onto meals contain a fibre called lignan, which helps to protect breast tissue.

- My favourite way to ingest a lot of nutrients quickly is by juicing. Blend some organic raw carrots, cabbage, apple, fresh root ginger, raw beetroot, radish and celery, add to this a teaspoon of any organic green food supplement and some aloe vera juice and you will feel really energized. In cancer, the only problem with juicing is that some of the live enzymes and nutrients and almost all of the fibre is left in the juicer. Scrape them out and add them to your juice, it makes it thicker but you then receive far more nutrients. Hence why I use my blender quite a lot as then you get the whole fruit including the peel. A great meal replacement is to chop a banana, an apple (remove the pips), a small box of blueberries, a teaspoon of soya lecithin granules, some green food powder with a couple of fresh or dried figs. I throw in some sunflower seeds and linseeds and a cup of organic soya milk and whiz this for a minute it makes the most deliciously healthy and filling shake.

- Replace margarines that contain hydrogenated and trans fats with healthier spreads such as Biona, Granose or Vitaquell.

- Many patients with cancer have low levels of the carotenes. Apricots, sweet potatoes, asparagus, French beans, broccoli, carrots, mustard and cress, red peppers, spinach, watercress, mangoes, parsley and tomatoes are all rich in carotenes. Fresh, organic carrot juice is a great source.

- Take extra fibre daily which keeps toxic wastes and old hormones from being absorbed from the colon into the bloodstream. The colon must be kept clean and bowels emptied regularly for healing to occur in the body. Start with a low dose and gradually increase –

mix one teaspoon increasing to one dessertspoon of psyllium husks in a full mug of lukewarm water – and take twice daily. Take at different times from other supplements, as it can cause bloating – this is why you start with a small dose.

■ Drink plenty of water to aid elimination of wastes.

Useful Remedies for Prevention and Healing of Breast Cancer

■ Active-H is a powerful antioxidant and when taken in larger doses, such as 6 x 250mg daily with food, has been reported by many cancer patients to be helpful (for details see *Antioxidants in Ageing*).

■ If you want to help prevent breast cancer, many companies make isoflavone supplements (see *Higher Nature Ltd* (page 13) or *Kudos* (page 14).Avoid taking them if you have cancer.

■ If you have cancer, you can take up to 5–10 grams of vitamin C daily in an ascorbate form for a few weeks. With such doses you may experience loose bowels – in which case cut the dose a little. For maintenance take 1gram daily.

■ Take a high-strength antioxidant formula that contains vitamins A, C and E plus zinc and selenium.

■ If you have breast cancer take co-enzymeQ10 x 200mg twice a day. This important co-enzyme has been shown to inhibit cancer cell growth and protect breast tissue. To aid prevention take 100mg daily.

■ Reishi, shitake and maitake mushrooms are available either as tincture or as tablets and should be taken three times a day. They have been shown to have great immune enhancing properties and to inhibit the growth and spread of cancer cells. For details call the *NutriCentre* (see page 14 for details).

■ Take a good-quality multivitamin/mineral.

■ Indole 3 Carbinol (I3C) is a phytochemical supplement isolated from cruciferous vegetables (broccoli, cauliflower, Brussels sprouts, turnips, kale, green cabbage, mustard, pak choy, etc). To ingest therapeutic quantities of indole would require eating enormous amounts of raw vegetables as cooking tends to destroy these phytochemicals. Take one tablet 2–3 times a day (see *The NutriCentre* details on page 14).

Helpful Hints

■ Examine your breasts once a month. If you find even the hint of anything unusual or any type of lump, see your doctor immediately. Remember, the earlier any problems are detected, the greater your chance of a complete cure. Many lumps are simply benign cysts, so the sooner you see your doctor the better.

■ Some scientists believe that antiperspirants may be linked to breast cancer. Many sprays contain chemicals that are absorbed into the body and they also stop you from sweating, which is nature's way of getting rid of unwanted toxins. The majority of breast cancers occur in the part of the breast nearest the armpit. Use natural tea-tree based anti-perspirants or aluminium-free deodorants such as Pit Rok Crystal or Crystal Fresh.

- In studies,women who wore a tight fitting bra for 14 hours or longer a day were 50% more likely to develop breast cancer. At the very least find yourself a comfortable loose-fitting bra that doesn't block lymph drainage. Some women who have had their breasts removed find that any remaining lymph glands, especially under the arms can be really painful. Manual lymph drainage can often relieve the discomfort (see under Useful Information and Addresses p.343).

- Keep your stress levels to a minimum (see also *Stress in Ageing*).

- As much as possible take regular exercise, but not to excess.

- Breast cancer is more common in people who are overweight and obese. Control your weight (see also *Weight Problems in Ageing p.330*).

- Oxygen therapies are well worth looking into (see also *Cancer* and *Oxygen in Ageing*).

- Patrick Holford has a great book called *Say No to Cancer*, Piatkus. If you have specific queries that you need help with, log on to www.patrickholford.com

- Read Dr John Lee's book *What Your Doctor May Not Tell You About Breast Cancer*, Warner Books.

- Read *The Breast Cancer Prevention and Recovery Diet* by Suzannah Olivier, Michael Joseph. To order call 0117 983 8851.

- Dr Rosy Daniel, the ex-Medical Director of the Bristol Cancer Centre, has written a wonderful book called *Living With Cancer*, published by Constable Robinson. Available from all bookshops or call 0117 980 9500.

- For advice, contact: Bristol Cancer Help Centre, Grove House, Cornwallis Grove, Bristol BS8 4PG. Helpline: 0117 980 9505, 9.30am-5pm weekdays. Website: www.bristolcancerhelp.org e-mail: info@bristolcancerhelp.org

- The Nutrition Cancer Therapy Trust (NCTT) have a network of practitioners all over the UK and elsewhere who can support you through their protocol for dealing with cancer without drugs and they report great success. Call 01483 202 264.

BREATHING

(See also *Lungs in Ageing* and *Oxygen in Ageing*)

The average person breathes in and out between 15 and 20 times a minute. That's around 22,000–30,000 times every 24 hours. When you breathe in, oxygen is taken in through the lungs and transported via the tissues into the blood. When you breathe out, carbon dioxide from de-oxygenated blood is exhaled via the lungs. Oxygen has an alkalizing (healthy) effect on the body, whereas carbon dioxide is acid forming (unhealthy). Every time you breathe out, you exhale toxic waste from your cells. This waste is highly acidic, hence why ancient monuments are now being closed to the public – our breath acts just like acid rain.

When you take a deep breath through your nose, you help re-alkalize and re-energize your whole body.

We can survive for days without food and water, but without oxygen your survival rate is shortened to a few minutes at most. After 10 minutes or so, brain damage can be irreversible and all body systems begin to shut down.

Most people tend to only use one-third of their lung capacity. Take a deep breath now through your nose and note what happens. If you are stressed then generally you breathe into your upper chest area. This type of breathing inhibits oxygen intake. You have heard the phrase "use it or lose it" and as you age, this definitely applies to your lungs.

Over time, if you shallow-breathe all the time, then lungs lose their elasticity and the more likely you are to suffer from conditions such as bronchitis, bronchial asthma and so on (see also *Oxygen in Ageing p.244*).

A healthy, anti-ageing way to breathe is to place your hands on your lower abdomen about 5cm (2in) below your navel. Then breathe in through the nose and watch as your hands rise as you breathe in, and go down as you breathe out. This type of lower abdominal breathing re-alkalizes the system, expands the lower lungs, energizes the body, encourages better digestion, brings more oxygen to the cells which inhibit chronic bacterial and fungal infections that thrive in low oxygen conditions.

Foods to Avoid

- Foods that are acidic, for example: meat, coffee and sugar, require more oxygen to process (see *Acid–Alkaline Balance*).

- Dense foods such as fats also require more oxygen to break them down completely so avoid too much full-fat dairy produce, creamy desserts, chocolates, full-fat cheeses, pastries etc.

Friendly Foods

- Water is 85% oxygen, so make sure you drink at least six glasses of water daily.

- Fruits can be up to 90% water and are therefore high in oxygen.

- Complex carbohydrates such as brown rice, vegetables, millet, buckwheat, seeds and nuts contain about 50% oxygen by weight – in terms of the make up of the carbohydrate structure.

Useful Remedies

- Too much exercise which involves extra breathing, increases lactic acid production – hence why you get sore muscles. If you tend to exercise very regularly then you need to replenish vital minerals that are lost when you sweat and over-breathe (pant). Take a multimineral in either a food state, colloidal or chelated form, which are more easily absorbed and help reduce sore muscles.

- Take 1000mg of calcium, 800mg of magnesium, 25–30mg zinc and 200mg of potassium. Take daily if you are exercising aerobically (see also *Exercise*).
- Potassium sulphate is the most important mineral for oxygenating cells, take 75mg a day.

Helpful Hints

- We also breathe through our skin, which is why it is called our second lungs. In the James Bond film *Goldfinger* when Shirley Eaton's character was sprayed with gold paint, she died because her skin could not breathe. Therefore to help your skin to breathe, avoid synthetic fabrics.
- Over the years, if I ever have mud wraps and beauty treatments in which my whole body has to be tightly wrapped, I have on occasion fainted. This could be caused by a combination of the heat generated, plus the fact that my skin simply could not breathe. The pores need to be open in order for us to perspire, which is nature's way of keeping the body cool.
- Sweat is full of unwanted acids and other toxins, therefore avoid as much as possible powerful antiperspirants, which prevent pores from eliminating these toxins. Use natural deodorants that are free from aluminium. Skin is a two-way mechanism and a scientist once suggested to me that if you can't eat or drink it, don't put it on your skin!
- Regular use of a natural bristle brush or loofah also aids elimination of toxins from the skin and removes dead skin cells, helping the pores to breathe more easily.
- If you over-breathe or hyperventilate, then you take in too much oxygen, and if left untreated the person would eventually faint which is nature's way of halting this process. This is why if someone has a panic attack, you should give them (if possible) a paper bag to breathe in and out from for a few minutes, which helps counterbalance the excess of oxygen.
- When you breathe deeply through the nose you promote easier digestion and elimination.
- Ideally we should breathe in through the nose, which warms and filters the air and breathe out through the mouth.
- Low tissue oxygen levels can exacerbate conditions such as candida and degenerative diseases like cancer.
- Yoga, t'ai chi and all gentle exercises encourage proper, regular breathing which improves skin tone, and increases resistance to disease.
- Every time you take a deep breath, which you should practise every 20 minutes or so, make sure you are standing or sitting upright and not in a slouched position.
- To increase your lung capacity and breathe more deeply, sing along to your radio (but not so you upset your neighbours!) or try chanting, which really encourages you to use your lungs more.

BRONCHITIS

(See *Lungs* in *Ageing*)

CALORIE RESTRICTION IN AGEING

(See also *Carbohydrate Control* and *Weight Problems in Ageing*)

Only one sure-fire way has been scientifically proven to delay ageing – food restriction. In the West, the average person eats 40% more food than they actually need and if we were to eat less, then our digestive systems and liver would not have to work so hard, our arteries would be less clogged, and we would have fewer toxins to eliminate. We would basically age far more slowly. This makes perfect sense, but personally I love my food too much and I'm already thin. If I lived on 800–1000 calories a day I would disappear and be very miserable indeed!

Dr Roy Walford, Professor of Pathology at UCLA and author of *Maximum Life Span*, has pioneered this work and he advocates a low-calorie diet to lose weight and lengthen your life.

His research, which has been replicated at other centres, has found that rats and monkeys fed half as many calories as those allowed to eat as much as they like, remained energetic for longer, have stronger immune systems and better memory. Their tissues suffered less oxidative damage and their tendons and ligaments stiffened more slowly. They lived to a greater age, with the longest-lived rats on low-calorie diets surviving up to 40 per cent longer than well-fed animals. However, some scientists question exactly what the rat studies mean.

Laboratory rats are very likely bored and just like bored humans they probably over-eat if their food supply is unlimited – think of a "couch potato" type person with an unlimited supply of crisps, cakes, biscuits, fizzy drinks, ice cream and chocolate bars. So perhaps this research is telling us not that under-eating will lengthen our lives, but rather that over-eating will shorten it.

During a two-year study of scientists, ecologists and workers living inside the huge man-made ecosystem called Biosphere 11 in America, Wolford found that the calorie-restrictive, mega-healthy diet that the inhabitants lived on for the two years, definitely improved and, in some cases, reversed many of the bio-markers (blood pressure, glucose levels, lean body mass) of ageing.

The obvious conclusion is that minimizing your calorific intake by eating what you need and no more is one of your best anti-ageing strategies. The source of these nutrients is vital, if you get them from foods that contain little or no nutrients, then you will age faster. You need to minimize your calories while maximizing your nutrient intake – and if you follow Roy Wolford's concept, almost everything you eat needs to be packed with vitamins and minerals, and refined, sugary or fatty foods clearly don't fit this advice. This is one of the key problems with junk food, they are not always harmful in their own right, for instance chocolate contains beneficial compounds, but it is also high in fat and sugar.

There are several reasons why excess calories can speed up ageing and shorten your life. More calories mean more energy metabolism, which involves burning more oxygen in your cells and therefore more oxidative, free radical stress (see also *Antioxidants in Ageing*). If this extra energy isn't used during exercise, it's stored in the body as fat, which leads to weight gain and eventually obesity, increasing your risk of heart disease (see *Weight Problems in Ageing*). Sugars increase your risk of diabetes, which increases your chances of heart disease – and an early grave. In other words the more we overeat, the more likely we are to suffer degenerative diseases and age faster.

Meanwhile, I'm very aware that some young women may read this and think "It's OK to be anorexic and to starve myself". This is definitely not what we are talking about here. We are talking about eating to live, not living to eat. People with eating disorders should always seek medical help and no one should even consider living on a serious calorie-restricted diet, unless it's under medical guidance.

We should restrict calories in an effort to lose weight, but calorie counting is so boring. If you want to age more slowly, you need to restrict your calories to just what you need, though this has to be pretty much for the rest of your life, especially if you want that to be a long time. Crash dieting, especially short-term calorie restriction, is for the most part a waste of time as your metabolism (the rate at which you burn calories) slows by as much as 45%, so you gain it all back very quickly when you stop dieting (see also *Weight Problems in Ageing p.330*).

Foods to Avoid

■ Avoid unnecessary fats by reducing meat, burgers, pizza, cheese and other full-fat dairy foods, plus crisps, fried food, cakes, biscuits, chocolate and fat-laden ready-meals or take-aways.

■ Sugar is the next obvious culprit. Avoid foods containing added sugar, cakes, biscuits, sweets, chocolate and ice cream. Treats are fine, but don't live on treats!

■ Remember that many low-fat foods are high in sugar or artificial sweeteners. Anything ending in "ose" – fructose, maltose, sucrose should be avoided as much as possible as should artificial flavourings or sweeteners, which burden your liver and pollute your brain.

■ Cut down on sodium-based salt.

Friendly Foods

■ You want to eat, as much as possible, only the most nutritious food you can (see *Diet – The Stay Younger Longer Diet* on page 114).

■ Remember that not all fat is bad, so be sure to include more healthy fats from oily fish, seeds, nuts and avocado (see also *Fats for Anti-ageing*).

■ There's another good reason to eat oily fish, seeds, nuts and the occasional egg – protein. Very low-calorie diets are often low in protein (because most animal protein comes laden with high calorie saturated fat) and the body can begin breaking down muscle, which is definitely not healthy.

■ Use an organic magnesium, potassium-rich sea salt and only add salt to the food once it's on your plate.

Useful Remedies

■ While you want to minimize your food intake, you also want to get optimum levels of nutrients. In practice, this means supplementing. Take a high-strength multivitamin/mineral and essential fats complex every day such as Kudos 24 (see page 348 for details).

■ If you are desperate for sugar, use a little fructose powder, which is many times sweeter than normal sugar and so you use less. Also fructo-oligo-saccarides, a white powder usually used to promote the growth of beneficial gut bacteria to aid digestive health, but it also works very well as a sweetener. Both are available from health stores.

■ The mineral chromium helps reduce sugar cravings – take 200mcg daily.

Helpful Hints

■ Try eating less food generally – you may be surprised to discover you're more energetic, not less.

■ Make a bowl with your hands. This is a rough guide as to how much to eat at each meal, every two to three hours (see *Carbohydrate Control p.80*).

■ Honey, syrups and malt spreads are still rich in sugar and are best kept to a minimum. You'll be surprised how your taste buds can change and become less dependent on sugar and sweetness.

■ For more information on calorie restriction read *Grow Young and Slim* by Nick Delgado. He also has a website: www.growyoungandslim.com or read the latest calorie-restriction research being done by Professor Stephen R. Spindler, at The University of California Riverside on www.lef.org

CANCER

(See also *Antioxidants, Breast Cancer, Essential Sugars, Mind Power* and *Oxygen in Ageing*)

One of the great concerns of ageing is the increased risk of contracting cancer. Although cancer can strike at any age, the great majority of cancer patients are 70 and over. Current figures show that almost one in every 2 men and one in 3 women will contract a type of cancer at some point in their lives. Cancer remains the second biggest killer in the Western world, ending the lives of over 6.5 million people annually. But there are plenty of things you can do to reduce your risk, and if you contract cancer, to help yourself. Without doubt, prevention is preferable to cure.

Newer screening methods and earlier diagnoses treatments have meant that surviving cancer (which technically means surviving for five years after diagnosis) is becoming far more commonplace. Thousands of people recover every year and there is always hope.

There are more than 200 types of cancer, but the biggest four killers are lung, breast, bowel and prostate. Cancer is a disease of the genes, this does not necessarily mean it is inherited, but it's a defect of the gene that controls cellular reproduction. Genes can be damaged by free radicals, radiation, viral infections and chemicals (see *Genes in Ageing*, *Antioxidants in Ageing*, *Radiation in Ageing*, *Cells in Ageing* and *Pollution Protection*).

Free radicals are unstable molecules that are formed within the body during normal metabolic processes, though more are produced by stress, excessive exercise, pollution, fried food, radiation and so on. Known risk factors for cancer are high-saturated fat diets, sunbathing to excess, exposure to toxic chemicals found in burnt food, petrol fumes, pesticides, preservatives, excessive hormones, multiple nutrient deficiencies and over-exposure to certain electromagnetic fields.

Eating healthily, staying physically active and maintaining a healthy weight, can cut your cancer risk by 40–90%, depending on who you listen to. Various cancers have been linked to over-consumption of specific foods, for instance, people who regularly consume overly processed foods, such as hot dogs and mass-produced burgers, are more likely to develop bowel cancer. And excessive intake of dietary animal-based fats results in higher levels of oestrogens, a known risk factor for cancers especially of the breast and ovaries.

Emotions affect our health too and tragic stories of people who suffer a major life, shock like the loss of a partner through death or divorce, and develop cancer within a few years, are common. My mother was angry and bitter after my father died aged only 50 from a heart attack. In later life, she developed a cancer that killed her, and I firmly believe it was her overall attitude to life that eventually caused her death. So it's imperative to heal emotional scars as well as physical ones. See Dr Caroline Myss' book under *Helpful Hints* in this section.

There are always exceptions. Some people eat healthily, exercise and really take care of themselves, but still develop cancer. Others smoke until they are almost 100 and are fine. We all carry within us our own genetic strengths and weaknesses, and if our genetic ability to adapt is exceeded by our diet, lifestyle, pollution overload and so on, then naturally occurring genetic errors can accumulate and overwhelm our body's ability to correct the damage.

The orthodox approaches to cancer treatment mainly rely on surgery (cut it out), chemotherapy (drug it out) and radiotherapy (burn it out). Unfortunately these approaches place a considerable additional burden on our bodies and often have negative side effects.

However, the picture has begun to improve. Dr Keith Scott-Mumby, a nutritional physician based in Manchester and London says, "At last there have been attempts to try and understand the mechanics of the life process, and tumour growth in particular, and how nature's wisdom can be harnessed to our advantage. One such idea has been to bond the damaging chemo-substance onto some inactive carrier that makes it harmless to the ordinary cells. But by using cancer cell antibodies (your natural immune response to cancer cells), the chemo-substance is delivered and released *only* in the tumour, which is where it is needed. It's like addressing a parcel bomb to the exact house you want to demolish, leaving the rest of the street intact. An even simpler idea is to set the 'bomb' to go off when oxygen levels drop, because cancer cells don't like oxygen and live only where there is less of it. Another idea has been to use the antibody weapon to trick the tumour into taking up a substance which sensitizes the cancer cells to light and then shining lasers on the tumour. As before, the ordinary cells are left unharmed. And in the next year or two these treatments will become more commonplace.

Meanwhile, don't leave everything to medical 'experts'. There are many steps which you can take if you are to have the best chance of surviving the crisis and going on to enjoy a happy, productive life.

Make no mistake, all cancers are a challenge, and surviving and thriving after cancer can mean that healing yourself becomes a full-time occupation. So a holistic strategy should include elements such as detoxification, an optimum diet, nutritional supplements, specific anti-cancer remedies, and mental, emotional and spiritual healing."

Dr Scott-Mumby adds, "The single most important thing you can do that offers you the best chance of avoiding or beating cancer is to eat a healthier diet – starting *today*. According to The World Cancer Research Fund (WCRF), eating at least 5 portions of vegetables and fruits each day could, in itself, reduce cancer rates by 20%. The WCRF asserts that half of all breast cancer cases, three out of four cases of stomach cancer and three out of four cases of colon cancer could be prevented by dietary measures alone. It must be your choice whether you go the natural route, the conventional route, or to try a combination of both. There are no guaranteed results; but the more right actions you take, the more positive reactions you are likely to see."

Foods to Avoid

- All non-organic meat, if you want to eat red meat then have no more than 3–4oz daily.
- Reduce or eliminate all dairy produce, especially from cows. If you do eat dairy, make it organic and low fat.
- No white flour, rice or pasta.
- Limit your alcohol intake, to say, one glass of organic red wine a day.
- Sugar, coffee, and any pre-packaged, tinned and mass-produced foods, such as burgers or take-aways.
- Don't re-heat pre-prepared foods in plastic containers, as the plastics they release into your food can have a negative effect on your hormones.
- Avoid fried, burnt or smoked foods. This is a good way to cut down on your exposure to

free radicals.

- Reduce your use of sodium-based table salts, use an organic sea salt and add a little to the food on your plate (see *Anti-cancer Diet* below).

Friendly Foods – Anti-cancer Diet

- Eat more organic foods, and if you have cancer, only eat organic. This is because many non-organic foods contain up to seven pesticides which are either carcinogens or hormone disrupters. They are allowed on food only because the levels are very low – and no negative effect is expected. This might seem reasonable except that we do not know of their accumulative cocktail effect.

- Most anti-cancer diets recommend juicing, but the pulp left in the juicer contains healthy phosopholipids, which are essential for healthy tissues. Therefore chop all the ingredients and use a blender instead, or if you have a juicer, then scrape out the pulp and add this to your juice mix, it will be thicker, but more nutritious.

- If you have a hormone-related cancer such as breast or prostate cancer, you need to avoid soya, but as a preventative measure you can have soya in its traditional form i.e., tempeh, miso,tamari soy sauce. **It should be avoided if you have a hormone related cancer.** Fermented soya contains anti-cancer compounds. A healthy amount is around 50–100 g in total a day. Fermented soya is without doubt beneficial to adults but it should not be given to small infants and children. Infant soya milk formulas give infants daily doses of phytoestogens, which help to protect adults against certain cancers, but for the infant the levels are too high. The obvious first choice is to breast feed infants for the first year. Soya lecithin granules are also a very good food for adults, lecithin lowers the bad cholesterol, (LDL),improves memory and helps protect against many cancers.

- Eat more Brussels sprouts, cauliflower, cabbage, spring greens, kale and garlic which all help to fight cancer. A great quick anti-cancer soup includes: 2 carrots, 2 heads of broccoli, half a pack of organic miso or tempeh, with a tablespoon of vegetable stock and some water in the blender for a flavoursome immune boosting soup. Add almond milk should you want it creamy, and spices such as curcumin if you like it hot. Heat and serve.

- Drink plenty of water as it helps to wash out toxins from the kidneys.

- Boil, steam or bake, eating most of your food raw or lightly cooked. Try "steam-frying" food using a watered down soya sauce, plus herbs or spices for taste. Barbecued and char-grilled foods, especially if fatty, are also best avoided because they contain relatively high concentrations of cancer-causing substances called carcinogens.

- Non-organic carrots, lettuce and many other healthy foods are overloaded with pesticides and herbicides that are associated with an increased risk of cancer. Throw away the outer leaves when preparing non-organic vegetables like cabbage or lettuce and always wash these vegetables thoroughly.

- Just one serving of crisp or raw cabbage each week can help reduce the risk of colon cancer by as much as 50%. Make more coleslaw: grate raw cabbage, carrot, apple, and add a few raisins, pumpkin seeds and a small amount of low fat mayonnaise.

■ Eat at least three pieces of fresh whole fruit a day. Vitamin C and natural beta-carotene and lycopene are potent anti-cancer nutrients. Lycopene is a carotenoid found in tomatoes which has been shown to reduce the risk of many cancers, especially prostate cancer but also reduces the risk of cancers in the colon, rectum, pancreas, throat, mouth, breast and cervix. If you are not allergic to tomatoes eat six to ten servings weekly. When the tomatoes are heated in a little olive oil more lycopene is released.

■ All foods that are rich in carotenes help reduce the risk of cancer. These include carrots, apricots, cantaloupe melons, asparagus, sweet potatoes, parsley, mustard and cress, red peppers, spinach, spring greens, watercress, raw mangoes, French beans and tomatoes.

■ A great way to take in a lot of nutrients quickly is to place your favourite fruits into a blender with a tablespoon of a good green food supplement powder, a teaspoon of mixed seeds (sunflower, sesame, flax and pumpkin), put it with a cup of organic rice or almond milk. I drink this every day either for breakfast or as a meal replacement at supper. My favourite blend is blueberries, apple, a pear and a banana. To ring the changes I add a kiwi, grapes or strawberries to the blend. It's delicious.

■ Strict vegetarians seem to develop fewer cancers than non-vegetarians. People who live in Thailand and Japan have much lower incidence of most cancers so adopting a Far Eastern diet may well be a good way of staying healthy – less refined foods and meat, and more fish.

■ Drink more organic green tea, it contains powerful antioxidant polyphenols that have been investigated for their cancer-protective effects and found to be even more powerful than vitamins C and E. It is believed that green tea consumption, on average three cups a day, may be another reason behind the relatively low rate of cancer in Japan.

■ Eat whole foods, unprocessed nuts, beans and seeds. Anything in its whole form, such as oats, brown rice, lentils, almonds or sunflower seeds are high in the anti-cancer minerals zinc and selenium. Buy a pack of each of the following: sunflower seeds, pumpkin seeds, sesame seeds, hazelnuts, Brazil nuts, almonds, walnuts and linseeds; whiz a tablespoon of each at a time in a blender and keep in an airtight jar in the fridge. Sprinkle daily over fruits, cereals, soups and desserts.

■ Wholegrains, such as brown rice, contain substances called phytates, which offer us protection against cancer. They are now available as an isolated substance called Inositol Hexaphosphate or IP6, which is extracted from brown rice. For details call The NutriCentre on 0207 436 5122. If you eat bran to keep your bowels regular, avoid wheat bran, which can irritate the gut. Try oat or rice bran instead.

■ Minimize alcohol. Alcohol is associated with an increased risk of cancer. Red wine does however contain antioxidant nutrients called polyphenols, which are associated with a reduced risk of heart disease. One glass a day is the recommended maximum. Red grape juice contains the same antioxidants without the alcohol.

■ Animal fats are a major contributing factor in cancers. Greatly reduce your intake of saturated fats from meat, full fat dairy produce, chocolates, cheeses, sausages, meat pies, cakes etc. Avoid any foods containing hydrogenated or trans fats. Once you start reading labels you will be appalled at how much saturated fat you are ingesting. Never fry with mass-produced, highly refined oils. Use only organic sunflower, sesame, walnut or olive oils for salad dressings. Eat more oily fish, which are rich in omega-3 fats, especially sardines, salmon, mackerel, herring and fresh tuna (see *Fats for Anti-ageing)*.

- Cut down on stimulants like sugar and caffeine. Sugar has been shown to lower your immune function for up to five hours after consuming it.

Useful Remedies if you Suffer from Cancer

- Some cancer specialists state that vitamins and minerals can stop the orthodox treatments from working, but numerous studies show that the right nutrients support your immune system and help fight the cancer.

- IP6, a substance extracted from brown rice, has been shown to inhibit the growth of certain cancers. There is 20 years' medical research behind IP6 and trials to date have proven very exciting. 6000mg (6 grams) daily needs to be taken on an empty stomach 30 minutes before food.

- Vitamin C, 3 or more grams a day, in an ascorbate (non-acidic) form.

- MGN-3 is a blend of the outer shell of rice bran with extracts of shitake, kawaratake, and suehirotake mushrooms. These three mushroom extracts are the leading prescription treatments for cancer in Japan. They increase natural killer (NK) cell activity. It is the activity of NK cells that determine whether you get cancer or a virus infection, rather than their number. In one study of 27 cancer patients, the NK activity increased from 100% to 537%, depending upon the kind of cancer, in only two weeks. If you have cancer, take 4 capsules three times daily with meals for two weeks, then 2 capsules twice daily for maintenance; 2 capsules twice daily may be taken for prevention. Available from The NutriCentre p.14.

- Maitake mushrooms available in capsule form have been shown to stimulate the immune system and seem to reduce the effects of chemotherapy.

- Read the section on *Essential Sugars*, a new food group called glyconutrients that are having an incredible (and well researched) effect on helping cancer.

- Take 200mcg selenium daily.

- A high-potency multivitamin/mineral without iron, as iron has been linked to cancer cell growth.

- Take 1200mcg of folic acid plus a daily B complex, which helps to stabilize genes.

- Try Essiac. Probably the most famous herbal cancer remedy. Essiac is named after Canadian nurse, Rene M. Caisse, who claimed it was an ancient Ojibway Indian formula. I've read many testimonials of its efficacy though, to date, no actual scientific studies. There are many sites devoted to this remedy on the Internet – but watch out for the cowboys.

Useful Remedies To Help Prevent Cancer

- Take IP6 – an extract of brown rice that has proven positive effects on cancers, most especially leukaemia – 2grams can be taken daily on an empty stomach (if you think you're at high risk) available from The NutriCentre (see page 14).

- Take a good quality high strength multi-vitamin/mineral, antioxidant, essential fats formula every day such as Kudos 24 see page 348.

- Active-H is a powerful antioxidant (see also *Antioxidants in Ageing*). Take 6 x 250mg a day if you have cancer or 2 x 250mg a day as a preventative measure.

- Take 1gram of vitamin C daily, more if you're stressed or ill.

- Take 200mcg selenium daily.

- Take 400iu of natural source vitamin E daily.

- Take alpha-lipoic acid 50mg daily.

- Also see details of MGN 3 (page 77).

Helpful Hints

- Firstly – detox your body (see *Detoxing*).

- If at all possible begin taking regular saunas as heat helps to eliminate toxins from the body. Don't use them if they are packed with too many other people, as you may pick up other people's toxins. Ask if you can have the sauna on a lower heat (120–140 degrees) and then you can stay in for a few minutes longer.

- Minimize your exposure to pollution. Remember, anything that is combusted produces free radicals, so reduce your exposure to car exhaust fumes. Only use mobile phones for 10–15 minutes at a time at most. Reduce your exposure to other electrical pollutants such as microwaves, TVs etc, and don't sleep with an electric clock by your bed (see *Radiation in Ageing*). Never use chemical pesticides and herbicides in your garden and home. Ask for environmentally friendly natural products. Greatly reduce or eliminate your exposure to non-organic foods, cleaning fluids, garden sprays, and insect sprays.

- If you smoke, give it up and stay away from smoke-filled rooms, as passive smoking has now been shown to trigger cancer.

- Curcumin, found in turmeric, used in most curries and Eastern dishes is a great anti-cancer spice. It enhances immune function and helps inhibit new blood vessel growth that occurs as tumours grow. It is especially useful for skin cancers, liver and colon cancers. It also helps remove toxic metals from the body and helps block pesticide-type pollutants from entering cells. Add to your diet or take in capsule form.

- Eat more pineapple and papaya, they contain the enzymes bromelain and papain. These enzymes help dissolve away the protective protein coating that surrounds most cancer cells.

- If you are already undergoing any type of cancer therapy, Dr Rosy Daniel (the former

Medical Director of the Bristol Cancer Help Centre) says that nutrition is vital to help bring back up the white blood cell count. She advises patients to eat plenty of organic fresh fruit and vegetables along with whole foods like brown rice and brown bread. All animal fats should be avoided. She also recommends that cancer patients take a good antioxidant formula, which contains vitamins A, C and E, plus a natural beta-carotene complex, zinc and selenium. Dr Daniel stresses that fear drains energy levels and advocates any therapy that can reduce anxiety, such as spiritual healing, Reiki, relaxation exercises, visualization, acupuncture or homeopathy. Dr Daniel has written a wonderful book called *Living With Cancer*, available from 0117 980 9500, published by Constable Robinson.

- If you're diagnosed with cancer and choose to follow the nutritional approach, or you've given up on orthodox approaches, or been given up on by the doctors, contact the Nutritional Cancer Therapy Trust (NCTT). The eminent biochemist Dr Lawrence Plaskett has "updated" the well-known Gerson Therapy (designed over 50 years ago) with modern knowledge of nutrient needs, detoxification and biochemical pathways, and made the whole process more manageable. The NCTT have trained practitioners all over the country (and some internationally) who are happy to discuss their therapies with you. Having started in 1995, they are noting that a very high success rate is obtainable with so-called terminal cancer patients. Call 01271 850 122. Check out www.defeatingcancer.co.uk or e-mail sarah@flower-iridol.freeserve.co.uk for more information or to arrange a consultation with a practitioner in your area.

- Laugh a lot. Watch films and programmes that make you laugh; laughter boosts your immune system. Stay as positive as possible, without doubt the patients with the more positive outlook heal and recover more quickly. This does not mean that you cannot shed tears, as tears release stress chemicals, and you are not meant to be a positive saint all the time! An inspiring book that uses this theme is *Love, Medicine and Healing* by Bernie Siegal, Rider at Random House.

- Oxygen therapies are well worth looking into. Dr Otto Warburg won a Nobel Prize for discovering that normal cells when deprived of oxygen for sufficient time turn into cancer cells. You can use an ozone cabinet and some doctors are working with hydrogen peroxide injections. Many therapists who offer these treatments have been harassed by various Government bodies. I can only surmise that some people would prefer people not to know that there is an inexpensive non-drug-based treatment that really does help.

- At The Hospital in Mexico, Dr Kurt Donsbach has used intravenous hydrogen peroxide for years and claims that the majority of his patients make a full recovery. For details log on to www.hospitalsantamonica.com

- In the UK, these therapies (as well as high-dose intravenous nutrients such as vitamin C) are used by Dr Patrick Kingsley in Leicestershire on 01530 223 622, Dr Fritz Schellander in Tunbridge Wells on 01892 543 535, Dr Julian Kenyon in London on 020 7486 5588 and Dr Keith Scott-Mumby in London and Manchester on www.alternative-doctor.com.

- Mark Lester uses ozone therapies that introduce ozone into the body via the rectum and vagina to treat patients. Call 020 8349 4730 or log on to www.thefinchleyclinic.co.uk

- For further information, I suggest you read *Oxygen Healing Therapies* by Nathanial Altman, Healing Arts Press, or *Flood Your Body with Oxygen* by Ed McCabe, Energy Publications www.misteroxygen.com

- The Cancer Alternative Information Bureau has been founded by Tina Cooke to help people who want more help on the holistic approaches available to cancer patients: Write to PO Box 285,405 Kings Road, London SW10 0BB. Call 020 7266 1505.

- Many associations offer help, counselling and advice. One of the best is the Bristol Cancer Help Centre, Grove House, Cornwallis Grove, Bristol BS8 4PG. Helpline: 0117 980 9505, 9.30am-5pm weekdays. Website: www.bristolcancerhelp.org E-mail: info@bristolcancerhelp.org

- An excellent book on the connection between emotional dysfunction and physical illness is *The Creation of Health* by Dr Caroline Myss, Bantam Books.

- Another helpful book is Patrick Holford's, *Say No to Cancer*, Piatkus or log on to www.patrickholford.com

CARBOHYDRATE CONTROL

(See also *Diabetes, Insulin Resistance,* and *Weight Problems in Ageing*)

Refined carbohydrates are killing us, and the more of them we eat, the faster we age. Of course food is also meant to be enjoyable and when there is a good, home- made apple pie on the table, I am the first to tuck in. We all need treats, but the problem today is that we are living on them. Everything in moderation.

We humans are effectively "solar-powered". Plants make carbohydrates by trapping the sun's energy in a matrix of carbon, hydrogen and oxygen. We're designed to run on carbohydrates, so we eat plants – fruits, vegetables and grains – to burn the carbohydrates they contain in each of our cells and release the stored energy to fuel our body and mind. If we eat complex, unrefined carbohydrates, such as brown rice, foods in their whole or natural state, this release of energy is a gradual process. Unfortunately, many of our refined foods, croissants, cakes, pastries and so on contain virtually no fibre that normally keep the whole system in balance and so when we eat them the sugar enters the bloodstream too quickly. You get an instant sugar hit, but you quickly need more and this becomes a vicious cycle. It's like burning a piece of paper, it quickly flares, and the flames are bright, but then the flames subside and you are left with a pile of ashes, and to keep the fire going you need to add more paper. This is what happens when we eat too much refined food.

This is why carbohydrates are the main killer in the average Western diet, not fat. Inuit and other aboriginal people with very high fat levels in their diet do not suffer degenerative arterial disease in the way we do in the "civilized world".

Refined carbohydrates are stressful to your body and sooner or later if you eat too many then symptoms such as diabetes, insulin resistance and obesity will result. The secret to avoiding these problems is to manage your blood sugar (see *Low Blood Sugar*).

Your body's main source of fuel is a sugar called glucose that it obtains by breaking down carbohydrates such as grains, beans, lentils, fruits and vegetables, which are rich in nutrients that the body needs for efficient digestion and metabolism. Their energy is released slowly, giving us optimum mental and physical energy. Your body has a mechanism for keeping its energy levels constant called "blood sugar balance" and by supporting this mechanism you can improve your energy, weight control, concentration, mood, memory, sleep and stress tolerance throughout your life.

Foods to Avoid

■ Make no mistake, white flour, white sugar, corn syrup, white potato and other starch-rich foods will shorten your life. Yet these are the ingredients commonly used in most mass-produced refined foods. Bread, cakes, biscuits, pasta, pastries and other confectionery items, French fries, food thickeners, coffee whiteners and white rice.

■ Avoid sugar and foods containing sugar such as fizzy drinks, chocolate, sweets and many processed foods (check labels), plus reduce your intake of honey, dried fruit and juices as they are all rich in fast-releasing sugars. Try diluting fruit juices. If you are desperate for sugar use a little fructose, which is many times sweeter than ordinary sugar, so you use less, and fructose has a lower glycemic index and therefore less of an effect on your blood sugar (see *Sugar in Ageing*). Keep in mind that sugar ages your skin and your cells.

■ Artificial sweeteners may seem like a good solution, but they do nothing to reduce your sweet tooth and they place a strain on the liver and can add to weight gain.

■ Caffeine found in coffee, tea and cola drinks is a powerful stimulant. A cup of coffee contains around 100mg of caffeine, cola 50mg, tea 60mg, and green tea 25mg, chocolate cake 25mg per slice and dark chocolate 30mg per ounce.

■ Replace chocolate with fresh fruit. Replace coffee and tea with coffee alternatives available in all health shops, and green, peppermint or fruit teas.

■ Alcohol is such a refined carbohydrate that much of it is converted to fat in the body. We are not suggesting you eliminate it altogether, but just be aware that it is fattening.

■ Note that many foods advertised as being low in fat are often high in sugar, which if not used up during exercise will turn to fat in the body and reside on your hips!

Friendly Foods

■ Make time for breakfast, this "kick starts" your metabolism for the rest of the day and is crucial for better energy balance. "In 6 years of advising people on how to improve their energy levels", says nutritionist Shane Heaton, "I've never met anyone who skips breakfast and has good energy levels for the rest of the day." He recommends a piece of fruit followed (15–30 minutes later) by muesli or porridge. Oats, rich in B vitamins and fibre, are ideal, providing good, slow-burn energy, though the most important thing is to choose breakfast foods you enjoy. By eating breakfast, your energy, concentration, mood and motivation will improve throughout the day. Any cravings for stimulants will decline, you'll sleep better and wake feeling more refreshed in the morning.

■ Eat more foods in their natural state. Complex carbohydrates and whole foods contain higher levels of nutrients and fibre, for example brown rice or even better brown Basmati rice, whole wheat/rye bread, porridge oats, fruits and vegetables.

■ Are you sitting down? Eat proteins and carbohydrates together. This flies in the face of the Hay Diet and Food Combining, which does make sense, as it's true these foods are digested at different rates, however if you have trouble balancing your blood sugar levels, eating carbohydrates alone all the time can constantly disrupt your efforts to stabilize your energy levels. Balancing carbohydrates and proteins (in a ratio of two to one, so twice as much carbohydrate as protein) at each meal or snack can help slow the release of sugars from the carbohydrates. For example, eat some nuts or seeds with fresh fruit, fish with rice, or lentil pate/houmous with rice cakes or amaranth crackers.

■ Choose more foods with a low "glycemic index". This is a guide as to how much and how quickly sugar is released for certain foods, compared to straight glucose, which is set at 100. Some foods are fast, others are slow, as explained above. For example, white bread scores 70, while rye bread is just 41. Bananas are 62, while apples are 39. You don't have to choose only low-glycemic index foods all the time, but where possible, choose alternatives with lower scores, and when you do eat high glycemic index foods, mix them with protein or low glycemic index foods to slow the sugar release. See the list of foods under *Sugar in Ageing*, for a longer list of foods and their glycemic index. For a complete list read *The 30 Day Fatburner Diet* by Patrick Holford, Piatkus (www.patrickholford.com).

■ Drink more water, aim for six glasses per day. Dehydration is a key cause of fatigue and can make you crave fast-energy foods that contribute to blood sugar imbalance.

Useful Remedies

■ Take a high-strength multivitamin/mineral.

■ The mineral chromium is the main constituent of "glucose tolerance factor", a substance that helps with the delivery of sugar to cells. It's used widely by nutritional therapists to help balance blood sugar and reduce cravings. Take 100–200mcg twice daily with meals. American research has shown that when people who tend to eat a high carbohydrate diet are given 200mcg of chromium daily, this one step helps reduce incidence of diabetes by 50%.

■ B vitamins, especially vitamin B3, are also important for glucose tolerance factor. As all the B vitamins work together, take a B complex daily.

■ Sucroguard contains a blend of nutrients, including chromium and B vitamins formulated by Dr John Briffa, specifically designed to help balance your blood sugar and reduce cravings. Take 1–3 daily with meals. Available from BioCare (for details see page 13.)

■ Vitamin C is involved with energy production, so if your energy levels are low and your stress levels are high, take 1000mg of vitamin C twice daily with food.

■ If stress is a real problem in your life consider trying the herbs rhodiola or Siberian ginseng.

They're both adaptogenic herbs, so help you adapt to stress and can really help improve your tolerance to stress of all kinds. Take 200–300mg of a standardized extract of either herb daily with meals.

Helpful Hints

■ Stress is a major hindrance to stabilizing blood sugar levels because the fight-flight mechanism floods your blood with sugar ready for action. If we constantly suffer from low blood sugar, we can sometimes learn subconsciously to use stress as a way of keeping us going. Staying in a stressful job, seeking out stressful situations (often subconsciously), taking too much on, doing things at the last minute, being late everywhere we go, etc. all add to the problem. Blood sugar imbalance itself is a major stress on the body and at the same time lowers your stress tolerance, so by improving your blood sugar balance your tolerance of other stresses in your life should improve. (See also *Stress in Ageing*).

■ Quit smoking – cigarettes are a stimulant, which many people use to keep themselves going, having one after meals to avoid the energy slump and at regular intervals throughout the day. If you find smoking relaxing, you're addicted. The feeling of relaxation is very likely the alleviation of withdrawal symptoms (commonly anxiety, stress, tension, nervousness, etc). Those who stop smoking and gain weight do so because they usually replace the cigarettes with other stimulants, sugar, or sugar-containing foods or drinks.

■ And finally some news you're really going to like. Snacking is good. The worst thing you can do if your energy levels are poor is go long hours without eating. So eat small, frequent meals throughout the day – every two to three hours or so – and avoid skipping meals. This isn't as hard as it sounds, breakfast, morning tea, lunch, afternoon tea, dinner, late snack for example. People who miss meals often experience hypoglycaemic (low blood sugar) symptoms. Obviously I'm not talking about junk food snacks, healthy snacks throughout the day may include fruit, nuts, seeds, rice or oat cakes with houmous or other spreads, raw vegetables such as carrots, rye crackers with lentil pate, alfalfa, etc.

■ Read *The X Factor Diet*, by Leslie Kenton, Vermilion 2002.

CATARACTS

(See also *Eyes in Ageing, Glaucoma* and *Macular Degeneration*)

A cataract is a gradual "clouding" of the normally transparent lens of the eye, which reduces the amount of incoming light, thus causing deterioration in vision. It is estimated that 20 million people worldwide suffer from cataracts and the majority of cataracts occur after the age of 50. In fact one out of every 2 people aged 65 or over has a cataract or cloudiness in the eye's lens.

In the Third World, cataracts are a common cause of blindness and they are becoming more common in the West with people who take too much sun.

There is plenty of research showing that the progression of cataracts can be slowed, or prevented, by the use of natural therapies and lifestyle changes.

Exposure to direct sunlight, smoking, diabetes, a poor diet lacking in antioxidants and overuse of steroids can all trigger cataracts.

If you have cataracts the most common remedy is laser surgery, but if you take more precautions from your 30s onwards then prevention is always preferable.

Friendly Foods

- Leafy green vegetables, especially spinach and kale are rich in the carotenoid lutein, found in the retina and the lens of the eye, that has been proven to reduce the incidence of cataracts. Vine-ripened tomatoes, are rich in lycopene, another carotenoid.

- Onions, apples, green tea, kiwi fruit, cherries, apples, pears, grapes, cranberries, red onions, green cabbage, leeks, peas, cos lettuce, garlic, mustard greens, yellow and orange vegetables, including yams, carrots and sweet potatoes, asparagus, butternut squash, pak choy, green peppers, mangoes, bilberries, blueberries, blackberries, cantaloupe melons and apricots are all great foods to support the eyes.

- Wheat grass juice and alfalfa sprouts are also great eye foods.

- Eat oily fish and calves' liver as they are rich in vitamin A.

- Wheatgerm, avocado, unrefined-organic sunflower, pumpkin and linseeds are rich in essential fats, vitamin E and selenium.

Foods to Avoid

- Reduce caffeine and soda-type fizzy drinks.

- Avoid the sugar substitute aspartame and man-made fats (corn oil and sunflower oil, trans- or hydrogenated vegetable oils including canola oil, and especially margarines). Eliminate deep-fat fried foods from your diet (see also *Fats for Anti-ageing*).

- Reduce all refined foods containing sugar and animal fats that speed up the oxidation process and leave you more vulnerable to cataracts.

- Limit your alcohol consumption. Alcohol interferes with liver functions, reducing protective glutathione levels in the eyes.

- Cut down on animal fats and full-fat dairy produce.

Useful Remedies

- Alpha-lipoic acid – studies showed that alpha-lipoic acid reduced cataract formation by 40% by protecting the lens of the eye from the loss of vitamin C, vitamin E, and glutathione. Take 250 mg daily.

- L-carnosine – is a powerful antioxidant that enters both the aqueous and lipid parts of the eye and helps prevent and repair light-induced DNA damage. Take 100mg a day.

- Multivitamin/minerals containing selenium, inositol, vitamins B2, B6, C and E, bioflavonoids and other antioxidants.
- Acetyl-L-carnitine is a powerful antioxidant that protects the lens from the damaging effects of excessive sugar intake and ageing. Take 500mg daily.
- Ginkgo biloba increases blood flow to the retina and can slow retinal and lens deterioration by its antioxidant activity. Take 120mg a day.
- Bilberry has been called the vision herb for its powerful effect on all types of visual disorders. Bilberry supports the structural integrity of the tiny capillaries that deliver oxygen and nutrients to the eyes. Take 240–300mg daily.
- Quercitin protects the eye from damage by solar radiation and works synergistically with taurine and vitamin E. Take 1000mg daily.
- Cysteine is important for a healthy lens. Taken as N-acetyl-cysteine (NAC), it increases production of glutathione, one of the most important antioxidants in the eye. Take 500–1000mg daily on an empty stomach.
- Taurine is another potent antioxidant that is highly concentrated within the eye, and is important for maintaining healthy eyes and regeneration of eye tissues. Taurine helps to prevent the formation of cataracts and may also protect cells in the retina from harmful ultraviolet light. Take 500mg daily.
- Vitamin C helps make collagen which strengthens the capillaries that nourish the retina and protects against UV light. The eye contains the second highest concentration of vitamin C in the body next to the adrenal glands. It is a powerful antioxidant and people who take vitamin C regularly are at a lower risk of developing cataracts. Take 500–3000mg daily.
- Note: most nutritional companies now make an eye health formula that contains most of the above (see pages 13 and 14).

Helpful Hints
- Natural sunlight is good for us – but it's like everything else – if you are exposed to too much then the eyes can be damaged. Therefore, when on holiday, wear a hat, stay out of the midday sun and make sure that you wear wrap around glasses that have guaranteed UV filtering abilities.
- Read *The Eye Care Revolution* by Robert Abel Jr MD, Kensington Publishing Corporation.

CELLS IN AGEING
(See also *Ageing*)

The average person manufactures 200–300 billion cells every day, but to make healthy cells you need the right raw material. In a perfect world, if we could breathe unpolluted mountain air, live on purely organic food, reduce stress, take regular exercise and so on, then the body could more easily repair itself. But in today's environment, new cells are often less than perfect which affects the body's natural repair processes. However, by eating more healthy foods and taking supplements proven to help repair cells, you can rejuvenate and increase their life span.

Your body is made up of around three trillion cells and each cell is basically a fatty bag of salty water. A tiny independently functioning unit, usually consisting of a nucleus surrounded by cytoplasm (the salty water) and enclosed by a membrane (the fatty bag). Within the nucleus in the center of the cell is your DNA – the instructions for how the cell should operate. In the cytoplasm are various structures involved in all the functions of the cell: protein manufacture, immune function, waste disposal and energy production. The latter occurs in tiny energy factories called mitochondria, which also contain a small amount of their own DNA. The membrane is responsible for allowing substances in and out of the cell depending on its needs, plus sending and receiving messages (including hormones) from the rest of organism. Each cell functions independently of others and can be likened to a little factory that produces goods (protein, hormones, etc.) and services (energy) in cooperation with all the other cells for the good of the whole organism – you.

We grow by single cells dividing into two new cells, which then continue to divide until they've created a bone, an organ like your liver or heart, blood vessel, skin, etc. And there are many types of cells – cells that divide all the time, like your gut lining which is replaced by fresh cells every 72 hours, blood or skin cells which, when you are young are replenished every month, and each year you make a new liver. The problem being that while our bodies are doing everything possible to keep us healthy, what do we do? We eat more junk foods, become stressed, are exposed to huge amounts of pollution and so on. This is like standing in the fire when you are trying to put out the flames!

And, it has been observed that cells appear to have a limited capacity to divide, around 50–70 times or so. With each cell division, your cells' ability to divide again is reduced, until it finally stops and enters a "twilight" or dormant state, which is known as senescence, which contributes to the ageing process. This limit is called the Hayflick Limit, after Leonard Hayflick who made this discovery in 1965.

However, Dr Keith Scott-Mumby, a nutritional physician who specializes in anti-ageing medicine says, "Some cancer cells are tough hardy brutes and go on indefinitely, thousands of times beyond the Hayflick Limit. Therefore, many of us believe there is no logical reason why ordinary cells cannot do the same, if they are given the right environment. Interestingly, recent science has shown that normal cells within the body survive longer than those in a test tube. Also, certain bone marrow cells have been shown to escape the Hayflick Limit and so the whole question is still very open. The really important point is that we could all live a long, long time, within the Hayflick Limit, if only we reduce the rate of cell damage and thus replacement."

The Russian researcher, Olovnikov, suggested in 1971 that the Hayflick "process" might be because of a reduction (with each successive cell division) in the length of the telomeres, the rounded protective ends of chromosomes, which are a bit like the ends of shoelaces that stop them from unravelling. Each time the cell divides, the telomeres get slightly shorter and when they reach a critical length, the telomeres stop working and the cells stop dividing. And we then develop saggy skin, weakened muscles and bones – we age. But if we could find a way to repair the telomeres, then we would have the keys to immortality. Within 10 years, this could be a reality.

Another theory involves those cells that cannot divide and have to depend on their own repair mechanisms. This repair is controlled by the DNA within the cells nucleus. DNA is rather susceptible to damage and it is thought that if damage to the DNA from toxins in our diet and environment begins to exceed the cell's ability to repair itself, damage to the DNA and the cell accumulates, until eventually the instructions within the DNA are so disrupted that the cells starts to malfunction – no longer producing their key products such as neurotransmitters, digestive enzymes, hormones and antibodies, etc.. Free radical damage to the DNA appears to be a key factor and studies suggest that antioxidant protection prevents or slows the start of ageing (see also *Antioxidants in Ageing*).

Meanwhile cell therapy for anti-ageing is really beginning to take off and there are two main types of cell therapies that often become confused. Stem cell and live-cell therapy are fast becoming the answer to many medical dreams and within the next 10 years, cell therapy will become commonplace. Life spans of 150 years will be normal. We will have the ability to restore movement in paralysed limbs, this is already happening at medical research centres in America.

Cell therapies now being refined will offer great hope and possible cures for Parkinson's disease, motor neurone disease, Alzheimer's disease, strokes, heart disease and even cancer.

Stem cell therapy is when immature cells taken from human embryos (from an aborted foetus or from embryos left over following fertility treatment) are engineered in such a way, that they can then grow into whatever organ, or specific cell, the scientists want them to become. For instance, if someone's liver is in need of repair, once the stem cells have been engineered, they can then be injected into that person, they will find their way to the liver and can then regenerate that organ. The same can happen with damaged nerves in the spine or in the brain. Although some people feel this work is unethical because of the source of the stem cells, I believe that we really should have the right to choose. If a woman freely chooses to have an abortion, or if she unfortunately has a miscarriage and then gives permission for the later removal of stem cells that have the potential to save lives, then why should she not have that option – I would do it.

Unfortunately, the stem cells that are present in adults, in bone marrow, skin, the gut, brain and liver, are more difficult to work with and less effective, though future research may overcome this and allow the field to move beyond the current ethical problem.

Christopher Reeve, the former Superman actor who was paralysed from the neck down when he broke his back in 1995, is a passionate supporter of stem cell research, believing it to be his best chance of recovery. Paralysed rats with similar spinal injuries have regained the ability to walk after their spines were injected with stem cells. The stem cells migrate to the area of damage and grow new cells to repair it.

Learning how to harness stem cells and direct them to safely regenerate tissues and organs, and to replace those that have worn out, is now happening. Once perfected, stem cell therapy will be one of the greatest miracles of anti-ageing and healing to ever be discovered.

In Europe **live cell therapy** has been used for over 50 years to help the body regenerate itself. This treatment usually involves removing cells from shark, sheep or bovine embryos, which are then treated to make sure that there is no possibility of transferring any disease. The cultured cells are then injected into the patient, which "wake up" and rejuvenate cells that are fast approaching senescence. After four to six weeks patients say they feel renewed and invigorated, their memory improves, joints no longer ache and skin looks fresher. It obviously worked for Sir Winston Churchill who abused his body and yet still lived to a ripe old age, with a very sharp mind. Clinique La Prairie was among the first to develop this treatment and their clinic is as popular today as it was 50 years ago. For details log on to www.laprairie.com or call (+41 21) 989 33 11 or contact Dr Claus Martin at the Four Seasons Clinic in Germany on + (49) 8022 24041, fax 8022 24740.

Foods to Avoid

■ See *Foods to Avoid* in *Ageing* and *Antioxidants in Ageing*.

Friendly Foods

■ See *Friendly Foods* sections in *Ageing* and *Antioxidants in Ageing*. See also *Diet – The Stay Younger Longer Diet (see page 114)*.

Useful Remedies

■ The best way to protect your cells is to take more antioxidants (for a full list see *Antioxidants in Ageing p.38*).

■ Carnosine is one of the most exciting supplements known when it comes to regenerating cells. It is made up from two amino acids and is naturally present in the body and food (mainly in lean red meat, organ meats and chicken). As we age, levels fall, but scientists have found that if you take carnosine as a supplement it has the proven ability to rejuvenate cells that are approaching senescence, which restores a normal appearance to cells and extends their life span. Carnosine acts like an antioxidant and as well as improving muscle tone, it helps remove toxic metals, rejuvenates connective tissue, speeds up wound healing, and best of all, it helps slow down cross-linking in all the body's cells, including the skin (see also *Sugar in Ageing*). The Russians have done a great deal of research into carnosine, and when the Cold War ended, it was confirmed by researchers in Australia, Japan and America. The Life Extension Foundation in America say that you need to take 500mg daily on an empty stomach for optimum results and I have been trying this dose for several months with no negative side effects. To order from them log on to www.lef.org. However, Dr Marios Kyriazis, a gerontologist in the UK, has been researching carnosine for some time, and he says he is seeing firmer muscles, younger looking skin and fewer grey hairs in patients who take 100mg daily and that it is more effective when taken with co-enzymeQ10 and vitamin E. Carnosine is available in the UK from The NutriCentre and Sloane Health Shop (see page 14 for details) and to order from all health stores.

■ For more information read *Carnosine and Other Elixirs of Youth* by Marios Kyriazis, Watkins Publishing.

■ Kudos 24 Multi-Active Age Management Complex is a multinutrient, up-to-the-minute formula, containing food state, GM-free, highly absorbable vitamins, minerals, antioxidants, amino acids, brain nutrients, essential fats, isoflavones, green foods and specific anti-ageing nutrients such as carnosine that both men and women of all ages can take once daily – for full details and a list of the ingredients see page 348.

■ See the section on *Essential Sugars* – which have also been proven to extend cell life.

Helpful Hints

■ Chelation therapy helps your body to make healthier cells (see *Chelation in Ageing*).

■ Live cell therapy for rejuvenating the skin is now available in the UK and America (see *Rejuvenation Therapies*).

■ For more information on Stem Cell Therapy see the National Institutes of Health website: www.nih/news/stemcell/primer.htm or log onto Dr. Robert Trosell's site: www.kmc-@rotterdam.nl, or call 0207 486 1095

■ For more information read *Ageing, Sex and DNA Repair* by Carol and Harris Bernstein, Academic Press 1991, or *Clones, Genes and Immortality* by John Harris.

CHELATION IN AGEING

Chelation therapy (pronounced key-lay-shun) has been used for 30 years in America and Europe and generally involves administering the amino acid EDTA (there are other types), intravenously, which not only removes toxic metals, a major factor in ageing, but also improves blood flow in blocked arteries in heart, diabetic and stroke patients, thus helping many patients avoid surgery.

The EDTA chelates or "grabs onto" ("chela" is Greek for "claw") toxic metals such as lead, mercury, cadmium and iron and eliminates them from the body. Lead and cadmium are linked to high blood pressure, too much iron can trigger heart attacks, mercury is linked to Alzheimer's and dementia and so on (see *Toxic Metal Overload*).

But during the last 20 years or so, medical researchers in America have gone one step further and shown that specific nutrients administered with the chelating agent, are set to become one of the most effective anti-ageing medicines currently available.

Dr Ralph Miranda, a spokesman for American College For The Advancement Of Medicine (ACAM), based in Laguna Hills, California says, "Free radical damage from toxins found in foods, water, prescription drugs and our environment, damages tissues, which eventually causes muscles and joints to stiffen, the skin loses its elasticity and you experience age-associated changes. However, nutrients such as glutathione, a naturally occurring substance that is vital for brain function, plus vitamins B and C and minerals such as magnesium, can help slow this degenerative process. And when these nutrients are combined intravenously with chelation therapy, then some of the processes associated with ageing can be greatly reduced and in some cases reversed."

This is because EDTA helps prevent the production of harmful free radicals in the body. It also has the proven ability to slow age-related skin damage, and Dr Keith Scott-Mumby, a nutritional physician based in London and Manchester, is one of a growing number of doctors in the UK using chelation and glutathione specifically for anti-ageing saying, "The key processes of ageing are free radical damage and progressive cell degeneration, due to inadequate nutrition. This dual-action treatment helps produce healthier cells which hold back the ageing process."

Dr Miranda agrees, "The average person manufactures 200–300 billion cells every day. But to make healthy cells you need the right raw material. If we breathed unpolluted air, lived on organic food, reduced stress, exercised and so on, then the body can easily repair itself. But in today's environment, new cells are often less than perfect which affects natural repair processes. The vast majority of our ACAM members are now using these two approaches in the same infusion. By removing toxic metals and quenching free radical reactions, this treatment encourages the body to repair itself." He continues, "Positive results are being reported by dozens of my medical colleagues treating patients suffering from age-related, degenerative conditions ranging from senile dementia, macular degeneration and impotence, to chronic fatigue, ME, arthritis, heart disease and strokes."

The reason I have used these expert comments in this section is because many orthodox doctors remain wary of chelation, as in general they are not up to date with the treatment results and research. In America, trials on 3,000 patients undergoing chelation are under way and the American medical establishment is at last accepting that this duel approach, often called intravenous antioxidant therapy, has great potential health benefits.

Before beginning this treatment, a full medical history is taken and various tests show the doctor the state of the patient's arteries. The drip is then tailored to individual needs and must be administered by a qualified doctor.

I have tried more than 15 of these treatments and have met stroke and heart patients, who after 20–30 treatments, have seen radical and positive benefits to their health. The amounts of nutrients such as vitamin C that can be administered intravenously are far higher than those that can be tolerated by mouth and are far more easily absorbed into the body. Dr Scott-Mumby is also having considerable success with younger patients suffering from ME, chronic fatigue and burn-out due to stress. For anti-ageing purposes, according to your overall health, diet and lifestyle, the number of treatments needed is between 15 and 20, but more are necessary for serious arterial conditions.

After 15 sessions, my skin looked more hydrated, I experienced renewed mental clarity and raised energy levels.

In certain areas, chelation is available on the NHS and private insurance companies are considering adding this treatment to their packages. But, it is worth a try if, like me, you just want to turn back the clock.

Foods to Avoid

- Most patients are told to eat normally prior to having chelation, but some doctors suggest that you eat a lighter diet on the day before the treatment so that the metals that are "chelated" by the treatment can more easily be eliminated.

- Chelation does not give you a licence to live on junk foods and is more effective if you eat a healthy diet (see *Diet – The Stay Younger Longer Diet on page 114*).

Friendly Foods

- On the day of the treatment make sure that you eat breakfast and take a banana, seeds, raisins, or a sandwich with you to eat during the process. This is because chelation also removes minerals from the body, which can affect your blood sugar levels.

- You will also need plenty of water, before during and after the treatment, which can trigger a dry mouth. Drink least six glasses daily.

Useful Remedies

- All the doctors that offer chelation should offer you an information sheet telling you all about chelation and an aftercare information sheet. If they don't – ask for one.

- As well as "chelating" toxic minerals and removing them from the body, chelation can also remove certain minerals and as the effects of the treatment last for several hours, you will need to take a high-strength multi-mineral approximately eight hours after the end of the treatment. Ask the doctor who administers the treatment for a specific list of supplements you will need.

- By adding glutathione to the chelation formula, positive results have been seen in Parkinson's, motor neurone disease and MS. Glutathione occurs naturally in the body, but levels fall as we age, and it is a powerful liver detox aid.

■ To raise levels of glutathione in the body you can take N-acetyl cysteine and alpha-lipoic acid in combination (see *Antioxidants in Ageing p.38*).

Helpful Hints

■ Dr David Perlmutter, a neurologist in Naples, Florida has pioneered the use of intravenous glutiathione and his book *BrainRecovery.com* makes fascinating reading. Published by the Purlmutter Health Centre. Available from the NutriCentre Book Shop, see page 14 or log on to his website: www.BrainRecovery.com

■ Dr Keith Scott-Mumby can be reached through his website: www.alternative-doctor.com.

■ The ACAM website carries a full list of doctors in the UK and worldwide who have been trained in their methods: www.acam.org

■ There are also several chelation clinics around the UK. For full details call 01942 886644 or log on to: www.chelationuk.com – a highly informative website that answers any queries you may have on chelation.

■ Dr Wendy Denning is at Dr Ali's Integrated Medical Centre at 43 New Cavendish Street, London also offer this treatment. She can be contacted on 020 7224 2423.

■ Dr Rodney Adeniyi-Jones also offers the treatment at the Regent Clinic in London on 020 7486 6354 or www.regentclinic.co.uk

■ The HB Health group in London also offer this and many other state-of-the-art therapies, call: 020 7486 1095. The website, www.hbhealth.com. I go to Dr Robert Trossell who works via HB Health in London at this number, 0207 486 1095.

■ Read *Everything You Should Know About Chelation Therapy* by Dr Martin Walker and Dr Hitendra Shah, Keates. Available from the NutriCentre Bookshop (see page 14).

CHOLESTEROL, HIGH AND LOW

(See also *Heart in Ageing* and *Strokes*)

While cholesterol levels have been used for many years as a possible way to predict our risk for heart attacks and strokes – it's only part of the story. In fact in more than 70% of cases of heart attacks, blood cholesterol levels have been found to be normal, while others who have high cholesterol have healthy heart function! It is no wonder that medical science is now beginning to re-think the role that cholesterol plays in heart disease and strokes.

The new kid on the block is your homocysteine level, which scientist's state is truly the most efficient indicator of risk for heart disease and stroke. Homocysteine is a toxic amino acid produced during the metabolism of proteins, and high levels are associated with an 80% increased risk for heart disease and strokes, even if you have a healthy cholesterol level. The good news is that there is now an easy way to test your own homocysteine levels (see *Helpful Hints* in this section), and you can lower levels naturally, by simply taking more B vitamins (see *Useful Remedies* in this section). If your level of homocysteine is high and you are taking B vitamins to lower it, retest your levels periodically to see if you are taking sufficient dosages.

High plasma levels of homocysteine cause damage to artery walls, then LDL cholesterol (the bad cholesterol) can easily stick to them, which triggers the cascade of events that leads to heart disease and strokes. It is also linked to numerous other age-related conditions from Alzheimer's disease and diabetes, to obesity and mental health problems such as schizophrenia.

But your cholesterol level is still an important indicator of health. These days instead of looking only at your total cholesterol level – doctors are more interested in the ratio of HDL cholesterol (the good cholesterol) which for good health needs to be raised, to the LDL cholesterol which should be lower. The HDL cholesterol should make up over 20% of the total cholesterol level, LDL should be no more than 60–70% of the total and the very low density lipoproteins (another "bad" type of cholesterol) should be around 10–15%.

Another important indicator of heart disease risk, is the level of LDL cholesterol. An ideal level would be less than 2.6 mmol/L. If your level is between 2.6 and 3.4mmol/L it is OK but a little high. If your level is 3.5 to 4.2 mmol/L, it is borderline high and between 4.21 and 4.89 is high. Levels of LDL cholesterol above 4.90 are too high and would need attention.

Cholesterol is a fatty substance made by the liver and is needed for healthy cell membrane production and the manufacture of hormones. It is also needed to help in the synthesis of bile acids for the digestion of fats and for production of vitamin D. Low cholesterol levels are linked to depression and in rare cases suicide, hence why fat-free diets are definitely not a good idea. For years we have been told to avoid certain foods, especially eggs, because they contain cholesterol. In fact, blood levels of LDL cholesterol, are more affected by eating too much fat and sugar, rather than foods like eggs which contain cholesterol (see *Friendly Foods* in this section).

Eating too many barbecued or burnt foods, especially meat, hard margarines or fried foods cause cholesterol to oxidize which makes it more dangerous, and once oxidized it begins attaching itself to artery walls. And as we age, cholesterol tends to oxidize at a faster rate, therefore the more antioxidant rich-foods we eat, the less cholesterol oxidizes, triggering health problems.

Around 20% of the body's total cholesterol is obtained from the diet, and the body manufactures the rest. Studies have shown that overweight people produce approximately 20% more cholesterol than people of normal weight for their age, usually triggered by eating too much fat and sugar, stress and smoking.

However, if you have a persistently raised cholesterol level but eat a healthy diet, you may have an under-active thyroid. Also, people with Blood Type A are more susceptible to high total cholesterol (see *Blood Type in Ageing*).

Optimum liver function helps you to make more good cholesterol, therefore the more you look after your liver, the more likely you are to have a healthy level (see *Liver in Ageing*). About one person in 500 has a genetic predisposition to high blood cholesterol levels and even this can be helped through diet and taking the right supplements.

Foods to Avoid

- Cut down on your intake of animal fats and full-fat dairy produce and eat more essential fats (for a full list see *Fats for Anti-ageing p.139*).

- Read labels – avoid foods and oils containing hydrogenated or trans-fats.

- Refined carbohydrates, white rice and pastas, processed white breads, cakes etc, can reduce the production of HDLs and white bread eaters usually have higher cholesterol levels than those who eat mainly wholemeal varieties.

- Sugar, if not burnt for energy during exercise converts to fat in the body and resides on your hips – and in the long run raises LDL cholesterol.

- Eggs contain cholesterol, but this is balanced by a high choline content (great for memory), which breaks down the cholesterol. However, some scientists say that if an egg is fried – this causes oxidative damage – and it's the frying that causes the problems not the eggs themselves. It makes sense then to boil or poach eggs.

- Alcohol and coffee (especially if microwaved) in excess has been shown to raise cholesterol levels.

- Greatly reduce the amount of sodium-based salt you use.

Friendly Foods

- Generally, you need to increase your fibre intake. Eat more oat or rice bran, rolled oats, wheatgerm, and any beans and peas such as soya beans, red kidney beans, lima beans, broad beans, chick peas and lentils. Wholegrains such as brown rice, wholewheat, barley, rye, millet and quinoa are great for controlling cholesterol.

- For even more fibre add one teaspoon of psyllium husks to a glass of warm water and drink daily in-between meals. It tastes awful, but these husks help to remove bile salts that in turn will lower LDL cholesterol levels.

- Increase your intake of fresh fruit and vegetables (raw, steamed, roasted or stir-fried, not deep fried or boiled). Green vegetables are especially rich in magnesium and potassium, as are cereals (also rich in B vitamins) honey, kelp and dried fruits like dates.

- A couple of raw organic carrots or apples per day can lower cholesterol levels.

- Eat porridge for breakfast. Make with half low-fat milk and half water. Add a chopped apple and a few raisins to sweeten, rather than sugar.

- Buckwheat is high in glycine, and has been shown to lower cholesterol levels. Buckwheat flour makes great pancakes.

■ Fermented soya products such as miso, tofu and tempeh can help raise HDLs and lower LDLs. Soya lecithin granules are a great way to help lower LDL and help to control the growth of kidney and gall stones. Sprinkle a tablespoon daily over cereals, in yoghurts and onto fruit salads.

■ Increase your intake of healthier fats found in olive oil, avocados, sunflower, pumpkin, sesame and linseeds, plus walnuts and Brazil nuts and their unrefined oils (see *Fats for Anti-ageing*).

■ Oily fish such as salmon, trout, mackerel, herring and sardines contain a fatty acid known as eicosapentaenoic acid (EPA). This helps to make the blood less sticky thus lowers the risk of coronary heart disease. Garlic and onions do the same.

■ Look for spreads that are free from hydrogenated and trans-fats such as Biona or Vitaquell.

■ Vegetarians tend to have lower cholesterol levels.

■ Use an organic, mineral-based sea salt available from all health stores.

■ Look for Columbus eggs, high in healthy omega-3 essential fats. Columbus chickens are fed on seeds that are rich in essential fats and therefore produce healthier eggs!

■ Use dandelion root tea which helps liver function and green tea which lowers cholesterol levels.

■ Globe artichoke and fennel stimulate liver function and cell regeneration and can help lower blood cholesterol.

■ Eat more live, low-fat, plain yoghurt containing lactobacillus acidophilus, as it lowers blood cholesterol levels by binding fat and cholesterol in the intestines.

■ A glass of red wine per day is also helpful.

■ Drink plenty of water – at least four to six glasses daily.

Useful Remedies

■ As a base, take a good-quality multivitamin/mineral antioxidant formula that helps prevent the cholesterol oxidizing (see *Antioxidants in Ageing p.38*).

■ One of the easiest ways to lower cholesterol is to take grapefruit pectin fibre such as Profibe, which has been shown to reduce LDL if taken daily, even in people who refuse to change their high-fat diets. For details contact The NutriCentre or Sloane Health Foods (see page 14 for details).

■ Take 1–2 grams of fish oil daily (see also *Fats for Anti-ageing p.139*).

■ Evidence has shown that taking garlic each day can help lower overall cholesterol blood levels and increase the levels of HDL over LDL cholesterol. Kudos make a high-strength one a day (see page 14 for details).

■ Co-EnzymeQ10, take 60–100mg daily. When it is combined with 100iu of natural-source full-spectrum vitamin E, it has been shown to be more effective in protecting LDL against oxidation, than vitamin E alone.

■ Folic acid, B12 and B6 all lower levels of homocysteine in the blood, thus reducing our risk of heart disease. A good B complex should contain 400mcg folic acid, 10–20mg B6 and 50–100mcg B12.

■ Taking 200mcg per day of the mineral chromium, can help elevate HDL levels while reducing cravings for sugary foods.

■ The minerals calcium and magnesium are useful for reducing cholesterol. Take 1000mg of calcium and 600mg of magnesium.

Helpful Hints

■ There is now an easy test to discover your plasma homocysteine levels. Made by York Laboratories and backed by The British Cardiac Patients Association – it's a simple pin-prick method that can be done by post. For details call York Labs on 0800 074 6185 or log on to www.yorktest.com

■ Exercise is vital for controlling cholesterol, it can raise HDL levels and lower LDL. Try and walk for at least 30 minutes daily and do some kind of aerobic exercise three times a week.

■ Smoking increases oxidation of LDL.

■ Eating smaller meals every 3–4 hours, rather than three big meals per day, can help lower cholesterol.

■ Stress thickens the blood! Therefore, if like me, you are a Type-A person, who wants everything done *now* – find a way to relax (see also *Stress in Ageing*).

■ A fantastic book, *The H Factor*, by Patrick Holford and Dr James Braly, tells you all you need to know about controlling Homocysteine Levels; from Piatkus Books, www.piatkus.co.uk

CHRONIC FATIGUE

(See also *Absorption, Energy in Ageing, Liver in Ageing* and *Stress in Ageing*)

How many times have you heard someone say that feeling tired is to be expected at "their" age?

Today I feel more energetic at 53 than I did in my 20s when I suffered from continual candida (a yeast fungal overgrowth) and numerous other conditions. If only I had known then what I know today! Know that it's never too late to turn back your biological clock.

As we age, our metabolic rate slows down, and consequently our ability to detoxify our system also slows. This is why most people tend to expand round their waistlines in middle age – but it does not have to be this way.

And if we also eat a poor diet lacking in nutrients then the liver can become toxic, which makes us feel sluggish, and our capacity to transport oxygen and nutrients within the blood is reduced. In addition to this natural ageing process, we are exposed to huge amounts of pesticides, chemicals, additives, preservatives, prescription drugs, pollution and junk and refined foods, therefore it's no wonder that a huge majority of us complain of feeling tired all the time.

Add to this our often rushed, stressed lifestyles and eating mass-produced, nutrient- deficient foods on the run, which hinder proper assimilation and absorption of nutrients. And it's an accumulation of some or all of these factors that can leave you feeling unnecessarily tired all the time.

The secret to remaining energetic for life is to look after your liver and bowels. Naturopath, Steve Langley, says, "If a patient has ME, chronic exhaustion, is tired upon waking even after a good night's sleep, or tends to feel exhausted by the middle of the afternoon, you can almost guarantee that their liver and bowel are overloaded with toxins. Once they clean up their diet for at least a month, huge improvements are noted. However, if there is no improvement after a month, then we investigate possible thyroid dysfunction (see also *Thyroid in Ageing*). Food allergies, anaemia and low blood sugar should also be investigated. Parasitic infestation is also a common cause of chronic tiredness."

To keep your energy levels in top form it's also important that you keep a correct acid–alkaline balance in the body (see also *Acid–Alkaline Balance*).

Also there are varying levels of exhaustion, but if you find you suffer from palpitations regularly during the day, chronic headaches, have an urgency to urinate regularly and experience a red flushing in your upper chest and throat area, this is most likely your adrenal glands telling you that your body is on limits. If you have low blood pressure, this may also denote your adrenal glands are struggling. You need to listen and take note of the signals, or worse is to come. Your immune system is lowered and you become more prone to infection. Rest is your best option at this point. Know when to walk away. It's not worth dying for … literally.

Foods to Avoid

- Avoid any foods and drinks containing caffeine, sugar or alcohol, all of which lower immune function, weaken the adrenal system, and play havoc with blood sugar levels. Unfortunately, these foods and drinks give a short-term energy boost but this soon wears off leaving you craving more sugary, refined foods.

- Reduce your intake of colas and fizzy drinks, chocolates, biscuits, cakes, snacks, croissants and mass-produced refined foods. Not only do they leave us feeling tired but they also deplete important nutrients like magnesium, and approximately 40% of ME patients have low levels of this vital mineral. They also deplete chromium, the mineral that helps reduce sugar cravings, and B vitamins.

- Some people use guarana and high-energy drinks as an energy source when they are very low in energy, but these products are usually high in caffeine and sugar, which can make the situation worse in the long-term.

- If you find yourself constantly craving foods such as wheat, sugar and snacks, feel bloated, have an urgency to urinate, are suffering mood swings and chronic tiredness you may well have candida, this should be investigated by a health practitioner.

- About 55–85% of people suffering chronic fatigue have a sensitivity to certain foods usually triggered by wheat, corn and dairy produce from cows' milk.
- Fats and sugar taken in one meal are hard to digest, so ease off the chocolate croissants which will make you feel even more tired.

Friendly Foods

- Eat more papaya and pineapples which are rich in digestive enzymes that will aid absorption of nutrients from your diet. Eat small amounts before main meals.
- Include plenty of low-sugar, high-fibre cereals, leafy greens such as cabbage, kale, spring greens, pak choy, broccoli and celery.
- Try wheat-free breads and use oat-based cereals and biscuits.
- Raw wheatgerm, Brazil nuts, walnuts, almonds, blackstrap molasses, raw honey and soya beans are rich in magnesium. All fruits and vegetables are rich in minerals, especially from organic sources.
- If you find you are intolerant to dairy, try oat, rice, almond or soya milk which can be used in place of cows' milk. Goats' milk is easier to absorb than cows' milk.
- Drink plenty of filtered or bottled water even if you are not thirsty to help detoxify your system. Dehydration can also make you crave more sugary foods.
- Eat sunflower, pumpkin and sesame seeds, packed with essential fats and fibre and use extra-virgin unrefined olive or sunflower oils for salad dressings.
- Eat more high-energy foods such as alfalfa, aduki bean sprouts or wheat grass.
- Generally by controlling your blood sugar levels, by eating small meals regularly instead of binging on junk foods, will help to conserve energy, as we use up to 50% of our energy to digest large meals (see also *Low Blood Sugar p.194*).
- Drink caffeine-free herbal teas.

Useful Remedies

- Siberian ginseng – take 1–3grams a day, as ginseng is an adaptogen, it helps the body to adapt to stressful circumstances and re-balances the system. Take for 60 days and then have 30 days off before you start again. Don't take this remedy if you are pregnant.
- The herb gotu kola supports adrenal function and helps recovery from stress. Take 500mg twice daily.
- Magnesium – take 500–1000mg per day, in a chelated, easy-to-absorb form, as the body burns up a lot of this mineral when we are exhausted.
- Co-EnzymeQ10 helps to raise energy levels, take 100mg daily with food.
- Milk thistle and dandelion are two herbs that support and detoxify the liver. Take 1ml, three times daily or 500mg twice daily.
- Take a high-strength multivitamin/mineral daily (see Kudos 24 on page 348 for details).

- Organic chlorella is packed with chlorophyll and minerals which help to clean the bowel. Take 500mg twice daily.

- Active-H is a very powerful antioxidant that really does help to raise energy levels (see *Antioxidants in Ageing p.38*).

- To encourage effective absorption, take a digestive enzyme complex with main meals.

- See the section on *Essential Sugars p.126*, a new food group called glyconutrients are having a profound effect on chronic fatigue.

- A great way to have more energy is to use liquid oxygen (for details of Life Support – Hydroxygen Plus see *Oxygen in Ageing p.244*).

Helpful Hints

- Exercise raises your metabolic rate, aids bowel function and helps drain the lymph system, so make sure you walk for at least 30 minutes daily.

- Make sure you are getting sufficient sleep.

- When you are tired, your muscles tend to ache. Try homeopathic Sarco Lactic Acid 6x twice daily for seven to ten days to reduce these symptoms.

- Many readers and people I have met and interviewed have been cured of chronic fatigue and ME by energy healers. One is Seka Nikolic. I know Seka personally and have interviewed many people (and their doctors) who are now free from ME thanks to Seka. At the time of going to press, Seka works from The Kailash Centre, 7 Newcourt Street, London NW8 7AA. For details call 020 7722 3939 or 020 8632 9466.

- The other is Kelvin Heard who suffered from ME for three years. After visiting a healer he was cured, and is a qualified, registered healer who specializes in ME. Again, I have interviewed a number of his patients who are now living normal lives. Kelvin Heard is on 07710 794627.

- Many people are sensitive to electrical equipment, especially mobile phones and computers. If your symptoms persist, try having your house dowsed for electrical or geopathic stress. To find a dowser, call The British Dowsing Society on 01233 750253, or log on to www.britishdowsers.org

- Read *Candida, ME and Allergies (The Way Back To Good Health)* by Jo Hampton, Kingston House. Available from all book shops, or call 020 7323 2382.

- If you suffer ME or severe fatigue then gentle exercise such as yoga, t'ai chi, qigong, or walking at leisure in nature helps to make you feel more positive and re-build energy levels.

- Find a practitioner who can really sort out your diet, such as a nutritionist or naturopath and make a determined effort to improve your food intake (see *Useful Information and Addresses* for details p.338).

- If at all practical, treat yourself to three days at a health spa to rejuvenate and rest.

CIRCULATION

If you laid out your blood vessels end to end, it is estimated that they would encircle the globe twice over – that's a lot of miles. No wonder we end up with so many circulatory problems. Our circulation becomes less efficient as we age and therefore less oxygen and fewer nutrients are delivered to the cells, which in turn reduces our cells' ability to eliminate toxins. Numerous conditions associated with ageing from leg ulcers and memory loss, atherosclerosis to cold hands and feet, are all linked to poor circulation. Hence why keeping your circulation in tiptop condition is vital to holding back the ageing process.

Our arteries make up a major part of our blood circulatory system and contain about 15% of our blood supply at any given moment. Healthy arteries have thick, muscular walls, which are necessary for the pressure of the blood moving through them. Your heart weighs just 280–310g (10–11oz) and it is about the size of a clenched fist. The left side of the heart forces blood into the arteries, which carry the bright red, nutrient rich, oxygenated blood through the body.

The oxygen (from the lungs) and nutrients (absorbed into the arteries via the gut) are taken up by the cells, before the blood (now a darker/bluish colour) is then returned to the heart via the veins, and the right chamber of the heart then pumps it through the lungs. Veins are more numerous and hold more of the body's blood (about 70%) and they transport blood laden with waste products and partly depleted of oxygen, back to the heart.

From the lungs the re-oxygenated blood returns, purified, to the left chamber, ready for redistribution and the whole cycle begins again.

Veins are forced to move against gravity much of the time. In order to maintain normal blood pressure, an adequate supply of blood must be returned to the heart from the peripheral vessels. Two main factors are responsible for this "uphill" flow from the legs and abdomen to the heart. Firstly, muscular contractions compress veins, thus squeezing the blood along. When a person stands still for a long time such as a soldier on sentry duty, the blood pools in the lower limbs due to the force of gravity and in the long-term, as the leg valves become weaker, can trigger varicose veins. This pooling of blood means that there is insufficient blood returning to the heart to maintain blood pressure, and less blood makes it to the brain. In extreme cases fainting can result, forcing the person into a horizontal position, which alleviates the problem.

Secondly, as we age, and thanks to a more sedentary lifestyle, we tend to breathe more shallowly which has a direct effect on our circulation.

Coronary heart disease is almost always due to a condition called atherosclerosis in which fatty deposits attach themselves to the insides of the arteries. Arteries that were once smooth and elastic become rough, inflexible and narrow (see *High Blood Pressure*).

With this narrowing, the volume of blood that the arteries can transport is reduced. Factors that contribute to atherosclerosis are high blood pressure, cigarette smoking, high cholesterol, a high-fat diet, excessive salt and so on.

Once an area has been damaged, fats from the blood, including cholesterol, accumulate and build up a thick fatty layer called plaque. This plaque narrows the artery and a clot may detach itself and if it causes an obstruction inside the coronary artery, a heart attack can occur. If it blocks an artery leading to the brain, it can cause a stroke.

This slow build up of plaque and consequent narrowing of the artery can also lead to a condition called angina which is very common after 50. The pain of angina (which can vary considerably) is generally felt when the person is under stress or more demands are put on the heart muscle during exercise.

The pain of a heart attack is a more "crushing" pain in the chest, which can radiate to the jaw or down the left arm.

Blood pressure tends to increase with age. Normal blood pressure depends on a number of factors including the elasticity of the arterial walls, amount and consistency of the blood, digestion, smoking, weight and stress. High blood pressure can trigger heart attacks and strokes.

An aneurysm can occur when there is where a weak spot in an arterial wall which balloons out and releases blood into surrounding tissues. Hence why looking after the integrity of your veins and arteries can help you to not only feel better, but look younger for much longer.

Foods to Avoid

■ Salt hardens your arteries (which need to be elastic) and although essential to life, most people consume too much inorganic salt in the form of sodium chloride. Too much salt can result in high blood pressure. It is found in most tinned, pre-packaged mass produced foods, burgers, crisps, laxatives, antacids and carbonated drinks.

■ Reduce your intake of animal fats such as red meat, full-fat milk and dairy produce, cheese and chocolates.

■ Pies, pastries, cakes and foods made with saturated/hydrogenated trans fats, such as lard and margarines, should be avoided or reduced (see *Fats for Anti-ageing p.139).*

■ Avoid or greatly reduce fried foods. Don't fry with mass-produced vegetable oils.

■ Avoid coffee, caffeine and other stimulants, which can ultimately lead to a constriction of blood vessels.

■ Avoid excessive alcohol. A glass of red wine with meals daily however, can be beneficial.

Friendly Foods

■ Try chopping seaweed such as kelp over your food instead of sprinkling salt.

- Use organic mineral-rich sea salt, but only over the food that is in front of you!

- Vitamin C is vital for healthy circulation. Foods naturally high in vitamin C include kiwis, blueberries, cherries and capsicum – and all fruits and vegetables.

- Garlic and onions help to thin the blood naturally.

- Wheatgerm, avocados, nuts and seeds are all rich in vitamin E, which also helps to thin the blood naturally.

- Foods rich in rutin help to strengthen the small blood vessels. So eat more buckwheat, the peel of citrus fruits, rose hips and apple peel.

- Silica-rich foods such as lettuce, celery, millet, oats and parsnips help to strengthen arterial and vein walls.

- Flax (linseeds), sunflower and sesame seeds and fish oils contain essential polyunsaturated fatty acids, known as omega-3 and omega-6 fatty acids, that have been shown to lower the bad fats and thin the blood. Try eating at least three portions of fish a week such as wild salmon, mackerel or tuna.

- Unrefined nuts: Brazil, walnuts, hazelnuts, almonds, seeds, and their unrefined cold oils, are excellent sources of essential fats and have one avocado a week, a rich source of mono-unsaturated fats.

- Sprinkle GM-free lecithin granules, which emulsifies fats, over your breakfast cereals.

- People on high-fibre diets are four times less likely to suffer from circulation problems and heart disease. Soluble fibre such as beans and lentils consists of compounds which bind to bile salts and this helps lower cholesterol levels.

- Psyllium husks are a good source of soluble fibre and a level tablespoon mixed into a large glass of water and taken each morning is a great preventative for high cholesterol. Make sure that you drink plenty of water throughout the day to help the psyllium work properly. If previously you have been on a low-fibre diet, begin with a teaspoon and gradually increase the dose.

Useful Remedies

- The herb gotu kola helps increase circulation to the extremities such as feet and hands through its vasodilatory action on peripheral blood vessels. Take 500mg twice daily.

- The herb butcher's broom is high in rutin, a bioflavonoid which helps to tone the vein walls. It is therefore very beneficial in treating varicose veins. As butcher's broom is a vasoconstrictor (the opposite to gotu kola), caution should be taken if you suffer from high blood pressure. Take 500mg twice daily.

- The herb horse chestnut has a similar action on varicose veins as its components help strengthen the small capillaries. Take 500mg daily.

- V-Nal contains butcher's broom, horse chestnut, B vitamins and rutin. It is made by Bional and available from all health stores. All the above herbs are usually used for varicose veins, as they strengthen veins, have anti-inflammatory properties, reduce swelling, thus making venous return to the heart more efficient.

■ The herb ginkgo biloba helps increase blood flow to the head. Poor circulation to the head can trigger hair loss, memory loss and eventually dementia. Studies have shown that patients suffering with visual and hearing problems linked to poor circulation have demonstrated improvements after taking ginkgo biloba for three months. To save taking several capsules daily, Kudos make a high-strength 900mg one a day formula (see page 14).

■ Vitamin C with bioflavonoids helps to strengthen capillaries. Take 1gram daily with food.

■ Vitamin E helps reduce stickiness in the blood, take 200iu daily of full-spectrum natural-source vitamin E.

■ Niacin (vitamin B3) increases circulation but can induce a "flushing" or reddening of the skin, so begin with 30mg and work up to 100mg daily.

■ Ginger helps to warm the body so make a ginger tea infusion three times daily and add grated fresh root ginger to stir-fries and fruit salads.

Helpful Hints

■ Exercise is a wonderful way to help increase circulation. Just taking a brisk walk every day can be very helpful. Skipping, dancing, rebounding and power walking all help.

■ Massage and reflexology are important, especially for people, who for health reasons, cannot exercise much or lead a more sedentary lifestyle. Aromatherapy massage using essential oils such as rosemary, black pepper or ginger can be very effective in aiding circulation.

■ Skin brushing also aids circulation. Work upwards from the feet and hands towards the heart, rubbing briskly and try to do this five times a week in the bath or shower.

■ Long-term stress constricts blood vessels which will impede circulation.

■ Magnets increase circulation by drawing blood to them. Magnetic insoles (placed in your shoes) can aid in circulation to the feet. As our peripheral circulation tends to lessen as we age, this can be very effective in winter. For further details call Homedics UK Ltd on 0161 798 5876, or write to them at Parkgates, Bury New Road, Prestwich, Manchester M25 0JW, or log on to: www.homedics.co.uk

■ If you smoke, give it up as it impairs breathing and hence circulation.

■ Acupuncture has a long history in the treatment of poor circulation and high blood pressure (see *Useful Information and Addresses*).

CONSTIPATION

(See *Bowels* and *Elimination*)

CREAMS – ANTI-AGEING
(See *Rejuvenation Therapies* and *Skin in Ageing*)

DEMENTIA
(See *Alzheimer's Disease, Brain in Ageing* and *Memory*)

DEPRESSION IN AGEING

There is a great deal of difference between being in a low mood for a few days – and suffering full-blown depression. People over 65 tend to suffer more incidence of depression due to poor nutrition, the loss of a loved one, feelings of no longer being useful and so on. Up to 15% of older adults have clinically significant symptoms of depression and 60% of these adults are not receiving the proper therapy. And persistent mild depression in older adults lowers immunity and the ability to fight off disease. Many people mistakenly believe that depression is a normal by-product of the ageing process. In fact, depression is not a normal response to growing older and there are lots of things you can do to help yourself to feel happier and more positive.

A truly depressed person has an all-pervading feeling of sadness. Other typical symptoms range from feeling worthless, inadequate or incompetent. And if you also suffer from loss of interest or pleasure in your job, family life, hobbies or sex, difficulty concentrating or remembering, insomnia, over- or under-eating, unusual irritability, a sense of humour failure, a feeling of being downhearted that just won't go away, frequent or unexplainable crying spells, recurrent thoughts of death or suicide – then you may be clinically depressed and you should seek help.

Depressed people often isolate themselves by withdrawing from friends and families. Not all symptoms denote clinical depression, for instance if you are feeling total apathy, such as you just don't want to get up in the morning, then such symptoms can be linked to adrenal exhaustion (see *Stress in Ageing*). Hormonal imbalances, low blood sugar and poor thyroid function can also trigger depressive-type symptoms (see under these sections for extra help).

Foods to Avoid
- Avoid or reduce alcohol, it can exacerbate depression, as it lowers levels of the feel good hormone serotonin, and depletes B vitamins needed for energy and nerve health.
- If you eat too much refined sugar, your blood sugar levels keep fluctuating which can greatly affect your mood (see *Carbohydrate Control* and *Low Blood Sugar*).
- Excessive consumption of refined, processed, fatty foods and caffeine can make your depression worse as they deplete vitamins B and C and the mineral chromium.
- Avoid the sweetener aspartame at all costs, which can have neurological side effects and

has been shown to interact negatively with anti-depressants. For further information log on to www.dorway.com

- Which foods do you tend to crave and eat the most? It could be flour-based, sugary foods and snacks. The foods you crave are usually the ones that make you worse. It takes discipline but for two days avoid these foods and replace with fresh fruits, vegetables and grains like brown rice and see how much better you feel.

- Lack of iron is also linked to depression, but as iron accumulates in the body and is linked to heart disease, find out if you are deficient.

Friendly Foods

- The brain is made up of around 60% fats, so eat more healthy fats including oily fish, linseeds (flaxseeds) and wheatgerm which are all rich in omega-3 essential fats. Walnuts, pecans, Brazil nuts and hazelnuts, as well as sunflower and pumpkin seeds, are all rich in omega-6 essential fats. Use unrefined nut and seed oils for salad dressings (see also *Fats for Anti-ageing p.139*).

- Increase your intake of fresh fruits, vegetables, wholegrains such as brown rice, pastas and lentils.

- To help raise serotonin levels eat more foods containing trytophan, such as fish, turkey, avocado, cottage cheese, organic meats, beans, lentils, tofu, soya milk, wheatgerm and bananas.

- Foods containing the amino acids phenylalanine and tyrosine can also help to raise mood, these include low-fat meats, fish, eggs, wheatgerm, dairy foods, oat flakes and chocolate. This is why eating chocolate often makes you feel good. If you are a chocoholic, to reduce the cravings, try taking 250–500mg of DLPA (DL-phenylalanine) with 2mg of vitamin B6 and 500mg of vitamin C on an empty stomach before breakfast.

- Spicy foods that contain cayenne pepper produce endorphins that help raise your mood.

- Drink six glasses of water daily to help remove toxins.

Useful Remedies

- Firstly begin taking a high-strength multivitamin/mineral such as Kudos 24 (see p.348 for details) to give you a good nutrient base.

- Various B vitamins play a major role in maintaining proper brain chemistry, and deficiencies of B vitamins are common in depressed people, take a 50mg B complex in addition to your multivitamin, twice daily. B vitamins turn your urine bright yellow – but don't worry, this is normal!

- Take 1gram of vitamin C daily.

- Omega-3 fats are vital for improving depression and have been shown in many cases to be more effective than anti-depressant drugs. If you are not eating oily fish three times a week then take an omega-3 fish oil capsule that contains 500–1000mg of EPA plus DHA daily.

■ 5-hydroxy tryptophan (5-HTP) helps raise serotonin levels in the brain. Extracted from the Griffonia plant from Africa, 5HTP helps balance mood, helps you to fall asleep more easily, reduces aggression, reduces appetite and creates a more relaxed waking state within 45 minutes. The recommended dose is: 50mg up to 200mg per day. Nutritionist Patrick Holford says for best results, start on a low dose at night and then gradually work up to 50mg up to four times daily. If your mood stabilizes, gradually lower the dose until you find how much you need. Taking more than you need will not be helpful in the long run. This supplement is more effective if taken with B vitamins and 10mg of zinc.

■ Try Patrick Holford's Mood Formula, which contains amino acids, zinc, B vitamins and 5HTP. It is available from all good health shops or call Higher Nature (see page 13).

■ In a study, DHEA hormone supplementation was tested on middle-aged and elderly patients with major depression for four weeks. Depression ratings and memory performance significantly improved. DHEA in other human studies significantly elevated mood in elderly people. Recommended dose: 50mg a day for men and 2mg per day for women – not available in the UK unless you have a prescription – but DHEA can be bought freely in health shops in America or log on to www.lef.org or www.pharmwest.com (See DHEA under *Other Vital Hormones p.239.*)

■ SAMe (S-adenosylmethionine) acts as a natural anti-depressant. It can give good effects within a week, but should be taken for five to six weeks for optimum results. 200mg twice daily.

■ Siberian ginseng has a tonic effect on the adrenal glands, which are usually struggling in people who are depressed. Take one capful daily in juice for a month, then stop for a month and take again, and so on.

■ The herb St John's Wort has been proven to help milder forms of depression. In over 25 double blind studies of over 1,500 people, St John's Wort demonstrated its effectiveness in improving mood, lessening anxiety and reducing sleep disorders. St John's Wort helps to reduce the sadness, stress and feelings of helplessness from depression. Do not take St John's Wort if you are pregnant or on the pill and avoid intense sun exposure while using it, since this herb can make the skin more sensitive to sunlight. Do not take St John's Wort with drugs such as Prozac, Zoloft and Paxil.

■ The herb rhodiola, grown in Siberia has been shown to help protect against the negative affects of the stress hormone cortisol, it increases energy levels and, most importantly for anyone suffering depression, rhodiola helps the brain to make serotonin a key neurotransmitter which makes you feel happier and more positive. Low levels of serotonin trigger depression and low moods. Kudos make a high-strength rhodiola (see page 14 for details).

■ A newly discovered antioxidant that is 10,000 times more powerful than vitamin C called Active-H helps to eliminate some of the free radicals in the brain that may interfere with the neurotransmitters in the brain (see *Antioxidants in Ageing p.38* for more details).

Helpful Hints

■ Natural sunlight helps to suppress production of the hormone melatonin and improves immune function. This hormone is produced by the pineal gland at night, hence why we tend to feel more depressed and sleepy during the winter months. Melatonin aids sleep and acts as an important antioxidant, but if you are depressed then you need less melatonin. Therefore get out into daylight as much as you possibly can, especially in the mornings and if you work in an office without full-spectrum lighting, make sure you use full spectrum light bulbs at home and at work. They last for ages and use less electricity. They are available from most stores or call Higher Nature (details on page 13).

■ Regular exercise is vital in the fight against depression. I know of one New York doctor who asks all his depressed patients to walk for 30 minutes in sunshine and then to tell him how they feel. This is because exercise and sunlight releases endorphins, natural anti-depressants, which raise your mood. Regular exercise can help you sleep better, feel better, look better, and provide you with an enhanced self-image. A German study showed a significant reduction in depression when patients walked for 30 minutes a day and other studies show that regular exercise is as effective as anti-depressants and more effective against relapse than drugs.

■ Studies have shown that having control over roles such as being a parent, grandparent or provider can add value to an elderly person's life. Also many companies are at last waking up to the fact that people over 65 are more committed, take less time off sick, and are more experienced workers who tend to be more cost effective than younger people.

■ Ask your doctor if you can see a counsellor – as a problem shared is a problem halved. And counselling is often more successful than taking anti-depressants. Talk your innermost fears through with a friend or relative, they may not even realize you are depressed. For details of your nearest qualified counsellor contact the British Association for Counselling, BACP House, 35-37 Albert Street, Rugby, Warwickshire CV21 2SG. You can also contact them by Tel: 01788 550 899, website: www.bacp.co.uk, E-mail: bacp@bacp.co.uk

■ Do volunteer work as helping others can boost self-esteem.

■ Watch videos, DVDs and films that make you laugh. Laughter produces natural mood boosting chemicals in the body.

■ Be sure to get enough quality sleep, but get up after eight hours or so.

■ Blend pure oils of bergamot, clary sage, geranium and neroli in a base of almond oil and ask a friend or relative to give you a massage. These aromatherapy oils help lift your mood.

■ Hypnotherapy and Neuro Linguistic Programming has helped many people (see *Useful Information and Addresses p.338*).

■ For further help read *Optimum Nutrition for The Mind* by Patrick Holford, Piatkus.

DETOXING

(See also *Bowels* and *Elimination*)

Detoxing brings huge anti-ageing benefits, such as clearer, younger looking skin, sparkling eyes, raised energy levels, faster elimination processes, healthier looking hair and so on. This is because all your internal organs, especially the liver, spleen (lymphatic system) and digestive system, are operating more efficiently and under less stress. For instance up to 50% of our energy is used in the digestive process, but by fasting, this energy is utilized in processes such as tissue repair and cellular regeneration which all helps slow the ageing process. Fasting also encourages toxins stored in fat cells to be moved into the bloodstream so that they are processed by the liver and eliminated out of the body.

Also, when you detox you also enable your lymphatic system to decongest. Your spleen is the largest body of lymphatic tissue in the body; other groups of lymph nodes are situated in the neck, groin and arm pits. Your lymphatic system removes toxins and microbes from the body's tissues and looks like a milky or transparent fluid; these toxins are filtered via the lymph nodes and spleen – and from there onto the liver and finally they are excreted by the bowel. Within the lymph nodes, lymphocytes (a specific kind of white blood cell that keeps your immune system in good shape) are also produced. Hence why a fully functioning lymph system helps you to fight off invading bacteria and viruses.

During an infection, the lymph glands can swell as they are producing more white blood cells – this is very common in cold and throat conditions for instance. If the lymphatic system becomes congested, the fluid thickens and becomes more gel like, which inhibits proper drainage and detoxification placing more pressure on the liver and kidneys.

So, if you decide to fast, but suffer an eating disorder such as anorexia, bulimia or mental illness, or any chronic conditions that requires medication, then always seek professional help before considering any type of fast. Also if you suffer diabetes or low blood sugar, only fast with the help of a qualified nutritionist or doctor.

You can devise your own fast for various periods from 24 to 72 hours, but if you are considering a lengthy fast, again, do this only with the advice of a health professional.

Foods to Avoid

- You can trigger a detox without fasting, by eliminating for one week any foods containing flour, sugar and dairy from any source and any foods or drinks containing caffeine.

- You may experience withdrawal symptoms such as headaches, aching joints, fatigue, skin rashes and sometimes diarrhoea, as toxins are released into the bloodstream, but these symptoms soon pass.

Friendly Foods

- Naturopath, Steve Langley, advises, "If you want to try a juice fast, then for a couple of days before you begin, only eat fresh fruits and vegetables, brown rice, lentils and pulses. This takes a load off the digestive system and helps avoid the symptoms which can be triggered if you detox too quickly."

- Juices are rich in vitamins and minerals that help to re-alkalize the body, they are also packed with enzymes that are often lost in the cooking process. Vegetable fasts are preferable for anyone suffering from candida, a yeast fungal overgrowth, or blood sugar problems. On average drink three 225ml (8 fl oz) glasses throughout the day – and greater benefits can be derived if they are freshly made with organic vegetables. Keep in mind that vegetable juices are the nutrient builders in the body and fruit juices are the cleansers.

- In general don't mix fruit and vegetables juices together, the exceptions to this are carrots and apples which are fine when mixed.

- Raw beetroot is a powerful blood cleanser and all green leafy vegetables, cabbage, kale, parsley, watercress, celery and celeriac help cleanse the bowel.

- Or you can make a fruit mix for breakfast and a vegetable mix for lunch and supper – just separate them.

- If you are really hungry on only juices, then blend raw wheatgerm, lecithin granules, linseeds, sunflower or pumpkin seeds or any organic green food powder into the mix to add bulk to the drinks.

- Drink herbal teas or dandelion coffee as often as you like. Burdock root or dandelion teas are very cleansing.

- If you cannot face a juice fast then for a couple of days try a mono diet – which is simply eating only one food such as grapes, bananas, melons or apples. Even one day of eating one fruit takes a huge strain off your digestion and helps promote some detoxification.

- Adding the juice of a lemon to a glass of warm water and drinking upon rising further helps support the liver.

- When detoxing or fasting it is imperative that you drink plenty of pure water throughout the day, preferably reverse osmosis or distilled. For details contact the Pure H2O Company on 01784 221188 or log on to www.pureh2o.co.uk who operate in 40 countries.

Useful Remedies

- Add a tablespoon of psyllium husks to a 225ml (8oz) glass of juice or water, and drink immediately. Best taken first thing in the morning to further aid elimination.

- The herb milk thistle aids regeneration of the liver. Take 500–900mg daily. Kudos make a high-strength one-a-day formula (see page 14 for details).

- Steve Langley makes a herbal blood and skin cleanser herbal formula containing burdock root and yellow dock root that can be used whether you are detoxing or not. This formula has proved especially helpful in reducing cellulite. Take one teaspoon is a glass of water three times daily preferably before meals. To order write to: Holos Health, PO Box 3063, South Croydon, Surrey CR2 7LZ.

■ BioFirm, developed in Denmark, contains citrus pulp, rich in flavonoids, which strengthens capillaries and helps to drain fluid from the system. It also contains pectin, which helps reduce cellulite and strengthens connective tissues. Try 2 tablets taken three times daily with water. For details call The NutriCentre (see page 14).

■ Organic spirulina helps to detoxify and re-alkalize the body and is packed with vitamins and minerals. Take one teaspoon three times daily. Available from Blackmores (see page 13).

Helpful Hints

■ There are so many fasts available, but the above suggestions, if followed, will trigger a thorough detoxification process.

■ Lymphomyosot – a complex homeopathic remedy – really helps lymphatic drainage. Take 10 drops three times a day in water, in-between meals. Available to order through chemists or call Biopathica on 01233 636678, www.biopathica.com

■ Other ways to support your digestive system would be to use Food Combining. Basically, proteins such as meat, cheese, eggs and fish should be eaten only with vegetables or salads. Conversely, if you eat potatoes, rice, bread or pasta, these should be eaten only with vegetables and not any proteins. Grains are more neutral and can be eaten at any time. Fruit should be eaten as a starter or in-between other meals.

■ Saunas, skin brushing and steam baths all aid detoxification of the skin.

■ A good massage such as shiatsu or manual lymph drainage all encourage lymph drainage (see *Useful Information and Addresses*). Your lymphatic system depends on exercise to remove toxic waste products, so make sure that you walk daily and take regular exercise.

■ Colonic irrigation helps to quickly detoxify the large intestine (colon). But anyone suffering from inflammatory bowel conditions, such as colitis or Crohn's Disease, should consult their doctor before considering a colonic. For your nearest therapist, log on to www.colonic-association.com or call 01442 827687. After any colonic you would need to take some acidophilus/bifidus healthy bacteria to replenish the bowel flora.

■ A good book to read is *The 20-Day Rejuvenation Diet Program* by Jeffrey S. Bland PH.D, Keates.

■ If at any time you begin to feel faint on any juice fast, break the fast and eat something like a couple of bananas as quickly as possible.

DIABETES – LATE-ONSET
(See also *Carbohydrate Control* and *Insulin Resistance*)

Type 2 Diabetes is also known as late-onset diabetes, which typically affects people after the age of 50, and accounts for 90% of diabetes cases. In America, 17 million people are estimated to be diabetic and The World Health Organization states that the number of people with diabetes will more than double from 120 million today to 300 million in just over one generation. The tragedy is that late-onset diabetes is now occurring in children as young as 13 who are eating too much junk food, and the disease has become a health time bomb. Make no mistake, late-onset diabetes can shorten your life – and it is totally preventable.

It is the fourth leading cause of death in the UK, which costs the NHS £5.2billion a year to treat. Three-quarters of cases are triggered by being overweight, resulting from the over-consumption of refined, sugar-based carbohydrate foods such as cakes, biscuits, sugar-filled fizzy drinks, fried potatoes and fried foods.

The rarer Type 1 diabetes is a life-long condition that usually starts during early childhood. Both types of diabetes involve too high a level of sugar in the blood. The hormone insulin is responsible for lowering blood sugar levels. Whereas Type 1 is caused by the failure of the pancreas to secrete adequate insulin, Type 2 diabetes is characterized by too much insulin being released, but the body becomes resistant to it and simply doesn't respond to the insulin as it should. Therefore, despite high levels of insulin, glucose is not properly transported into the cells and it increases to unacceptable levels in the blood. The body tries to get rid of excess sugar in the urine, hence why doctors test for diabetes through urine.

Diabetes can trigger heart, brain, eye and arterial problems that accelerate the ageing process. The life expectancy of an individual with diabetes is therefore considerably below what it should be and the risk of heart disease in diabetics is two to three times greater than in those who do not have the disease. While diabetes can have a hereditary link, your genes do not usually predetermine your health, but rather they interact with your environment (including your diet) to either improve or worsen your health (see *Genes in Ageing*). We can inherit more from our parents than just their genes; their eating habits are often passed on too.

The main symptoms of diabetes are excessive thirst, frequent urination, increased appetite, fatigue and loss of weight. Other symptoms, though less common, include muscle cramps, blurred vision, itchy skin and poor wound healing. If you are diagnosed as diabetic by your doctor with blood and urine tests, you will very likely be offered various courses of action. In mild cases, late-onset diabetes can be kept in check by diet alone. If severe, the diet is accompanied by oral medication or injections to either increase the production of insulin or improve your sensitivity to insulin. It's worth noting that if you suffer thrush regularly – you may be diabetic.

Foods to Avoid

■ See also diet under *Carbohydrate Control* and *Insulin Resistance*.

■ Avoid sugar and foods containing sugar, such as fizzy drinks, chocolate, desserts and sweets, which release their sugars too quickly into the bloodstream.

■ Avoid all refined, mass-produced white flour–based foods such as pizza, pastas, white breads, cakes and biscuits and white rice that are usually high in sugar and saturated fats.

- Honey, maltose, dextrose are still sugars and can exacerbate the problem.
- Beware that most foods advertised as being low in fat are often high in sugar.
- Don't drink concentrated shop-bought fruit juices. Make fresh juices or dilute no-added-sugar juices with two parts juice to one part water.
- Reduce saturated fats from animal sources to less than 10% of daily food intake.
- Basically cut out red meats or eat only occasional lean steak and lamb.
- Reduce your use of sodium-based table salts, look for magnesium-rich sea salts and add only a little to the food on your plate.

Friendly Foods
- Eat more unrefined, high-fibre carbohydrates such as wholemeal bread, brown rice, buckwheat, oats (especially porridge), jacket potatoes plus low-fat proteins such as beans, pulses, lentils and barley.
- Fruits and vegetables are high in antioxidants and soluble fibre, eat them raw as much as possible.
- Fish oils have been shown to improve the pre-diabetic condition, insulin resistance and help to prevent full-blown late-onset diabetes developing, therefore eat more oily fish and fresh fish. But don't fry it – poached or grilled is best.
- Eat more unrefined sunflower, pumpkin, sesame and linseeds and their unrefined oils, which are rich in omega-3 and 6 essential fats. Blend these oils half and half with extra virgin olive oil for salad dressings.
- Vitamin E-rich foods help to lower the risk of many conditions associated with diabetes, such as circulation and eye problems. Food sources are soya beans, raw wheatgerm, sprouting seeds, green vegetables, eggs, unrefined and unprocessed nuts especially almonds and hazel nuts. Look for a low-sugar muesli that is rich in nuts, oats and sprinkle raw wheatgerm onto the muesli.
- Eat fresh bilberries, blueberries and blackberries when in season, or use frozen, as these fruits help to protect the eyes.

Useful Remedies
- A high-strength multivitamin/mineral complex taken every day provides a good baseline of nutrients, such as Kudos 24 (see page 348).
- The mineral chromium is vital for helping to control and prevent late onset diabetes. Scientists in America found that taking 200mcg of chromium daily helped reduce the incidence of late-onset diabetes by up to 50%. Chromium also helps to reduce cravings for sweet foods. And in time, chromium should enable you to reduce your medication, which you would need to discuss with your doctor.
- 1000mg of Vitamin C taken twice daily can lower glucose response.

- Magnesium, which is needed to process insulin, is usually lacking in diabetics. Take a multimineral daily that contains 300–450mg of magnesium, 20mg zinc and a trace of copper.

- B complex vitamins are useful as diabetic patients are usually deficient in B vitamins, needed for energy production and nerve health.

- If you don't eat oily fish regularly then take a 1-gram fish oil capsule daily and make sure it's free from PCBs and dioxins. BioCare, Higher Nature, FSC and Seven Seas all make pure fish oil capsules (see pages 13 & 14 for details).

- Alpha lipoic acid (ALA) is a powerful antioxidant (see also *Antioxidants in Ageing*) ALA has also been shown to improve insulin action. Take 50–60 mg daily.

- The hormone DHEA (see also *Other Vital Hormones*) helps to lower insulin levels, and protect vital organs, particularly the kidneys against damage due to high blood glucose. Never take hormones unless you have been shown to need them.

- Aloe vera juice helps to lower blood sugar levels in non-insulin dependent diabetes.

- **Note: taking supplements can affect blood sugar levels. Diabetes must be supervised by a medical practitioner, so any supplement regimen should be undertaken only with the help of a medical doctor and/or a nutritionist.**

Helpful Hints

- If you are overweight, you greatly increase your risk for diabetes, especially after 50 (see *Weight Problems in Ageing*).

- Exercise is vital because it reduces the need for insulin, reduces blood cholesterol and prevents obesity. It doesn't have to be intense exercise, but try and walk for at least 30 minutes daily, as regular walking has been shown to improve insulin sensitivity and glucose management. If you have been a "couch potato" for a long time, just start gently, walk for 15 minutes a day and then build up to 30 minutes daily, and then to 45 minutes to an hour.

- Don't go overboard on sweet foods that claim to be suitable for diabetics. It's very likely your attraction to sweets that got you into this mess, so it's time to retrain your taste buds and kick the sweet habit. A little of these foods on occasion is fine.

- Have regular eye checks, and see a chiropodist regarding your feet, as both can be affected by diabetes.

- Have regular reflexology on your feet, which improves circulation (see *Useful Information and Addresses p.338*).

- Most health shops now sell small wooden foot rollers that you simply roll your feet on for a few minutes each day to increase circulation.

- The actor Terence Stamp has developed a range of organic foods, that are sugar and dairy free. For your nearest stockists of Stamp Collection call Buxton Foods on 0207 637 5505, website: www.buxtonfoods.com.

- For further help, contact Diabetes UK, 10 Parkway, London NW1 7AA. e-mail: info@diabetes.org.uk

DIET – THE STAY YOUNGER LONGER DIET

It's not your last meal that kills you – it's your last 1,000.
Dr Udo Erasmus

Many doctors still perpetuate the myth that if you eat a healthy balanced diet, you will receive all the nutrients you need. In reality only 5% of people in the Western World actually eat a healthy, balanced diet. The vast majority take meals on the run, eating pre-packaged, fast food that is lacking in nutrients. And for the most part, unless you can prepare a meal in under 30 minutes, you often don't want to know. Elderly people and singles who live alone are equally at risk of nutrient deficiency. Up to 30% of school children don't eat a single piece of fruit in a week and the same can be said for many adults. For any parent who wants to offer their child a long, healthy life the best thing you can do is teach them that their bodies are made of what they eat. If everyone started eating well when young, their cells would be healthier for life and much illness associated with ageing could be reduced or eliminated.

Meanwhile, for those who make an effort to try and balance their diet, by eating some fresh fruits and vegetables believing they are high in vitamins and minerals – think again.

Of course it's healthier and preferable to eat plenty of fresh fruit and vegetables – but thanks to intensive farming that uses tons of pesticides and herbicides, air travel, and our ability to store produce for longer – a great majority of "fresh" produce is very depleted in nutritional terms. For instance a serving of spinach can contain anything from 158mg of iron to 0.1mg, depending on where it's grown. Store an orange for more than a week and its vitamin C content can be halved. Refined white flour generally contains 80% less of the anti-ageing minerals: zinc and chromium than its unrefined wholewheat counterpart.

Then what about taking extra vitamins and minerals to make up for what is often lacking in our diet? Well, the EU sets RDAs (recommend daily allowances) that are said to be sensible and safe levels of each nutrient needed daily. In the EC, RDAs and RDIs (recommended daily intake) currently exist for 13 nutrients – but there are 45 needed for health. And the RDAs vary greatly from country to country.

If you are feeling confused – join the club. These bureaucrats take no account of your height, weight, age, gender, your current health, nor what amounts of nutrients might be left (or not) in our fruits and vegetables.

You can buy a packet of painkillers and if you swallow the packet you could die. And yet if you were to swallow too much vitamin C – the worst that could happen is loose bowels, which for most people would be a welcome change! Water can kill you if you drink enough of it but at least we still have the right to choose whether to drink it or not.

Make no mistake, your freedom to buy truly healthy produce, plus vitamins, minerals and essential fats – which is what your body is made of – or herbs that are proven to help many conditions, is being eroded every day.

Having said all this, there is now absolutely no doubt that eating the right diet makes us healthier, and barring accidents, definitely helps us to stay younger longer for much longer.

Over the years, I have read pretty much every fad diet going. Some say, only eat protein – oh no say others, only eat carbohydrates – oh definitely not say others, eat grilled liver for breakfast, cabbage soup for lunch and wheatgerm for supper. Give me a break! Do any of these people have to get to work? Are they lonely, sick or living alone? I seriously doubt it.

Governments advise us to eat three pieces of fruit daily, plus five servings of vegetables. I'm a health writer and there are many days when even I have trouble reaching these targets.

Therefore, I'm simply going to offer what I believe to be balanced dietary options that should help you to stay younger longer. In the introduction to this book, I invited you to live consciously – to know what's good for you and what is not - and to find a balance between the two. After all, food is also a pleasure and I adore my treats, hence why I walk a middle road. If I eat a "naughty meal", I thoroughly enjoy it, but then I eat really healthily for a few days before my next treat.

If you choose to live on seeds, nuts, fruits, vegetables and so on because you want to live a younger life until 120, then that is your conscious choice. Conversely, if you want to live on burgers, chips, chocolates and colas – you can do that too, but when you have your first heart attack, or develop diabetes, don't moan at the Government for not offering you 5-star health treatment when you have been filling your body with 1-star fuel. When your car breaks down, you can easily replace the parts, the same for the moment, is not true of our bodies.

- There is now *no* doubt that eating a well-balanced, nutrient-dense diet is the simplest and easiest way to live a longer, healthier life.

- Unless you suffer eating disorders and you regularly eat far more than you need, one of the simplest ways to prolong your life is to eat less. Serve meals on smaller plates. Stop eating when you are full. Ask for smaller portions of highly nutritious foods.

- Eat when you are hungry. When you are really hungry, don't just eat a quick-fix doughnut, which contains lots of empty calories and few nutrients, as junk-type foods will fill you for a short while, but you will soon be hungry again.

- Quality proteins such as chicken, fish or organic tofu will keep you satisfied for longer.

- Eat locally grown, organic, fresh foods as much as you can. This is because all nutrients (vitamins, minerals and essential fats) work synergistically (together) in the body.

- On average 85% of our diet comes from just 19 foods, so begin experimenting a lot more. The greater the variety you can eat, the more nutrients you will ingest.

- Really enjoy treats, but don't live on them.

- As much as possible, eat only certified organic foods, which have been proven to contain more vitamins and minerals and fewer pesticides than non-organic food.

- Wash all fruits and vegetables thoroughly before eating.

- Eat 40% of your diet as alkaline forming foods. These include fruits, vegetables, sprouted seeds, almonds, millet and buckwheat. By eating more alkalizing foods you can help avoid many degenerative health problems (see *Acid–Alkaline Balance p18*).

- Avoid foods containing hydrogenated or trans-fats such as cakes, biscuits, breakfast bars, refined oils and hard margarines. Look for non-hydrogenated spreads such as Biona and Vitaquell.

- Avoid fried foods – as frying converts fats into dangerous forms. Stir-frying is fine with a little olive oil, but never heat the oil to smoking point, which turns it into a dangerous form. Add a little water to the pan once your vegetables are added and this "steam fries" which is healthier (see *Fats for Anti-ageing p139*).

- Eat more essential fats found in unrefined sunflower, hemp, pumpkin and linseeds and their unrefined oils (for a full list see *Fats for Anti-ageing p139*).

- Don't barbecue or burn foods and avoid smoked foods. The more "burning" that is involved the more free radicals are produced which add to the ageing process (see *Antioxidants in Ageing p38*).

- Cut down on full-fat dairy produce from cows – sesame seeds contain more calcium than milk. Try rice, oat, almond, low-fat goat and sheep milks ... Experiment.

- Eat more raw foods, which are higher in nutrients and fibre. I make a salad every day when I'm at home and grate into it a selection of vegetables, which makes them easier to chew.

- Make time for breakfast. A boiled egg with wholemeal toast is ideal, as proteins keep you satisfied for longer. Fresh fruit with live yoghurt helps to re-alkalize the system, and porridge balances blood sugar, which stops you craving those mid-morning snacks.

- When you need a snack, have an apple, a banana, some grapes, a low-fat yoghurt with added fruit, raisins, or muesli. Look for healthier snacks bars such as organic Mother Hemp Bars that are high in seeds and free from hydrogenated fats. Keep oat, rice and amaranth crackers handy and use a low-sugar spread or jam. Make up a small container with whole seeds, raisins and dried apricots and snack on these instead of chocolate biscuits.

- Don't add sodium-based salt to your food and reduce your intake of crisps and highly salted foods. They are dehydrating, causing the skin to become prematurely dry and wrinkly and they can increase high blood pressure and cause hardening of the arteries. Ask at your health store or supermarket for an organic mineral rich sea salt. I love Herbamare, an organic blend of sea salt and herbs from Bioforce, available from all health stores.

- Greatly reduce your consumption of sugar. It's highly addictive and *very* ageing. Use a little fructose instead. Remember that any excess sugars, from whatever source if not burned up during exercise will sit on your hips (see also *Sugar in Ageing p302*).

- Avoid the artificial sweetener aspartame, also known as Canderel. The manufacturers are now thinking of calling it Neatame. If they succeed – avoid it.

- Cut down on your intake of "white foods": white bread, rice, pasta, cakes, biscuits etc.

- Keep in mind that the foods you crave and eat the most are usually the ones that trigger many of your health problems. The biggest culprits are usually wheat, cows' milk and sugar.

- If you have a chronic running nose, suffer coughing after eating certain foods, catarrh, itching behind your ears, eczema or wheezing then you most probably have a food intolerance. It can be as diverse as garlic or wheat to bananas or oranges. Know your "enemy". Allergy specialists note that once any "offending" foods are removed, the person starts to look younger. This is because food intolerances set up an inflammatory response in the body and inflammation is one of the key factors in ageing.

- Cut down on caffeine in foods and drinks. Caffeine is a burden on the liver and if the liver becomes congested, this can lead to digestive problems, high blood pressure, skin problems, lack of energy, headaches, and dark circles under the eyes. Caffeine triggers calcium to be leeched from bone, contributing to the risk of osteoporosis and it taxes the nervous system by over-stimulating it, contributing to stress and exhaustion.

- Enjoy an alcoholic drink – but achieve balance in all things.

- As you age, the mechanism that makes you feel thirsty becomes less effective, so keep sipping water even when you are not thirsty. Make time to drink at the very least four large glasses of water a day, preferably six (see also *Water in Ageing p325*).

- Avoid too much liquid with meals, which dilutes stomach acid you need to digest your food.

- Walk for five to ten minutes after a meal to aid digestion and absorption of nutrients.

- Chew your food – this is a great way to aid digestion and absorption of nutrients.

- Eat as slowly as you can, preferably sitting down and not on the run.

- Cut down on your intake of red meats, if you love meat, eat organic and only eat lean cuts.

- Cut down on the amount of processed, fast foods, TV dinners and tinned foods you eat.

- Steam, bake or lightly grill foods. You can even buy steam ovens that guarantee less vitamins and minerals are lost during cooking.

- Make the effort to eat at least two pieces of whole fruit a day: apples, grapes, pears, peaches, nectarines and bananas are so easy to carry with you.

- Cut down on fizzy drinks, which are high in sugar and phosphorus – which can trigger mineral and bone loss.

- Increase your intake of fibre from raw fruits and vegetables, nuts and seeds, cracked flaxseeds (linseed), oat and rice bran.

■ Eat quality protein at least once a day. Fresh fish, or organic chicken are fine. If you enjoy red meat then as much as possible eat organic or free-range game. Gentlemen keep your protein intake to around 100gm (about 4oz) in any one meal and ladies 50–75gm (2–3oz). Unless of course you are a six footer who does manual work all day! Protein is a vital food for good health, but when eaten to excess, it depletes minerals from the body.

■ Fermented soya–based foods are a good source of vegetarian protein, help prevent hormonal cancers and cardiovascular disease, and can also help reduce menopausal symptoms. Kidney beans, chickpeas, lentils, peas, whey and eggs etc are all good sources of protein. Nuts and seeds are also high in protein and provide essential fatty acids and minerals. Try eating pumpkins seeds, sunflower seeds, sesame seeds, hemp seeds, linseeds, almonds, cashews, Brazil nuts and hazelnuts.

■ Wholegrains also contain some protein: brown rice, quinoa, millet, barley, oats and rye.

■ The most anti-ageing foods are those that help to mop up free radicals in the body. They are known as ORAC foods – which stand for Oxidant Radical Absorbance Capacity. These include, prunes (dried plums), raisins (dried grapes), blueberries, blackberries, strawberries, raspberries, plums, oranges, red grapes, cherries, kiwi fruit and pink grapefruit; kale, steamed spinach, Brussels sprouts, alfalfa sprouts, broccoli, beetroot, red bell peppers, onion, corn and aubergine; green leafy vegetables, lettuce, cantaloupe melons, apples, sweet potatoes, tomatoes and carrots.

■ Baked beans (buy organic) and kidney beans are also great anti-ageing foods.

■ Eat more fresh root ginger, pineapple and papaya, which aid digestion.

■ Include more fresh herbs in your diet, such as basil, sage, coriander and rosemary, which are packed with antioxidants.

■ If I had to put all this in a final anti-ageing nutshell, I would say: reduce refined carbohydrates such as white bread, rice etc; eat more complex carbohydrates such as fresh fruit, vegetables, brown rice, barley, lentils and pulses. Cut down on your sugar intake, eat quality protein at least once a day, eat more healthy essential fats and make the effort to drink more water.

DIGESTION

(See also *Absorption, Acid Indigestion, Acid-Alkaline Balance* and *Low Stomach Acid*)

As we age, our digestive system becomes less efficient, generally due to a reduction in enzyme production. Enzymes are found in and produced by saliva, the stomach, pancreas, small intestine and liver, which aid digestion and absorption of foods.

If we don't digest our foods properly then we cannot absorb the vital nutrients that are needed to keep our cells healthy and young.

Stomach acid levels also tend to decline as we age. Unfortunately, many people mistakenly believe that they make too much stomach acid, but in most cases it's not enough (see *Acid-Alkaline Balance* for a great way to find out whether you are making too much or too little).

Healthy digestion is upset by stress, eating too much at one sitting, drinking too much liquid with foods, eating on the run, and eating foods combinations that compete with each other during digestion. Even the most robust digestive system cannot in the long-term continually cope with a typical meal of meat, alcohol, cheese, tea, coffee and sugar.

Foods to Avoid

■ Saturated fats found in meat, pizzas, full-fat dairy produce, especially cheeses and chocolates are particularly hard to digest. Melted cheese is the worst.

■ As we age, the combination of fat and sugar we eat also places a great strain on the digestive system, so avoid those chocolate croissants!

■ Fried foods are very hard on digestion, so grill, poach, steam or bake. Stir-fries are fine as long as you use a little olive oil and add a little water as soon as you add the foods.

■ Fizzy drinks and waters produces gas in the stomach, which impedes proper digestion.

■ Avoid drinking too much black tea with foods, as the caffeine and tannin content interfere with proper digestion. Generally avoid too much liquid with meals.

Friendly Foods

■ A glass of red wine with food helps to stimulate stomach acid production; apple cider vinegar or lemon juice in a little water will do the same.

■ Foods such as porridge, millet-based desserts, tapioca, goats' or sheeps' milk are easier on the digestive system.

■ Eat a little pineapple or papaya before meals as they are rich in digestive enzymes.

■ Peppermint, meadowsweet, lemon balm and dandelion herbal teas, if sipped after a meal, will aid digestion.

Useful Remedies

■ Take a digestive enzyme capsule with all main meals, but if you suffer from active stomach ulcers or conditions such as colitis, then consult a health professional.

■ Take a multivitamin/mineral, as many nutrients are required for digestive processes.

■ Swedish bitters, made from herbs, help increase bile flow from the gall bladder. Take according to instructions, it is generally a teaspoon in water before a meal. They are available from most health stores.

Helpful Hints – see also *Hints* and *Diet* under *Absorption p16*.

■ Digestion begins in the mouth – so chew all foods thoroughly. As much as possible sit down to eat in a relaxed setting.

■ Walking for even 15 minutes after a meal really aids digestion.

■ For more help, read Good Gut Healing by Kathryn Marsden (Piatkus Books), which is one of the best guides to bowel and digestive disorders I have ever come across.

ELECTRICAL POLLUTION AND AGEING
(See *Radiation in Ageing*)

ELIMINATION
(See also *Bowels, Detoxing* and *Liver in Ageing*)

We are not only made of what we eat and absorb, but to a huge degree our health also depends on our elimination processes. If the bowel becomes overloaded then toxins can be re-absorbed back into the bloodstream. Parasitic infestations are more likely when you are constipated as you create a great "soil" for them to thrive in. There are more than 1,000 types of parasites that can infect humans from water, food, insect bites, pets or when you walk in tropical countries without shoes (hook worm). These parasites not only deplete nutrients from the body, but you get the added toxicity from their excrement. Naturopath Steve Langley says, "Parasitic infestation is very common, and almost 50% of irritable bowel and ME (chronic fatigue) patients have at least one parasite (see *Useful Remedies* in this section). Other symptoms include tingling in the fingers, extreme fatigue, grinding of teeth, anaemia, itchy skin rashes, headaches, muscle pain, bloating after eating and blurred vision that changes during the day."

This situation can create a self-intoxification process, in other words, the body begins poisoning itself and when cells can no longer efficiently eliminate toxins then the ageing process is accelerated.

Even if you do not have parasites, but are chronically constipated, then the toxins that are re-absorbed into the system cause the liver to become congested and so it dumps excess toxins into the skin. Up to a third of our waste can be eliminated by the skin. This results in conditions such as acne, acne rosacea, eczema and dry skin, which will make you age faster! Therefore it makes sense to look after your liver (see *Liver in Ageing*).

Also, if you suffer chronic constipation, even though your diet is good, you may have an underactive thyroid – this is especially true of women between 45 and 65 (see *Thyroid in Ageing p313*).

Foods to Avoid
■ All animal products, especially red meats, have a long transit time through the bowel and

should not be eaten more than once a week.

- Many people do not have the enzyme needed to break down lactose, the sugar in milk, which can also lead to putrefaction in the bowel. This is especially common in African and Caribbean people.

- Reduce your intake of dairy-based foods, which are mucous forming, as they add to the mucoid plaque in the intestines. However rice, oat or goats' milk are generally better tolerated.

- Refined sugars found in cakes, biscuits, desserts and highly-processed foods ferment in the gut causing gas and bloating as healthy bacteria are destroyed by candida overgrowth. These bacteria help break down digested foods and aid in the manufacture of certain vitamins, especially B group vitamins. If these healthy bacteria are missing, your digestion and elimination are impaired.

- Parasites also love sugar … so cut it out.

- When you mix flour and water it makes a gooey paste, it does the same in the bowel, therefore cut down on pastries and flour-based foods.

- Low-fibre foods such as jelly, ice cream and soft desserts, all white flour products and refined breakfast cereals which contain virtually no fibre.

- Also avoid foods to which you have an intolerance, for instance cows' milk has been found to be responsible for a lot of infant constipation.

- Cut down on full-fat cheeses and don't eat melted cheese over food – it sets like plastic in the bowel.

- Kerrin Booth, naturopath, says, "Although potatoes and bananas are healthy foods, if eaten to excess they can aggravate constipation in some people".

Friendly Foods

- Bran is good to eat, as it is an insoluble fibre derived from rice, soya or oats. The insoluble fibre is needed to stimulate the bowel to work properly. Wheat bran is fine so long as you don't have an intolerance to wheat, otherwise it can actually aggravate the problem.

- Try eating more brown rice and beans such as black-eyed beans, kidney, haricot, butter and cannellini beans.

- Linseeds are a blend of insoluble and soluble fibres which bulk the stool, encouraging it to move gently through the bowel.

- Wholewheat rye bread, Ryvita-type crispbreads, rough oatcakes, or amaranth crackers can be eaten as an alternative to wheat bread.

- Other high-fibre foods are fresh and dried figs, blackcurrants, ready-to-eat dried apricots and prunes, almonds, hazelnuts, fresh coconut and all mixed nuts.

- All lightly cooked or raw vegetables and salads will add more fibre to your diet.

- Eat more, live, low-fat yoghurts which contain healthy bacteria, a lack of which can exacerbate constipation.

- Drink at least six to eight glasses of water daily.
- Psyllium husks are a great way to add bulk to the stools. Take a tablespoon of psyllium husks in water before breakfast to help keep things moving.

Useful Remedies

- Take 1–2 teaspoons a day of Dr Gillian McKeith's Living Food Energy powder. This blend of fibres and nutrients helps improve bowel function and digestion. It is available from all health shops. Or buy a chlorella in powder form and take 500mg, four times daily.
- Acidophilus and bifidus are healthy bacteria which can be taken after a meal, particularly if constipation has started after antibiotics.
- Take 1 level teaspoon two to three times a day of vitamin C powder with added calcium and magnesium for a few days to help soften the stool and increase the frequency of bowel movement; magnesium helps to tone the bowel muscles.
- One of the best ways I have found to eliminate constipation is to replace one meal a day with a fruit and vegetable blend whilst eliminating all flour from any source for at least two days. I put half a cup of aloe vera juice, a banana, an apple, blueberries and any fruit I have to hand, plus a teaspoon of any good green food mix, a teaspoon of sunflower seeds, a dessertspoon of linseeds and a teaspoon of olive oil into my blender. To this I add half a cup of organic rice milk and blend. It's delicious and packed with fibre. On alternate days I make a vegetable juice to which I still add the aloe vera juice but not the rice milk.
- The mineral silica can tone the bowel wall and help relieve constipation. Take 75mg daily.
- Arabinogalactan (AG), a fibre from the larch tree, is very useful in the treatment of constipation. It acts as a stool softener which helps to normalize bowel movements. Also when AG enters the colon, it reacts with existing bacteria to produce short chain fatty acids (SCFAs). These are a good food source of friendly bacteria in the gut and promote a lower pH in the colon, which in turn promotes peristaltic movement. Try one capsule twice daily. For details call The NutriCentre on 0207 436 5122 or log on to www.nutricentre.com
- If you think you have parasites you should consult a qualified practitioner, but you can try a herbal formula such as Paraguard, which includes wormwood, black walnut and berberis, that help to kill the parasites. For details call the NutriCentre as above.

Helpful Hints

- It is very important that you eliminate any underlying causes for your constipation. Visit your GP and make sure there is nothing more serious going on.
- A lot of people complain of constipation and I tell them to stop eating anything containing any flour from any source for three days and to increase vegetables, fruit and salads. They often say, "Oh I hardly ever eat bread" and then you go through their diet and it's flour-based cereals for breakfast, biscuits mid-morning. pasta for lunch and a toasted sandwich for supper! Try a totally flour-free diet for just three days and I'll bet this helps.

- Use a natural skin brush and brush in the direction of the heart which helps encourage lymph elimination, so brush from the feet and ankles up the legs, and up the arms from the hands. From the lower trunk brush up towards the heart and so on.

- Have a warm bath with added Epsom salts, ginger root or Alkabath by Bestcare (see below for details) which help to open the pores and eliminate toxins from the skin. Always after such a bath, drink 2 glasses of water.

- Squatting to pass faeces helps to encourage elimination, as it is a more natural position for the colon.

- Over-use of laxatives makes the bowel lazy.

- Do not strain when you have a bowel movement as this places a strain on the vascular system and can, over time, lead to varicose veins or piles. Remember rather than fall asleep after every meal, go for a leisurely walk.

- When you feel the need to pass a motion, be sure not to ignore the signal; take the time to read a magazine on the loo!

- For healthy bowel movements you need about a pint of fluid in-between each meal to get waste moving through successfully.

- Stress is a major factor as it slows down the peristalsis movements.

- When you add more fibre to your diet and you're not used to it, it is essential that you drink more water. Adding fibre without more fluid can actually aggravate constipation.

- In the elderly a lack of folic acid can be the cause of constipation, therefore, supplementing with folic acid in the form of a good-quality multivitamin/mineral should help.

- For severe constipation, especially after surgery, and with your doctor's permission, try colonic irrigation. I have a colonic two or three times a year as a thorough cleanse especially if I am forced to take antibiotics, which cause me real problems! For your nearest practitioner send an SAE to Colonic Association, 16 Drummond Ride, Tring, Hertfordshire HP23 5DE, call 01442 827687 or log on to www.colonic-association.com

- You can also use a lukewarm water enema at home. Available from Best Care products on 01342 410303, www.info@bestcare-uk.com

ENERGY IN AGEING

(See also *Carbohydrate Control, Chronic Fatigue, Detoxing, Exercise,*
all *Hormones* sections *and Low Blood Sugar*)

Lack of energy is one of the most common complaints of ageing. And yet when I was younger, I was so riddled with candida (a yeast fungal overgrowth) triggered by too many antibiotics, I was always tired. My diet was also a disgrace. White breads, cakes and chocolate snacks lacking in nutrients, but full of sugar and fats were for a time my staple diet. In consequence my blood sugar levels were all over the place, which triggered severe chronic fatigue.

Highly-refined carbohydrate diets are killing us and they greatly drain your energy. These days I know a lot more about the body and thankfully I have more energy at 53 than I ever did in my 20s. Father Time does not automatically steal your energy and there are plenty of ways you can help yourself.

Firstly, if you eat too much, too often, you place a huge strain on your digestive system and liver. After a hearty Sunday lunch, you want to lie down and rest; too much food in one sitting wears you out (see *Digestion* and *Liver in Ageing*).

Secondly, if your body is full of toxins, then you will definitely feel very sluggish and have low energy (see *Bowels*).

Toxins equal more free radicals in the body and the more free radical reactions within the body, the less energy you will have (see *Antioxidants in Ageing*).

An obvious way to raise energy is take make sure that you have sufficient quality sleep. Also if you tend to be a "couch potato" and hardly ever do any exercise, then it should come as no surprise that you are tired all the time as you need oxygen for energy and you need to move. Unless you are poorly or totally exhausted, then exercise is vital for energy production.

All of these factors, plus depression, loss of a loved one or a job, an illness, constant pain and so on will all contribute to lack of energy.

A hormone imbalance can also drain your energy levels, therefore if you are over 45, or feel that your hormones might be in flux, have a blood or saliva test and find out what's happening. Hormone supplementation with DHEA (see also *Other Vital Hormones*) can greatly increase your energy levels.

Foods to Avoid

- Sugar and caffeine, refined carbohydrates, cakes, fizzy drinks, snacks, breakfast bars, croissants and so-called energy drinks, all of these provide us with a quick burst of energy but then you get a low blood sugar slump and you'll be craving even more.

- Read the labels on breakfast cereals, you will be amazed at just how much salt and sugar they contain.

- Reduce white foods: breads, pastas, cakes, biscuits and so on.

- If you are desperate for something sweet, use a little honey, brown rice syrup or fructose in your foods and drinks.

- Avoid mass-produced hydrogenated or trans-fats and fried foods that drain your energy.

- Wheat is best kept for the evenings, as wheat makes some people feel sleepy.

Friendly Foods

- The easiest way to have more energy is to eat a hearty breakfast, which helps to keep your blood sugar levels on an even keel. Porridge made with skimmed milk or rice, soya or almond milk, is a great way to start the day. Otherwise, protein helps to wake up your brain, so boil or poach an egg and enjoy with rye bread toast.

- Eat more fresh fruit, vegetables and complex carbohydrates such as beans, brown rice, wholemeal pasta and millet.

- For sustained energy, eat more protein foods, such as lean meat, eggs, goats' or sheeps' milk cheese, tempe, oily fish which will keep you satisfied for longer. Vegetarian proteins are barley, brown rice, rye, oats, peas, beans, lentils, nuts, seeds and fermented soya-based food.

- Hi-energy snacks are organic dried figs, dates and apricots, pumpkin and sunflower seeds. Low-fat (low sugar) live yoghurts are also fine, add wheatgerm and raisins for more energy.

- Dehydration can make you crave more fast-energy high-carbohydrate foods, therefore make sure you drink several glasses of water during the day.

- Begin juicing, as fresh juices are packed with energy. Add aloe vera juice to the vegetable or fruit juices and stir in some spirulina or chlorella powder or freshly juiced wheat grass for that extra boost.

Useful Remedies

- A useful high-energy supplement is organic dried spirulina (available from Blackmores, see page 13) or wheat grass. They are neat energy, take up to 10 tablets/capsules daily in-between meals.

- As we age, our ability to manufacture co-Enzyme-Q10 (an enzyme produced in the liver, found in organ meats) is reduced. This enzyme is essential for the production of energy in our cells, it acts like a spark plug in a car – without that spark, the car won't start! Hence why I recommend that anyone over 40 should take between 40–60mg of CoQ10 daily.

- Take a good quality multivitamin/mineral that contains B vitamins, a lack of which can cause low energy; see details of Kudos 24 on p348.

- Ginseng is great for boosting energy. Add to juices daily. Ginseng works best when taken for one month and then stopped for a month, and so on.

- If you fall asleep easily, but find it hard to stay asleep you may be lacking in magnesium, take 600mg of calcium and 600mg of magnesium before bed.

Helpful Hints

- Eating smaller meals regularly keeps our energy levels constant, whereas relying on one or two large meals overloads the body and often makes people feel tired.

- Try and walk in the fresh air, away from main roads, for at least 30 minutes every day. The more daylight you are exposed to, the more energy you should have.

- Take regular holidays, or at least odd days out that are your very own.

- Do something that you really enjoy. Recently I attended a pop concert and when I left I was so energized that I could have danced all night!

- Don't hang around with really negative people, they drain your energy. Make friends with people who make you feel good.

- Have some Reiki healing which really relaxes you and improves energy levels (see *Useful Information and Addresses p338*).

- Try nutritionist Jan de Vries' wonderful Vitality Essence, available from all health stores or e-mail: enquiries@bioforce.co.uk

- There are, of course, times when you feel totally without energy, but if you get some rest, eat more of the right foods and think as positively as you can, things usually improve within a few days. But if you are still lacking in energy after a month, then see a doctor and have have your thyroid checked, plus a thorough check-up (see also *Depression in Ageing*).

ESSENTIAL SUGARS

(See also *Sugar in Ageing*)

Until recently, it has been accepted that to survive, the human body needs 50 factors. These are 13 vitamins, 21 minerals, 9 amino acids and 2 essential fats – plus carbohydrates, fibre, air, water and light.

But now researchers have isolated and begun to understand the importance of glyconutrients (also known as saccharides and essential sugars), an essential food group, without which we cannot sustain optimal health. This is big news.

The story began in Russia during the 1940s. Eminent scientists were given a blank cheque by the National Science Academy to find something that would boost their athletes' performance – thus demonstrating the superiority of Communism. After more than 30 years they came up with glyconutrients, sugars that are found in breast milk, fruits, vegetables, some mushrooms, tree barks and herbs.

Meanwhile in America during the early 80s, and knowing nothing of the Russian findings, Dr Reg McDaniel, then the Professor of Clinical Pathology at Fort Worth Medical Centre in Dallas, was researching immune support for patients with advanced cancers and Aids. From various sources he heard about people who were seeing measurable health benefits from taking aloe vera juice. Eventually, he and other scientists began researching what specific ingredients the aloe contained that was having such beneficial effects. It was a natural sugar called mannose.

Dr Reg takes up the story, "For over 5,000 years the aloe has been prized for its healing capabilities, but now we know why. We began testing Aids patients with the isolated mannose sugars and were astonished to see a 71% improvement in just 90 days." Various scientists went on to find that there are eight essential sugars, mostly found in human mothers' breast milk and vine ripened foods, without which our immune cells cannot function at optimal levels. And once they began giving patients a full spectrum of essential sugars, they were astonished at the results.

Dr Reg has witnessed cancer patients with inoperable tumours who by taking 7 tablespoons of essential sugars daily are now well. He is hearing similar results from all over the world in Aids, Parkinson's disease, cancer and hepatitis patients, and also improvements in people suffering from auto-immune diseases such as lupus.

This all sounds too good to be true and yet Dr Reg says that the huge body of evidence now available (including the original Russian research) shows that essential sugars are a vital "missing link", a lack of which is contributing to a myriad of modern diseases and accelerating the ageing process. He continues, "Researchers around the world have shown that when people take a teaspoon or two of these essential sugars every day, then the bio-markers (blood cholesterol, lean body mass, insulin levels, aerobic capacity etc) of ageing can be greatly slowed or reversed. These essential sugars help cells to function more efficiently and can extend cell life" (see also *Cells* in *Ageing p85*).

He adds, "It soon became obvious that because most modern foods, especially fruits and vegetables, are picked way before they are ripe, that many essential vitamins, minerals, plus the essential sugars are missing. It's rather like trying to drive a car without a clutch or a braking system. We have become deficient at a cellular level and so we keep breaking down."

This makes sense for anyone who has tasted locally grown, vine-ripened fruits and vegetables, they have more depth of flavour and colouring.

But even after reading hundreds of pages of research about glyconutrients, I remained sceptical. Then I spoke with Jenny Yates, aged 42, from Church Down in Gloucester. Jenny is a clinical haematologist who was diagnosed with lupus in March 1999. This is an auto-immune condition, in which your immune system starts attacking itself. Symptoms include aching muscles and joints, chronic and severe fatigue, memory loss, a severely underactive thyroid, and hair loss. The only orthodox medicine is steroids and certain anti-malarial drugs. After having seven months off work and taking prescription drugs that made no difference, a friend told Jenny about the essential sugars. Coming from a medically trained background she was highly sceptical, but began taking 2 teaspoons of the powdered essential sugars daily. After six months her "mind" became clearer, her energy levels were restored and the pain in her muscles disappeared.

Jenny then stopped taking the sugars and gradually her symptoms returned, so today she takes them every day and her blood tests are now clear. This is an amazing story and yet I have heard similar results from people suffering with a multitude of conditions from arthritis to Parkinson's disease.

Dr Reg now lectures on essential sugars globally and is determined to educate his more orthodox colleagues as to the benefits of this newly discovered food group.

Foods to Avoid

- The commonest sugar is sucrose, which is definitely an unhealthy sugar (see *Sugar in Ageing p302*).

- Fructose is common in fruits and table sugar, but it is not an essential saccharide.

- Glucose – many of the foods we eat contain various sugars, which our bodies convert into glucose for brain fuel, but this does not mean we need to eat more refined sugars (see *Sugar in Ageing p302*).

Friendly Foods

- Eat more locally grown, preferably organic vine-ripened fruits and vegetables.

- N acetyl-neuramic acid is found in human breast milk, as human breast milk contains five essential sugars that help give babies a stronger immune system. It also helps improve memory and lowers LDL (the bad cholesterol).

- Mannose – drink more stabilized aloe vera juice containing mannose from the inner gel to boost immune function and aid skin healing.

- Xylose is a gum extracted from tree bark that is often seen in sugar free gums, but otherwise we don't ingest this in our everyday diet. It is anti-bacterial and anti-fungal and may help reduce the incidence of cancer of the digestive tract.

- N-acetyl–glucosamine is not readily available in our diets, but is a well-known amino sugar that aids cartilage regeneration, usually extracted from crab and lobster shells.

- Fucose is found in human breast milk and medicinal mushrooms, such as shitake and reishi.

- N-acetyl-galactosamine is found in milk.

- Galactose and lactose are found in milk sugars. Most people have plenty in their diet, unless you suffer from a lactose intolerance. (But Dr Reg says that after taking glyconutrients for a period of time, a number of people have found that they are now no longer lactose intolerant.)

- Other foods and herbs that contain one or several essential sugars are garlic, astragalus, echinacea, tree saps, coconut meat, husks, maize, fruit pectins and algae.

Useful Remedies

- The only supplement that I know of that contains a full spectrum of essential sugars is called Ambrotose. For details call 0800 028 6071. Take 1 to 2 teaspoons in water or juice daily for life! Remember these are an essential food group like essential fats; they are not a supplement you just take now and again.

Helpful Hints

- We do have the ability to manufacture certain glyconutrients, but stress, toxins from our diet and environment, can inhibit their conversion.

- Subscribe to Dr Reg's Newsletter: DrReg@drreg.com.

- Visit www.glycoinformation.com for a good introduction and www.glycoscience.com an American Virtual Library.

- I strongly suggest that you read *Sugars That Heal* by Emil Mondoa MD, Ballantine Publishing, or *Miracle Sugars* by Rita Elkins, Woodland Publishing. To order, call 0207 323 2382.

EXERCISE

(See also *Joints in Ageing, Muscles in Ageing, Osteoporosis* and *Oxygen in Ageing*)

Taking the right amount of exercise really helps to slow the ageing process. You would be amazed at how many people in their 70s and 80s can still run a marathon. I have met people who have learned to swim and practise yoga in their 80s and I stress that it is never too late to start doing some form exercise.

Conversely, the media is full of stories telling of children and adults who are total couch potatoes, which in time results in blocked arteries, heart disease and diabetes. Being a total couch potato could take ten years off your life.

So, if you really want to add life to your years, reduce depression, feel more positive, have younger looking skin, more supple joints and extend your life span, you need to take regular exercise.

There are many days when I wish that someone could do the exercises for me, and of course there are machines that will make your muscles contract and relax, like the Slendertone and Ultra Tone Systems, (see *Muscles in Ageing*). These types of treatments will help firm your muscles but they are not aerobic, they don't make your heart pump faster and they don't bring more oxygen into your lungs. And one of the most important biological markers of ageing is your aerobic capacity, which basically means how much air you can comfortably take in and exhale, which brings more oxygen into your blood and every cell in your body (see *Lungs in Ageing p202*).

However, there are people who become addicted to exercise, and some women exercise until their periods stop, which is not only ill-advised, but increases the risk for infertility and osteoporosis in later life.

Foods to Avoid

- When we exercise, our muscles produce a toxic substance called lactic acid, which causes us to feel stiff, most especially the day after strenuous exercise. The more junk, refined, sugary foods you eat, the more lactic acid you will produce.

- Don't eat heavy meals before exercising. If you eat a large meal, wait two hours before exercising, however a walk can aid digestion.

- See under *Diet – The Stay Younger Longer Diet (see page 114)*.

Friendly Foods

■ Foods that have a low glycaemic index, which release their natural sugar content more slowly than high-sugar foods, help you to exercise for longer. For instance lentils will help you to exercise longer than potatoes (see *Sugar in Ageing p303* for a full list of low-glycaemic foods).

■ If you practise aerobic exercise and you become dehydrated, this can also trigger cramps. Drink plenty of water and take a pinch of sea salt to help replace lost mineral salts.

■ An intense workout requires complex carbohydrates such as brown bread, pasta and rice.

■ For lengthy exercise of two hours or more, your body will need carbohydrates and fats.

■ For muscle growth and repair you need good-quality proteins from fish, meat and beans.

Useful Remedies

■ All health shops and chemists sell electrolyte-based vitamin C type powders. An electrolyte is a chemical capable of carrying or conducting an electrical charge in solution. Electrolytes are basically minerals such as sodium, potassium and magnesium. The best sachets I have found are sold worldwide in health stores called Emergen-C. These are also great when you are travelling long haul to help prevent dehydration.

■ See also *Muscles in Ageing p227 and Joints* in *Ageing p181*.

■ A lot of sports drinks are high in sugar, artificial sweeteners, colourings and extras such as guarana. Unless you exercise to a very intense pace, these drinks in the long-term can do more harm than good.

Helpful Hints

■ If you have any serious health conditions such as heart disease, angina, high blood pressure, or are overweight, check with your doctor and take his/her advice on which exercise would be best for you.

■ Begin walking for 15 minutes daily and over seven days build up to 30 minutes and more.

■ Otherwise join a local gym or a health club and in this way not only will you receive professional help, but you will make new friends.

■ Make sure that you change your regimen regularly, as the body gets used to a certain type of exercise, it helps to try something new every 6–10 weeks.

■ Regular exercise increases the body's production of SOD, superoxide dismutase, an anti-ageing enzyme that fights free radicals. However, excessive exercise increases cellular metabolism and therefore free radical production, so if you exercise a lot, make sure you take extra antioxidants.

■ Lactic acid is toxic and a build up of lactic acid in the body can make muscles ache and cramp. If you suffer these types of symptoms, you will need to rest for a moment while the blood brings more oxygen to the muscles.

■ Regular exercise helps to raise levels of the anti-ageing hormone, DHEA, and the feel-good hormone serotonin (see *Other Vital Hormones*). It also produces endorphins in the body, which act as nature's painkillers.

■ Exercise is vital for keeping your lymphatic system in good shape, which not only helps to remove toxins but also transports the fat-soluble vitamins such as vitamin A, E, K, D and co-EnzymeQ-10 around the body.

■ Regular exercise makes ligaments and tendons stronger, thickens joint cartilage, which helps bones to absorb more shock. However, long-term impact exercise, such as running, can overwhelm the body's ability to repair itself – as in all things a balance is needed.

■ If you begin shivering, this is your muscles working to try to produce heat in order to raise your body temperature.

■ Stretching increases range of movement at the joint and helps you remain more supple for life. And the more you stretch before a workout the less likely you are to suffer muscle and ligament injuries. Ideally any exercise session should end with some form of relaxation.

■ Regular exercise increases your metabolic rate, which means you can burn your stored fat faster – even when at rest – as your muscles become more efficient at burning fat for energy during exercise, so you stay slimmer.

■ Regular weight-bearing exercise keeps your bones stronger for longer and it helps relieve stress and tension.

■ Your resting heart rate falls as you can supply the same amount of blood with fewer heartbeats and after exercise your heart is more able to return to its normal resting rate faster. In general (obviously depending on your age etc), the fitter you become, the lower your resting pulse rate, and your circulation works more efficiently. You produce more red blood cells to help oxygen delivery.

■ When you breathe in, your rib muscles and diaphragm grow stronger so the chest cavity gets bigger, which allows the lungs to expand further and take in even more air. More oxygen can be picked up with each breath and more carbon dioxide can be expelled, so you will have more energy.

■ As you age, swimming, walking, dancing, stretching, yoga and Pilates all help to keep you supple – flexibility is the first thing to go.

■ If you don't support your body by working your muscles regularly, then joint and back problems become more common.

■ Crucial muscles to look after as you age are the spine and the abdominal muscles, as your stomach and lower back muscles help to support and strengthen your trunk.

■ Posture is vital, otherwise your shoulders can become rounded, which impairs digestion. I see so many women with rounded shoulders who are only in their late 30s. Don't slouch as this causes the shoulders to become more rounded and when you slouch, you look shorter and older. When you walk try to imagine that you have a rope attached to the top of your head and think of it pulling you upwards. Allow your shoulders to go back and your neck to fall into alignment with your spine. This not only helps posture in later life but also makes you look more confident.

■ Practise this simple exercise all the time – as you are walking, standing or sitting. Place your hands by your side, with your palms facing your side and your thumbs facing forward. Then simply rotate your palms outwards until the thumbs are facing backwards. This simple movement will help keep your shoulders back.

■ Muscles work in pairs, so if you practise stomach crunch exercises for instance, you move forward – then make sure you, work the opposite muscles in your back, which extend the body. This keeps the body in balance.

■ If you over-exercise when you have not had sufficient rest, then the stress hormone cortisol can be released and instead of repairing muscle, this hormone can begin to break down muscle, this is why rest is so vital.

■ People who are fit tend to recover faster from all illnesses, from colds to major surgery.

■ An excellent book called *GCSE PE for Edexcel* by Tony Scott, although written for secondary schools contains a wealth of easy to read and informative information on all aspects of exercise and diet. Log on to www.heinemann.co.uk

EYES IN AGEING

(See also *Cataracts, Glaucoma* and *Macular Degeneration*)

One of the most vulnerable areas to ageing is the eyes. It begins with not being able to read small print – especially menus in dark restaurants! Most people can see at distances, but close reading becomes difficult as the years pass. At this point, you really need to begin looking after your eyes, and start by having regular eye tests.

Over half of the population over 75 years old has either cataracts, glaucoma or macular degeneration.

Ultraviolet rays in sunlight create free radical reactions in the eyes, which in time cause the gradual destruction of retinal cells if there are not sufficient antioxidants present. Lack of antioxidants in the eyes is a major factor in ageing eyes.

If you look in the eyes of a child or teenager, who eat a good diet, the whites of their eyes are a pure white and their eyes look really clear and sparkling, but, as we age, toxins accumulate in the body and the whites of our eyes begin to yellow. But if you go on a detox, you will notice that your eyes begin to clear and look youthful again (see also *Detoxing p108*).

Consistently red-rimmed eyes even after sufficient sleep can be a sign of malnutrition or lack of B vitamins. It can also be a sign of malabsorption of nutrients within the gut from your diet, which is extremely common in the over-60s (see also *Leaky Gut* in *Ageing p187*).

Dry eyes can occur at any age, but seem more common after 40. The tear film that covers the eye's surface is made up of three layers, secreted by glands in the eyelids and around the eyes. Its function is to keep the eyes wet which helps inhibit bacterial growth. Deficiency in any of these layers caused by ageing, central heating, too many hours staring at a computer, dust, regular air travel in dehydrated conditions and so on can trigger dry eyes. Symptoms range from gritty to itching or burning eyes, which can be very painful and red and even the lids can become red and inflamed. To alleviate this problem, buy some "natural tear drops" from your pharmacy and use regularly. You should also drink plenty of water and take essential fats (see *Fats for Anti-ageing*).

Foods to Avoid

- Full-fat dairy foods, plus meats, hamburgers, mass-produced pies, sausages, cheeses, chocolates and sugary, fatty foods – all the usual suspects.

- Definitely avoid too many fried foods and hydrogenated/trans-fats found in most margarines and mass-produced vegetable oils (see *Fats for Anti-ageing p139*).

- Cut down or eliminate sodium-based salt. Use a natural mineral salt available from all good health stores.

- Avoid monosodium glutamate (MSG) which is a potential retinal toxin.

- Avoid excessive alcohol, but the occasional glass of wine is fine. Too much alcohol interferes with liver function and reduces levels of protective glutathione levels in the eyes.

- At all costs, avoid foods and drinks containing aspartame, the artificial sweetener.

Friendly Foods

- The most important foods for healthy eyes are carotenes (especially lutein and zeaxanthin). Lutein is found in all dark green leafy vegetables such as spinach, kale, broccoli, spring greens, cabbage and so on.

- Zeaxanthin is found in yellow/orange fruits and vegetables such as carrots, yams, peaches, persimmons, pumpkin, sweet potatoes, mangoes, apricots and cantaloupe melons.

- Other great eye foods are onions, apples, green tea, cherries, pears, grapes, cranberries, red onions, garlic, mustard greens, alfalfa sprouts, asparagus and butternut squash.

- Eat more dark purple foods, like blueberries, bilberries and blackberries, which are rich in flavonoids that help protect and strengthen the eyes.

- Generally, eat more wholefoods such as brown bread, rice and pastas, lentils, barley and so on. Experiment with pulses and grains rather than eating wheat all the time.

- Eat oily fish, which is rich in vitamin A, to help prevent dry eyes, plus other fish rather than meat.

- Add more sage to your meals, as it has tremendous antioxidant properties.

- In addition, green drinks of organic grasses, blue-green and sea algae, herbs and other nutrients are very helpful.

- Vitamin E-rich foods are great for the eyes, these include hazel nuts, almonds, cod liver oil, raw wheatgerm and tomato purée.

Useful Remedies

- Take a high-strength multivitamin/mineral daily as a base. Also most vitamin companies now make excellent all-in-one eye formulas, ask at your health store or call one of the companies listed on pages 13 and 14.

- See Active-H under *Antioxidants in Ageing p38*.

- Bilberry has been called the vision herb for its powerful effect on all types visual disorders, take 200–300mg daily.

- Bioflavonoids like quercitin and rutin are neither vitamins nor minerals, but antioxidant plant pigments that protect the eyes from sunlight damage, and fight free radical damage. Take 1,000mg of bioflavonoid complex daily.

- Cysteine is important for a healthy retina. Taken as N-acetyl-cysteine (NAC), it increases production of glutathione, one of the most important antioxidants in the eye. Take 500–1,000mg daily on an empty stomach.

- Taurine is another potent antioxidant that is highly concentrated within the eye, normally found in high concentrations in the retina. A deficiency of this amino acid alters the structure and function of the retina. Take 500mg daily on an empty stomach.

- Lutein protects against macular degeneration, and free radical damage from UV light. Studies have shown it helps prevent retinal eye conditions. Take 6–20mg before bedtime.

- Take a natural-source carotene complex, which converts to vitamin A in the body.

- If you don't eat oily fish regularly, take a 1-gram fish oil capsule or a 1gram linseed oil capsule. Both are rich in omega-3 essential fats.

- Take 1gram Vitamin C daily to help make collagen, which strengthens the capillaries that nourish the retina and protects against UV light. The eye contains the second highest concentration of vitamin C in the body next to the adrenal glands.

Helpful Hints

- As we age, the lens becomes less flexible. If you exercise, you strengthen the muscles that control the shape of the lens, and can delay near-point fuzziness to some degree.

- To keep your eye muscles fully flexed, hold out your thumb at arm's length. Move it in circles, then in figure eights, closer and farther away. Follow it with your eyes.

- Switch frequently from near to far. If you keep your eyes fixed for long periods on a computer screen, for example, your eye muscles can temporarily become stuck. This slows focusing when you try to zoom from near to far and back again. To keep your eye muscles in shape, look up every 10 minutes and focus on a picture or poster located about 2.5m (8ft) away. Then look back at the words on the computer screen. Shift your focus back and forth repeatedly for 30 seconds, do this several times daily.

- Invest in full-spectrum light bulbs. As your eyes age, you need more light for everyday activities. By the age of 60, most people need six times as much light as they did at 20 to perform the same tasks. If you have better lighting, the pupils become smaller, and the amount of blurring you experience may be less. For instance I now use reading glasses for close work, but if I am reading in bright sunlight I don't need my glasses at all. Full spectrum light bulbs are available from Higher Nature (see page 13).

■ Be sensible in the sun, sunlight is great for your health, it improves our sense of wellbeing but too much direct sunlight on the eyes is damaging in the long-term. A great way to make sure you are getting sufficient full-spectrum light is to stand in the sun, close your eyes and face the sun for one minute and allow the light to wash over you. There is a difference between exposing yourself to natural light and being in full sun.

■ If you work in the sun or are on holiday, by all means allow natural light into your eyes, but don't continually expose your eyes to full sun. Wear a hat, and use wrap around sunglasses with a high UVA and UVB blocking protection.

■ Avoid cigarettes. Smoking produces cyanide, a retinal toxin. Cigarette smoking among women has been shown to more than double the risk of macular degeneration.

■ Try a detox twice annually and you will be amazed how much clearer your eyes look (see *Detoxing p108*).

■ Traynore Pinhole Glasses help to take the strain off the eyes and encourage them to focus properly. They are sold at all good health stores or contact Traynore Pinhole Glasses, Thornhill Farm, Moor Lane, Batcombe, Shepton Mallet BA4 6BS, or call 01749 850822.

Dark Circles Under The Eyes
(See also *Liver in Ageing*)

You don't need to be "old" to suffer dark circles, but they are more prevalent as we age. The most obvious cause of dark circles is lack of sleep, but they can also be a symptom of an under-active thyroid, excessive stress (as the adrenal glands become exhausted), food intolerances/and or allergies and smoking. Dark circles can also be a hereditary trait. The kidneys are linked to the adrenal glands (which sit on top of the kidneys) and if you tend to burn the candle at both ends, have too much stress in your life and are a Type-A person, who always has to be on the go, then the adrenals get tired of pumping so much adrenalin and eventually become exhausted. And if the adrenals are always under pressure, then food intolerances are more likely, which in turn triggers dark circles.

Foods to Avoid
■ Cut down on alcohol and salt and drink plenty of water to flush toxins from the body.
■ If you are sleeping well but still have circles after three or four good nights' sleep, then eliminate wheat for four days and see if this helps. Then try eliminating cows' milk. These are the most common triggers.

Friendly Foods

- The cleaner your diet and bowel, the less likely you are to suffer dark circles, unless you are simply lacking in sleep (see *Friendly Foods* under *Eyes in Ageing p133*).
- Drink plenty of water to eliminate toxins and generally eat a clean diet avoiding too much refined food and sugar.
- If you decide to try the wheat-free diet for a few days, then it may be a good idea to eliminate all flour from any source during this time and see what happens.

Helpful Hints

- Steve Langley gives facial acupuncture. When I have this treatment, any dark circles disappear instantly for a couple of days. Steve works at the Hale Clinic in London on 0870 167 667, or see *Useful Information and Addresses* to find your nearest practitioner.

Puffy Eyes

Puffy eyes are triggered by fluids that get trapped in the tissues under the eyes. This problem is common when you first wake up, when you cry, and if you have a hangover. But if you have puffy eyes all the time, then you most probably have a food intolerance, again the most common triggers are wheat and dairy from cows. Puffy eyes are also nature's way of telling you that your kidneys may not be working as well as they should. Puffy eyes can also be related to an under-active thyroid. If after trying the suggested dietary advice and supplements, your eyes are no better, then consult a nutritionist or your doctor.

Foods to Avoid

- You almost certainly have sensitivities to various foods so keep a food diary and notice when the puffiness is worse. The most common food triggers are wheat, dairy from cows, citrus fruits, eggs and nuts.
- Salt is a major trigger, which definitely exacerbates any water retention and increases swelling in all parts of the body if you suffer fluid retention.
- Mass-produced breakfast cereals often contain more salt than the average bag of crisps.
- Dairy products from cows, cheese and cottage cheese are high in sodium.
- Most pre-packaged, refined foods will have additional salt, and a lot of foods that are naturally sweet have salt added, partly as a preservative, but also to take the edge off the sweeteners.

Friendly Foods

- Drink plenty of water to keep your kidneys flushed.
- Eat plenty of green vegetables, fish, sunflower seeds, black treacle, almonds, tomato purée and organic dried fruits, especially apricots which are rich in potassium.

Useful Remedies

■ Puffy eyes can denote that your sodium–potassium ratio is out of balance, in which case take 100mg of potassium daily for 14 days and see if this helps.

■ Celery-seed extract aids drainage of excess water from your body, take 500mg twice daily. Available from BioCare (see page 13).

■ Place raw cucumber, potato or apple slices on closed eyes and lie down for 5 minutes. If you use potatoes they will also help take the dark circles away.

■ Soak a couple of black tea bags in cold water, then hold one on each eye for 10 minutes. The tannic acid content is the key to reducing swelling. Gently press from the inner to outer corners of your eyes to hasten drainage.

Helpful Hints

■ Try facial acupuncture or manual lymph drainage, to reduce the swelling (see under *Useful Information and Addresses p338*).

■ Eyebright herb or tincture can be made into a tea and when cooled, used as an eye lotion. It has anti-flammatory, astringent and anti-catarrhal properties.

■ The homeopathic version of eyebright, euphrasia, can be used for bathing the eyes and is very soothing. Always dilute with sterile water. Most good health stores should stock this.

■ Don't use anyone else's face cloth or towel just in case the problem is infectious. If your eyes are inflamed, chloride compound is useful to reduce redness around the eyes. It is available from Blackmores (see page 13).

■ As the years pass, fat can deposit under the eyes and if all else fails you may choose to consult a qualified plastic surgeon who can advise the best course of action (see under *Plastic Surgery*).

FACIAL HAIR IN AGEING

(See also all *Hormones* sections, *Liver in Ageing* and *Menopause*)

Except for your lips, the palms of your hands and soles of your feet, your entire body is covered with hair follicles and all women have hair follicles below the skin surfaces of their face. Facial hair growth is completely normal and natural.

Every woman has a normal amount of male hormones (called androgens) in her body but around the menopause the body produces more of these androgens. Androgens cause beard and moustache growth in men, which is totally acceptable. But in women androgens can trigger an increase in darker, thick hairs or longer fine hairs on the chin, upper lip, upper cheeks or neck area, which most women find unacceptable and unsightly.

Women who have a history of Polycystic Ovarian Syndrome (PCOS) are generally more prone to this problem.

Also, as we age, we tend to hang onto fat more easily and fat retains androgens, so the more overweight you are, the more likely you are to experience facial hair.

The liver is vital for hormonal regulation, it breaks down any excess hormones, such as androgens. Therefore if the liver is not functioning optimally, hormones are not broken down quickly enough and a higher amount of hormones will be circulating throughout the body (see *Liver in Ageing p189*).

Foods to Avoid

- Help your liver by limiting alcohol and coffee, and avoid foods containing artificial colourings, flavourings and preservatives.

- Try to avoid non-organic food containing pesticides as man-made chemicals stress the liver, and pesticides can have an oestrogen-like effect in the body, which can trigger facial hair (and hormonal cancers).

- Keep your weight down by avoiding saturated fats (meat and full-fat dairy) and refined carbohydrates: white sugar, white flour, white rice. Stick to complex carbohydrates contained in wholegrains (see *Weight Problems in Ageing p330*).

- Don't cook ready-made meals in plastic containers, as the plastics contain oestrogen-like compounds that can leach into your food.

Friendly Foods

- Foods that help to regulate hormone imbalances are traditional fermented soy foods such as miso, tamari soy sauce and tempeh – plus chickpeas, fennel, beans and lentils.

- Eat plenty of leafy green vegetables plus peas, broccoli, cauliflower, cabbage, alfalfa sprouts, fresh watercress, artichoke, radiccio and beetroot, which all help to balance your hormones and cleanse the liver.

- Eat more omega-3 fats found in oily fish and linseeds (and unrefined linseed oil), which also help your hormones (see *Fats for Anti-ageing p139*). Generally, eat more sunflower, pumpkin, sesame and hemp seeds and use their unrefined oils for salad dressings which are all rich in omega-6 fats.

- Avocado, wheatgerm and nuts, especially almonds and hazel nuts, are rich in vitamin E.

- Drink herbal teas, such as sage (but not if you are pregnant), red clover and alfalfa, which will help to regulate your hormones.

- Drink plenty of water to help cleanse the liver.

Useful Remedies

- The most effective herbs for reducing the level of androgens in the body are: vitex agnus castus and dong quai. Take 500mg of either or both daily. Most health companies make a blend of both. Try agnus castus in the first instance.

- Another hormonal balancing nutrient used to balance oestrogen levels is soya-isoflavines. take approximately 40 mg daily

- Sodium sulphate is specific for helping the liver detoxify and break down excess hormones. It is contained in Blackmores Sodiphos at 200mg per tablet, take three times a day.

- Help the liver to detox and regenerate by taking milk thistle. You will need 1000mg daily. Kudos make a high-strength one-a-day milk thistle (see page 14).

Helpful Hints

- The Pill and HRT can place a greater burden on your liver and are linked with facial hair.

- Stress can have a very negative effect on your hormones (see also *Stress in Ageing*).

- Have your hormones checked. If you take hormones like DHEA, and take too much, then facial hair (and spots) can result (see also *Other Vital Hormones p237*).

- Natural progesterone cream derived from yams has helped many women with this problem. It is available on prescription in the UK or you can order it for your own use by calling FREEPHONE 00 800 8923 8923, or log on to www.pharmwest.com and www.immunalive.com.

- For a list of doctors in the UK who work with natural progesterone, or a Women's Information Pack, send a first-class stamp to NPIS, PO Box 24, Buxton, SK17 9FB.

- Electrolysis is an effective way to remove unwanted hair permanently, it can take several visits and costs vary, depending on the salon and the length of your treatment.

- You can also use waxing and depilatory creams, which can trigger rashes in some people Beauty therapists suggest that you should not pluck these hairs out saying they will grow even thicker – well I have been plucking my few stray dark hairs for years and they have never regrown thicker!

- You may also choose to have the unwanted hairs lasered away. This is not cheap, but many women say it's highly effective. Laseraesthetics based in Wigmore Street in London have a useful website with a free consumer guide on www.laseraesthetics.co.uk, or call 020 7935 3366. Medical lasers emit a beam of light which is absorbed by the pigment in the hair follicle. This light passes through the skin for a fraction of a second: just long enough to disable the hair follicle without causing damage to the surrounding skin. Once the hair follicle is damaged, hair regrowth is significantly reduced or stopped.

FATS FOR ANTI-AGEING

If you want supple, hydrated skin with fewer wrinkles, more energy, and a healthy brain and arteries into your 80s and beyond, then one of the most vital foods you need to eat more of is essential fats. After all, your brain is almost 60% fat, but it needs more of the right type of fats to function effectively.

Essential fats (EFAs) are essential to life, hence their name, and as we cannot manufacture them in the body we must take them in from external sources through our diet. Most people consume approximately 42% of their calories from fat, but unfortunately it's usually the wrong type.

Dr Udo Erasmus, a Canadian-based bio-chemist, and world renowned authority on fats and oils, says "A huge proportion of degenerative ageing conditions, are triggered not only by eating excessive animal fats, but also over-consumption of mass-produced fats and oils. The majority of vegetable oils found in supermarkets, have been refined, bleached and deodorized and then used for frying, which introduces huge amounts of ageing free radicals into the body."

To compound the negative health affects, a commercial practice called hydrogenation, in which liquid oils are turned into spreadable fats called trans-fatty acids, found in most margarines, mass-produced cakes, biscuits, cereal bars, flapjacks, chocolates, crisps and so on, are also unhealthy fats.

Erasmus adds to this list sweet and starchy foods: desserts, high-sugar fizzy drinks, pastries, chocolates etc, which tend to be high not only in sugar but also saturated fats. And if not used up during exercise, sugar converts to fat in the body and you'll wear them on your hips, thighs and stomach.

But before sugar turns into fat, it triggers cross-linking in the skin, which means you develop wrinkles faster. Bacteria also thrive on sugar which will impair your immune system, and sugar increases inflammation in the body, and inflammation can trigger practically every disease of ageing from arthritis to Alzheimer's disease, cancer to Parkinson's disease. And as the average person in the West consumes around 14kg (30lb) of sugar annually, it's no wonder that so many people age more quickly! (See also *Sugar in Ageing p302*).

Having said this, some children, especially young girls, are becoming obsessed with eliminating all fat from their diets – this is really dangerous. If the body becomes too low in fat, then chronic depression and a host of skin disorders, such as eczema, can result. Children (and adults) need fats for vital functions such as the manufacture of hormones and energy. That said, I would not encourage really overweight children, who do little or no exercise, to eat lots of junk-fatty foods; but I would never recommend that normal weight children give up all fats. We all need treats, but we do need to stop living on them. The body also needs essential fats to encourage weight loss, as EFAs, help to burn stored fat. There are two main types of EFAs, omega-3 (alpha-linolenic acid) and omega-6, which comes in two forms, linoleic acid and gamma-linolenic acid (GLA). More about GLA *Useful Remedies* in this section.

One of the best sources of omega-3 is oily fish, which contains EPA and DHA (easily utilized types of omega-3 fats), this is why Inuit people rarely suffered heart disease until they began eating a Western diet.

Linseeds, walnuts, hemp seeds and pumpkin seeds also contain omega-3 fats, which the body then converts into the useful EPA and DHA forms – in fish oil this has already been done by nature.

There are a few people who cannot easily convert the essential fats in seeds and nuts into EPA and DHA, which is known as atopic tendency, and common characteristics of this condition are asthma, eczema and hay fever. Therefore if you suffer these conditions take fish oils as your first line of defence.

Omega-3 fats help to transfer oxygen around the body, relax blood vessels, are vital for hormone production, healthy eyes, gut function, weight loss, reducing inflammation, speeding wound healing, and so on. Unfortunately, because we eat 80% less oily fish now than we did in the 1940s, 60% of people are now deficient in omega-3 EFAs.

The second type of EFAs, omega-6, are found in evening primrose, starflower, blackcurrant, walnut and sesame oils. Walnuts, Brazil, pecans, almonds, sunflower, pumpkin and sesame seeds are also rich in omega-6 EFAs. These fats help to lower blood pressure, thin the blood, help insulin to work, which keeps blood sugar levels in balance, and helps reduce the cravings for sweet foods.

We need twice as much omega-6 as omega-3. But today most people ingest some omega-6s from nuts and non-hydrogenated vegetable oils and margarines, but insufficient omega-3s. Therefore, to address our modern dietary deficiencies Dr Erasmus suggests a ratio the other way around – two parts omega-3 to one part omega-6.

Another beneficial fat, omega-9 is found in unrefined, extra-virgin olive oil, a monounsaturated fat which is far more stable for cooking, but never heat this oil until it spits and produces smoke.

Polyunsaturated fats (also found in seeds, nuts and their oils) are healthy in their cold, unrefined form and they are rich in omega-6 EFAs. So if you use sunflower, walnut, sesame seed or grape seed oils in their unrefined forms in salad dressings they are healthier.

But once polyunsaturated oils which you find in most biscuits, flapjacks margarines and mass-produced vegetable oils are heated, this makes them unhealthy.

Many people cook (mostly fry) with oils and margarines labelled "polyunsaturated" believing them to be healthier, but it is not so. If the oils that you buy are mass-produced, all the processes I mentioned earlier will have long ago destroyed the majority of any health benefits.

Butter is actually better for cooking at low temperatures, as it does not turn rancid like the essential fats. Butter contains vitamin A and butyric acid, which has anti-cancer properties, and a little butter, preferably organic is OK, if you have sufficient EFAs in the body.

All essential fats should be kept cool and not heated, as heat destroys delicate EFAs. The same applies to all oil-based supplements which need to be kept in the fridge.

Typical symptoms of insufficient EFAs are dry skin and eyes, cracked lips, water retention, increased thirst, physical and mental exhaustion, mood swings, inflammatory conditions such as eczema and arthritis, frequent infections, hay fever, allergies, mental health problems, poor memory and learning difficulties and cardiovascular disease. Most of these conditions we tend to accept as we age, but if you take sufficient EFAs then you should avoid such symptoms for many more years.

Foods to Avoid

■ I don't want you to stop enjoying your food and if you like red meat, just eat lean meats once a week. Generally, you need to cut down on all meats, meat pies, sausages and so on and if you eat meat choose a lean cut. With chicken, turkey, duck, quail, or other game, always cut off the skin. If you eat bacon, make it only a once a week treat, then grill it and cut off the fat.

■ Reduce your intake of full-fat milk, cheeses, chocolates, crisps and refined mass-produced cakes and biscuits. These are usually high in hydrogenated or trans-fats and which are not good for your health.

■ Avoid as much as possible all refined vegetable oils typically found in margarines, biscuits, cakes and shortening and of course mass-produced vegetable oils.

■ Eliminate or greatly reduce the amount of fried foods you eat.

■ Remember sugar, if not used up during exercise, turns to a hard fat inside the body and many foods advertised as being low in fat are usually packed with sugar!

Friendly Foods

■ Look for non-hydrogenated spreads such as Vitaquell and Biona.

■ If you need to shallow-fry use a little olive oil or butter. Although butter is a saturated fat it does not turn rancid like vegetable oils when heated. I also use a little butter for baking cakes. For biscuits and flapjacks, I use extra-virgin olive oil.

■ Nutritionist, Gareth Zeal, recommends blending extra-virgin olive oil with butter to use as a healthier alternative to hydrogenated-trans-fat-based margarines, also for spreads and making cakes and biscuits.

■ If you like stir-fries, use a little olive, canola, ground nut (peanut) oil or grapeseed oil. Heat through but not until spitting or smoking then add vegetables etc and stir for a minute. Then add a little water and "steam fry" for a couple more minutes. This helps to reduce the amounts of free radicals that are produced when you fry food.

■ Oily fish, like mackerel, wild salmon, sardines, tuna and herring are all rich in omega-3 fats.

■ Soya and kidney beans also contain some omega-3 fats, but try and use only GM-free and organic tempe, miso and natto.

■ Walnuts, pecans, almonds, but not peanuts, are all rich in omega-6 fats.

- If you use linseeds to increase your omega-3 intake, either buy them ready cracked such as Linusit Gold, available from most supermarkets. Or, grind them first. Use a coffee grinder which breaks them up in seconds, or simply crush them with a pestle and mortar. Otherwise, chew linseeds really well or they will mainly pass through your system whole and you miss out on the omega-3 health benefits.

- Seeds like sunflower and pumpkin, can be eaten as a snack or sprinkled on soups, salads and added to meals.

- Hemp seed is now readily available and is a good blend of omega-3 and 6 fatty acids.

- Eat more (but not to excess) mono-unsaturated fats, such as those found in avocados and olive oil – as they are still fats.

- Eat more raw wheatgerm and rice bran, rich in vitamin E, which helps you to absorb the EFAs more effectively.

- Buy good-quality, unrefined and preferably organic sunflower, walnut and sesame oils and mix them half and half with olive oil to make delicious salad dressings or drizzle them over cooked foods (once they are on your plate). Keep them in the fridge to protect the EFAs.

- Once a week, I pop a tablespoon each of sunflower, pumpkin, sesame seeds and linseeds, walnuts, almonds, Brazil and hazel nuts, into a food mixer and pulse for a few seconds. I then place them in a glass jar in the fridge and use them over breakfast cereals, yoghurts, desserts, fruit salads and so on. This is a great way to get more EFAs.

Useful Remedies

- If you are not vegetarian, then take 1–3grams of fish oil capsules daily. Many people no longer take fish oils as they worry about the concentrations of toxins, such as PCBs and dioxins, but Higher Nature, BioCare (see page 13), FSC and Seven Seas One a Day fish oils are all guaranteed to be free from toxins. Cardinova Eskimo 3 stable fish oil capsules are especially pure and are distributed by PPC Galway Ltd, Mulvoy Business Park, Sean Mulvoy Road, Galway, Ireland. Tel: 00353 91 753222, fax: 00353 91 753471, or e-mail ppc@iol.ie

- GLA is an omega 6 EFA and can be found in evening primrose oil, blackcurrant oil and borage oil. It has anti-inflammatory properties and helps increase your metabolic rate, and reduces symptoms of PMS-PMT. Most supplement companies sell GLA and you can take around 250mg daily.

- If you want pure flax (linseed oil) try Omega Nutrition from Higher Nature (see page 13).

- Udo's Choice Oil is made from organic flax, sunflower and sesame seeds, plus rice and oat germ oils, in the correct ratio for good health. Dr Udo Erasmus says we need approximately 1 tablespoon for every 23kg (50lbs) of body weight and we need more EFAs in winter than in summer. It is available either as an oil that can be blended with other oils for salad dressings, or a little can be drizzled over cooked dishes. It is also available in capsules. These oils are highly unstable, should never be heated and need to be kept in the fridge. Udo's Choice is available from health stores worldwide, or to find your nearest stockist in the UK contact Savant Distribution Limited, Quarry House, Clayton Wood Close, Leeds LS16 6QE, or call 0845 0606070, website: www.savant-health.com or e-mail: info@savant-health.com

- Another good blend of omega-3 and 6 oils in capsule form is Efalex from Efamol.

- When supplementing with fatty acids, either in capsule or liquid form, it is important to take extra vitamin E at least 100iu a day.

- For anyone who has had their gall bladder removed, suffers Crohn's disease, colitis, has a sensitive gut or irritable bowel and cannot tolerate too much oil (as the liver has to metabolize all fats and oils) use Dri-Celle Omega Plex essential fatty acid powder by BioCare (see page 13). The EFAs have been micro-encapsulated into water-soluble fibre and then freeze-dried using no oxygen or heat. This powdered formula is therefore stable, which increases absorption. It bypasses the liver and is 100% absorbed in the intestines.

- For those who want to know more about this subject Dr Udo Erasmus has written *The Fats That Heal and Fats That Kill*, Alive Books. He has also written an EFA cookbook. To order, call 0845 060 6070, or log on to www.savant-health.com

GALL BLADDER

The gall bladder is a storage unit for bile, which is needed to break down or emulsify all fats, and it helps to mobilize toxins out of the bowel. The gall bladder is a small pear-shaped organ/sack, which sits underneath and is connected to the liver. Gallstones may produce pain on the right side of the stomach, or in the right shoulder area. In some cases the pain can be so severe that the patient feels nauseous and faint.

Removal of the gall bladder is becoming extremely common, even in younger people, but in the majority of cases surgery could be avoided by a change in diet.

As we age, the gall bladder is somewhat impeded by a build up of stones – 20% of adults over the age of 65 suffer gall stones but only 20% of people with gall stones experience symptoms. A build-up of stones will increase the ageing process due to a reduction in the bile flow and therefore the detoxification process from the bowel.

This condition tends to affect women who are fair, overweight and in their 40s.

Foods to Avoid
- High fat and fried foods, which put an extra load on the gall bladder and its ability to digest fats (see *Fats for Anti-ageing p139*).

- Alcohol and coffee place an extra strain on the liver, which can make the problem worse.

- Avoid red meat and full-fat dairy produce, especially melted cheese.

- Eat no more than one avocado a week; although healthy, avocado is high in mono-unsaturated fats which place extra strain on the liver and gall bladder.

Friendly Foods

- People who eat more beans such as butterbeans, kidney beans and so on, plus lentils, are much less likely to end up with gall bladder or liver problems.
- Artichokes, celeriac, radiccio, rocket, bitter lettuces and beetroot are excellent for liver and gall bladder function.
- Black cherries, kale and pears are all good for the gall bladder.
- Try making fresh vegetable juices daily with celery, artichoke, parsley, raw beetroot, apples, carrots and any green vegetables that you have in your fridge. Add this to half a cup of organic aloe vera juice and drink daily to help detoxify your liver and gall bladder.
- Regular consumption of small amounts of unrefined extra virgin olive, walnut, or flax oil diminishes the risk of developing problems. Use for salad dressings and drizzle over cooked vegetables and rice dishes.
- Drink at least six glasses of water daily.
- Drink lemon juice in warm water every morning before breakfast to stimulate the liver and gall bladder.

Useful Remedies

- Milk thistle and dandelion root are very effective for maintaining a healthy gall bladder. They both have the ability to enhance bile production, flow and activity. Take 1ml of tincture 15 minutes before each meal, or try a high-strength milk thistle capsule made by Kudos (see page 14 for details).
- Sprinkle one tablespoon of lecithin granules over breakfast cereals, fruit whips and yoghurts, which helps to emulsify fats within the body.
- Artichoke is a bitter tonic which enhances bile flow.
- Sodiphos contains sodium sulphate and sodium phosphate which helps the flow of bile. Take 3 tablets daily. It is available from Blackmores (see page 13).
- See also *Useful remedies* for *Gall Stones p147*.

Helpful Hints

- Eat small meals regularly rather than large meals which stress the gall bladder.
- Generally, to avoid gall bladder problems you need to control your cholesterol and stress levels. See also *Cholesterol, High and low* and *Stress in Ageing*.

Gall Stones

Although up to 25% of the population have gallstones, only 15–20% eventually develop symptoms. Gallstones are twice as common in women especially after 40. People who tend to eat high-saturated fat and sugary diets that do not include sufficient fibre, obesity, constant dieting with rapid weight gain, or suffer Crohn's disease are at a higher risk. Multiple pregnancies, the Pill and HRT are other factors, as is a high stress level. The gall bladder gets rid of unwanted substances such as cholesterol and bilirubin into the bile duct, which in turn drains into the intestine. Most gall stones consist of a sediment made up primarily of cholesterol, bilirubin and bile salts and occur in individuals with excess cholesterol in the bloodstream or as a result of stagnation in the gall bladder. Small gall stones often produce no symptoms, but if they become large enough to obstruct the bile duct they can cause jaundice, inflammation, intense pain and vomiting. Symptoms tend to be much worse after high-fat meals or foods to which the individual has a sensitivity, such as eggs. Constipation can be linked to the risk of gall stones so it is very important that adequate fibre is eaten to reduce the risk of developing gall stones.

Foods to Avoid

- Greatly reduce your intake of animal fats from any source.
- Low fibre foods such as white bread, cakes, biscuits, ice cream, most puddings and pre-packaged meals should be avoided as much as possible.
- Foods like eggs, pork, onions, pickles, spicy foods, peanuts, citrus fruits and sometimes coffee are likely triggers.
- Ironically, regular coffee drinkers (that's real coffee, not decaffeinated) have a much lower risk of developing gallstones, but if you have a sensitivity to coffee then you need to avoid it completely.

Friendly Foods

- Drink plenty of water, at least six glasses daily, to prevent the bile from becoming too concentrated.
- Small amounts of lamb plus brown rice, peas, pears and broccoli are usually no problem.
- Other foods which help the function of the gall bladder include beetroot, artichoke, dandelion, dried beans and legumes, linseeds, oat bran and psyllium husks, all of which are high fibre foods. Sprinkle a tablespoon of lecithin granules over a low sugar, oat-based muesli or cereal, as soya lecithin helps to break down the fat in foods.
- Drink dandelion root tea three or four times a day. It's rather bitter so add a little honey or ginger to make it more palatable; it helps to cleanse and stimulate the gall bladder.
- Use wholemeal bread and pastas made from corn, lentil, rice and potato flour. Include fresh fish, a little chicken without the skin, plenty of salads and fresh fruit in your diet.
- Replace full-fat milks with skimmed, or use rice milk, or try herbal teas.
- Enjoy one glass of wine daily, but if you drink to excess, especially on long flights, again you could be in trouble!
- Use organic, extra-virgin olive, sunflower and walnut oils for salad dressings, these are all rich in essential fats, which help to dissolve stones.

Useful Remedies

■ Milk thistle and dandelion root in combination as tablets or capsules or dandelion formula. Take 1 or 2 tablets/capsules with every meal or measure 10–20 drops of tincture.

■ People with gall stones tend to be deficient in vitamin C and E. Take 1 gram of vitamin C daily with food, which is needed for the conversion of cholesterol to bile acids and 200–400iu of natural source vitamin E.

■ Silica and calcium fluoride tissue salts can help to break down and expel the stones. Take 4 of each daily.

Helpful Hints

■ Homeopathic Chelidonium 30c – take three times daily if you are in pain.

■ As multiple food sensitivities are linked to gall bladder problems, consult a qualified nutritionist or naturopath who can sort out your diet. The initial few weeks may be hard but there are plenty of foods you can eat (see *Useful Information and Addresses* for details).

■ A reader sent the following gall bladder "flush" remedy to me after being advised by a top American nutritionist. Only attempt this remedy after discussing it with your GP and it should not be tried by people who suffer Crohn's disease, colitis or irritable bowel. If you have chronic liver problems, this remedy should not be taken.

1. For 5 days prior to "flush", drink 2 litres (3 1/2 pints) of fresh, organic apple juice daily. Eat normally but avoid all saturated fats.

2. On the sixth day: have no evening meal. At 9pm take 1 or 2 tablespoons of Epsom salts (a laxative) dissolved in 1–2 tablespoons of warm water.

3. At 10pm mix 115g (4oz) unrefined olive oil with 50g (2oz) lemon juice. Immediately upon finishing the olive oil and juice go to bed and lie on your right side with your right knee drawn up towards your chin. Remain in this position for 30 minutes before going to sleep. This encourages the olive oil to drain from your stomach, helping the contents of gall bladder and/or liver to move into the small intestine.

4. Next morning the stones should pass. They should be green in colour and soft like putty.

GENERAL ANTI-AGEING HEALTH HINTS

■The single most important thing you can do to help slow the ageing process, is to think more positively. Scientists at Yale University in America have found that people who are more positive and adaptable in their outlook, have generally happier, more fulfilled lives, and on average live eight years longer than everyone else. Remember that what you expect tends to be realized – always, always, trust that things will turn out for the best and if you really believe this – they usually do (see *Mind Power and Ageing p224*).

- Change your attitude. When you are feeling low or angry, just look at things from a different perspective. For instance instead of just saying, "Oh my back hurts", think "In what ways am I not supporting myself?"

- Add more laughter to your life. Laughter enhances your immune system, raises mood and helps slow the ageing process. In an hour you could laugh off as many as 300 calories. When you laugh your body releases endorphins, hormone-like substances that act as natural painkillers – they also help muscles to relax. Laughter, gives your lungs a work out and you take in more oxygen – which not only boosts energy levels but also encourages your internal organs to work more efficiently. Laughter reduces production of the stress hormones cortisol and adrenalin, it releases pent-up anger and tension, which can be so destructive and ageing.

- Being in love and giving love makes you look and feel younger. Happily married couples live longer. Even if you are alone, join a class or club with activities or hobbies that give you a chance to interact in a positive way with others. Researchers have found that when people watch classic love stories, more immune protective antibodies are produced. Another study showed that people in love have less toxic lactic acid and higher levels of feel-good endorphins in their blood. But probably the best proof came from a famous study of 10,000 male heart patients in Israel in 1976. Researchers found that patients were far less likely to have dangerous heart symptoms if they could answer "Yes!" to the simple question: does your wife show you she loves you?

- Spend more time thinking about what you *do* want in your life and less time focusing on what you *don't* want. Learn to say *yes* to what you do want and *no* to what you don't – this point alone could take years off the way you feel.

- Learn to meditate (see *Meditation*).

- Think young. Wear younger looking clothes. Knock 10 years off your chronological age and every day say, "I only look and feel..." (see also *Mind Power p224*).

- Keep your weight within sensible limits (see also *Weight Problems in Ageing p330*).

- *Stop worrying* – As Dale Carnegie once said, 85% of the things we worry about never actually happen and worrying ages you. Long-term negative stress is a major factor in ageing (see *Stress in Ageing p293*).

- Enjoy occasional days when you don't have to look at a watch – people who are continually "running out of time" will eventually do just that. Keep saying "I have plenty of time".

- One day a week or more – don't read the papers. They are often so full of bad news, it drags you down. Create your own positive reality and watch it expand into your life and environment.

- Anger affects your liver and your heart, not being able to speak up for yourself will affect your lungs and throat. Never under-estimate how emotions can affect your health.

- Help someone every day without expecting anything in return and believe me, magical things will begin to happen. More right actions bring about more right reactions.

- Spend one hour in daylight (full-spectrum light) every day – or use full spectrum light bulbs in your office and home.

- Reduce your exposure to mobile phones, microwaved food and electrical equipment, especially in the bedroom (see *Radiation in Ageing p265*).

- Don't overeat. Eat what you need and no more, as this has been proven to slow the ageing process. But as balance is needed in all things, if you overeat now and again, enjoy the food, be grateful you had it and visualize it doing you good.

- Live consciously – accept more responsibility for what you eat, think and do. For instance, if you chose to sunbathe to excess, then live consciously by eating more foods that will nourish your skin, take the right supplements and use organic sunscreens.

- Get sufficient sleep – this is the cheapest and most effective way to turn back the clock. While you are sleeping, cells and your immune system can repair and rejuvenate. Your digestive system and brain get much needed rest (see *Sleep – Insomnia p286*).

- Sleep on your back– a plastic surgeon recommended this years ago. At the time I had just had my overhanging eyelids removed and while the stitches healed, the only way I could sleep was on my back. It really made a huge difference. Unfortunately, I soon returned to sleeping on my side and have never managed to master the art of sleeping on my back – but women who can, look much younger and have fewer wrinkles, not only on their faces, but also on their chests and neck.

- Eat as great a variety of fresh foods as possible, preferably locally grown and organic, which contain less pesticides and higher levels of nutrients, than foods flown thousands of miles. In this way we can improve our health and also the health of the planet.

- Eat at least three anti-ageing foods every day and increase your intake of green foods from alfalfa to cabbage (see under *Diet – The Stay Younger Longer Diet (see page 114)*.

- Avoid chemicals, food additives and heavy metals that greatly accelerate ageing. From insect sprays and car exhausts, to cadmium in cigarettes and chemicals in cosmetics. For a full list and more information about chemicals in our everyday creams and cosmetics read *Drop Dead Gorgeous* by K. Erickson, Contemporary Books (also see *Toxic Metal Overload*).

- Take a full-strength anti-ageing multivitamin/mineral, essential fats formula (see *General Supplements for Anti-ageing p150*).

- Make time for breakfast which is the most important meal of the day. You are literally breaking a fast and to keep your blood sugar levels on an even keel you need to eat, or you will end up craving sugary snacks by mid morning.

- Drink at least six glasses of filtered, bottled or distilled water daily (see *Water in Ageing*).

- Cut down on tea, coffee, alcohol and caffeinated soft drinks, which dehydrate the body. For every caffeinated or alcoholic drink you need 250ml (8fl oz) of water.

- Additives, artificial sweeteners (especially aspartame) and sugar in soft drinks and foods can cause hyperactivity, mood swings, and sugar will age your brain and skin faster. Forget low calorie drinks, they place a strain on your liver, which slows weight loss (see also *Essential Sugars* and *Sugar in Ageing*).

- Remember it's the foods and drinks you tend to crave the most that are often causing most of your health problems.

- Do not become fanatical about fad diets. Everything in moderation and keep a balance of foods at all times for good nutrition.

- Avoid smoking and smoky atmospheres.

- Get plenty of fresh air and learn to breathe deeply, which aids relaxation. Deep breathing also helps to alkalize the body. Stress makes it too acid (see also *Acid–Alkaline Balance* and *Breathing*).

- Sunlight is great for your health. Moderate sunbathing is fine with organic-based sun screens, but avoid the midday sun (see also *Sunshine in Ageing*).

- Take regular, sensible exercise, which is one of the best favours you can do for your health and to slow ageing. Don't exercise to excess (see also *Exercise*).

- Get into blending and juicing. This is a fantastic way to ingest huge amounts of nutrients quickly. Buy yourself a blender and a juicer and twice a week try the following blended anti-ageing cocktail; 1 tablespoon of organic sunflower, pumpkin or flax seeds, 1 teaspoon of a green powder mix such as Dr Gillian Mc Keith's available from all health shops, 1 dessertspoon of organic lecithin granules, 1 teaspoon of raw wheatgerm, 2 ready-to-eat prunes or apricots, half a box of blueberries, a fresh or dried fig, a chopped apple (without the pips), a banana, or any fruit you love. To this, add half a cup of aloe vera juice and a cup of organic rice or low fat goats milk. Blend all of it for 30 seconds or so and drink as a meal replacement (this should be sufficient for 2 servings). It is rich in fibre, vitamins, minerals, protein and essential fats which will all help to turn back the clock.

- With a juicer, on alternate days make yourself fresh raw vegetable juices. I adore organic carrots, celery, apple, raw beetroot and cabbage with a little fresh root ginger. Again I add extras such as aloe juice, green powder, a few drops of any herbal tinctures like dandelion and burdock, which cleanse the liver. Drink immediately after juicing while the beneficial enzymes are still alive. Also add all the "left overs" which are rich in fibre to soups, stews etc. Or add them to the juice and eat with a spoon!

- No-one ever had engraved on their tombstone, "I wish I had spent more time at the office" – get a balance in your life.

- Enjoy the journey.

- See also *Diet – The Stay Younger Longer Diet (see page 114)*.

General Supplements for Anti-ageing

(See also *Ageing* page 25)

- KUDOS 24 Multi-Active Age Management Complex – a multinutrient, up-to-the-minute formula, containing food state, GM-free, highly absorbable vitamins, minerals, antioxidants, amino acids, brain nutrients, essential fats, isoflavones, green foods and specific anti-ageing nutrients, that both men and women of all ages can take. For full details and a list of the ingredients see page 348.

■ See also *Supplements* under the *Ageing* section p28.

■ Take one acidophilus/bifidus capsule daily. This replenishes the good bacteria in the gut and helps prevent many problems like candida, yeast infections, constipation and an over-acid system, caused not only by our diet but the chemicals we inhale from the air. Acidophilus/bifidus capsules mostly need to be kept in the fridge and taken with meals for 4–6 weeks, periodically.

GENES IN AGEING

(See also *Cells in Ageing*)

Genetics is the latest medical buzzword being touted as the explanation and cure for everything, from arthritis to cancers to increasing our life span. Scientists, Richard Weindruch and Tomas Prolla from the University of Wisconsin in America, have developed tiny anti-ageing gene chips, which they are implanting into mice and rats to regulate other genes and restore youth. Within 10 years these gene chips should be available to us all. Meanwhile, by looking after our diet and lifestyle we can change which genes are expressed. Let me explain.

Within the nucleus of every one of the 100 trillion cells that make up your body, are chromosomes that carry your personal genetic code in the form of molecules called DNA. This code, which is unique to you, and according to current research contains approximately 40,000 genes, is inherited from both of your parents.

Genes transmit characteristics from one generation to the next, your eyes, skin, and hair colour for example. Some diseases are known to result directly from genetic defects, such as cystic fibrosis, Down's Syndrome and other rare conditions.

But for the most part, just because your mother, grandmother or other relatives contracted or died of a certain disease, it doesn't automatically mean that you will too. Nutritionist, Patrick Holford, says, "It isn't simply the presence of certain genes that determines our risk but whether or not these genes are activated or not. For instance a woman (or man) might inherit a BRCA1 and BRCA2 gene, in which case breast cells are likely to grow larger or more quickly if they are exposed to chemicals that have an oestrogen-like effect in the body. These range from plastics, pesticides, foods, drinks and polluted air, which may then trigger over-growth of breast tissue.

So, you don't inherit a breast cancer gene per se, you inherit a gene for breast cell growth, which means you inherit a greater probability of contracting breast cancer. But if you eat the right diet and change your environment then you can greatly reduce this risk." (See also *Breast Cancer p64*).

In 2000 a major trial on 45,000 pairs of twins set out to find what was the percentage risk of inheriting breast cancer and the answer published in the *New England Journal of Medicine*, says that no more than 15% is inherited.

Your lifestyle, diet and the right supplements can determine whether a gene is switched on or off. Hence why I find it crazy that some women are being tested and told that they have inherited these genes and are then offered mastectomies.

My mother died of breast cancer and I personally don't want to know if I have this gene, as I would most probably worry so much, that it would give me cancer. And unless I was diagnosed with cancer, I would never consider having my breasts cut off as a "just in case" measure.

The World Cancer Research Fund recently studied 6,000 people and found that you can halve the risk for cancer just by changing your diet. The three main factors were eating more fruits and vegetables, reducing red meat and not drinking too much alcohol.

Patrick Holford continues, "Also people believe they inherit, say, arthritis – but we all have inflammation genes and arthritis and inflammatory conditions occur when the inflammation gene is switched on, because the person eats too many of the wrong foods etc. But the gene can be de-activated by giving that person the right essential fats and a better diet and lifestyle (see *Arthritis p42*). The same would be true of breast cancer and most diseases."

So, understand that you don't, in the majority of cases, inherit the disease, just a tendency – and Patrick says that with more "nutritioneering" you can change which genes are expressed. You can stack more of the genetic cards in your favour. This is great news. You are born with one set of genes, but there are millions of different possible combinations of which ones are switched on or off. According to American medical biochemist, Dr Jeffrey Bland, "Those codes and the expression of the individual's genes, are modifiable. The person you are right now is the result of the experiment called 'your life' in which you have been bathing your genes with experience to give rise to the outcome of that experiment. If you don't like the result of the experiment that makes up your life thus far, you can change it at any moment, whether you are 15 or 75 or 90."

Where does all this leave us in anti-ageing science? Professor Stephen R. Spindler, Professor of Biochemistry at the University of California, has shown that specific diets (see *Calorie Restriction in Ageing*) have an anti-ageing effect on the expression of some 11,000 age-related genes in animals. His results were published in the *Proceedings of the National Academy of Sciences* (September 11, 2001). Basically by restricting their diets to a really light, but very nutritious diet, even old animals became young again.

Foods to Avoid

(See also *Diet – The Stay Younger Longer Diet (see page 114)*)

- Reduce your consumption of foods we know increase free radical damage to cells and DNA, especially fried foods and alcohol.

- Don't eat excessively – restricting your calorific intake to just what you need and no more has been shown to dramatically lengthen maximum lifespan in tests with animals (see *Calorie Restriction in Ageing p70*). The easiest way to do this is to avoid foods high in calories but low in nutrients: cakes, biscuits, burgers and processed foods, white rice, bread and pasta, sugar, fizzy drinks, chocolate, ice cream, etc.

Friendly Foods

(See also *Diet – The Stay Younger Longer Diet (see page 114)*.

- Antioxidant-rich foods are able to help prevent oxidative stress and damage to your DNA, so eat plenty of fresh fruits and vegetables every day, especially Brussels sprouts, watercress, tomatoes, berries, grapes, broccoli, cabbage, peppers, carrots, garlic and olives.

- Drink 2–3 cups daily of green tea, without milk – which is also high in powerful antioxidants.

Useful Remedies

- Antioxidants work best in combination with one another, as one antioxidant can "recycle" another after it's done its job. So while vitamins A, C, E, selenium and zinc are all good antioxidants in their own right, it's best to supplement them in combination with one another in an antioxidant complex.

- Other powerful antioxidants such as quercetin, N-acetyl cysteine, alpha-lipoic acid, CoQ10, lycopene and pine bark extract have also been shown to prevent DNA damage and improve immune function. You needn't necessarily take them all, though the more stress and toxins you're exposed to, the more you need (for a full list of anti-ageing antioxidants see *Antioxidants in Ageing p38*).

- For a full-spectrum multivitamin/mineral/essential fats/antioxidant formula – see details of Kudos 24 – Multi-Active Age Management Complex on page 348.

Helpful Hints

- Reduce your exposure to pollutants by stopping smoking, avoiding traffic and busy roads as much as you are able, and using organic food where possible.

- Use a water filter to remove unwanted chemicals from your drinking supply. Reverse osmosis filters remove 99.999% of all known chemicals; it also removes minerals, so if you only drink RO water you will need to take a multimineral daily. RODI water will even filter out anthrax bacteria. For details of reverse osmosis water contact The Pure H2O Company on 01784 21188, or www.pureH20.co.uk or the Fresh Water Filter Company on 0870 442 3633, or www.freshwaterfilter.com (For details, see *Water in Ageing p325*).

- Take holidays in areas of little pollution. Athens, London and Los Angeles would not make the clean air list!

- Forget the "it's all in the genes" mentality and remember that you can to a large extent control how they are expressed.

153

- Reduce stress – it's a sure way to an early grave, as it accelerates ageing by hindering your immune function and leaving your body less protected from the constant attacks of pollutants and toxins, including those produced naturally in the body (see *Stress in Ageing*).

- Genetic profile tests are available in the UK. These tests show which foods and supplements we specifically need for our body based upon our own genetic code, to help prevent many diseases of ageing (available from Great Smokies Laboratory via the Society for Complementary Medicine, on 0207 487 4334). For more advice and information on genes log onto www.genovations.com. You can also contact Diagnostic Services Ltd on 01663 718860, or write to them at Meridian House, Botany Business Park, Macclesfield Road, Whaley Bridge, High Peak SK23 7DQ, e-Mail: info@diagnosticservices.co.uk

- To learn more about genes and ageing and the work of Dr Stephen R. Spindler, visit: www.lifespangenetics.com His work has been funded by the Life Extension Foundation: www.lef.org

- On a final note, I need to mention genetically modified foods. The large food and seed companies will tell you that GM food is a great way to feed the world. But we need to keep in mind that once these genes are spliced and released into our atmosphere, they can never be taken back. Many scientists now believe that GM food could be another BSE/CJD scenario in the wings. For now, I would never knowingly eat GM foods, and try as much as possible to only eat organic. To keep abreast of the latest developments in GM foods and many other environmental/health issues, subscribe to the *Ecologist Magazine*, which is sold worldwide. Tel: 01795 414963 e-mail: theecologist@galleon.co.uk

GLAUCOMA IN AGEING

(See also *Eyes in Ageing* and *Macular Degeneration*)

Glaucoma is a group of eye diseases that cause vision loss through damage to the optic nerve. Glaucoma is the leading cause of blindness worldwide, which affects more than 60 million people, mostly after the age of 50.

It was once thought that high intraocular pressure (IOP – when the pressure within the eye is elevated due to a blockage of the normal flow of fluid between the cornea and the lens) was the main cause of this optic nerve damage. Although IOP is clearly a risk factor, other factors are involved because even people with "normal" IOP can experience vision loss from glaucoma. Researchers now believe that other factors such as low blood pressure, insufficient blood flow to the optic nerve head and retina, and the effects of excitotoxins (substances that "excite" cells to death) such as aspartame, may all contribute to glaucoma. Early-onset glaucoma is usually linked to an inherited gene.

Symptoms of glaucoma differ depending upon the type of glaucoma diagnosed. In the majority of cases, typical symptoms would be progressive loss of side vision, followed by reductions in central vision plus watering eyes, headaches, an inability to adjust the eye to darkened rooms, difficulty focusing on close work, and a frequent need to change eyeglass prescriptions. If you have a family member who suffers glaucoma, or you have any of these symptoms, consult an optician immediately who can test the pressure in your eyes and if necessary refer you to a specialist.

Foods to Avoid

■ Reduce or eliminate drinking caffeine and cola-type drinks.

■ Avoid the artificial sweetener aspartame and greatly cut down on your sugar intake (see *Sugar in Ageing p302*).

■ Avoid all mass-produced vegetable oils including canola oil, and especially hard margarines. Eliminate deep-fat fried foods from your diet.

■ Avoid monosodium glutamate (MSG), which is a potential optic nerve toxin.

■ Limit your alcohol consumption. Alcohol interferes with liver functions, and reduces levels of protective glutathione in the eyes.

■ See also *Foods to Avoid* under *Eyes in Ageing p133*.

Friendly Foods

■ See *Friendly Foods* under *Eyes in Ageing p133*.

Useful Remedies

■ Vitamin C (ascorbic acid) helps to stabilize intraocular pressure and plays an important role in the prevention and treatment of glaucoma. Take 2 grams daily with food.

■ High-strength ginkgo biloba has demonstrated some improvement in reducing IOP, while improving visual field. Call Kudos (see page 14 for details).

■ The mineral magnesium has been shown to improve blood supply and visual field, as it relaxes constricted blood vessels. Take 200mg per day.

■ The mineral chromium not only helps to balance blood sugar, but also helps the eyes to focus and low levels of vitamin C and chromium are associated with IOP. Take 200mcg daily.

■ Essential fats, especially fish oils, are also vital for healthy eyes (see *Fats for Anti-ageing*).

■ For all other great eye supplements see *Eyes in Ageing p132*.

Helpful Hints

■ Glaucoma is linked to stress, which thickens the blood and constricts circulation. Avoid emotional upsets and upheavals, for external pressure increases internal ocular pressure (see *Stress in Ageing p293*).

■ Climates with great temperature variances are thought to be detrimental. Temperate, even climates and temperatures appear better tolerated by the glaucoma patient.

- Don't smoke, as smoking constricts blood vessels, reducing the blood supply to the eye.

- Avoid prolonged eye stresses, such as long movies, excessive TV viewing, or excessive reading and staring at computer screens for hours on end. Take regular breaks, preferably outside.

- There is now a new type of implant surgery that has been developed in America that helps presbyopia (another eye condition in ageing) and primary open-angle glaucoma. It has proved so successful, that this surgery is now available in the UK and Europe. For details see www.cibavision.co.uk or www.cibavision.com

- For more help and to find details of where to have laser surgery, log on to the Glaucoma Research Foundation website at www.glaucoma.org

GROWTH HORMONE

(See also *Men's Hormones, Other Vital Hormones* and *Women's Hormones*)

Human growth hormone (Hgh), secreted by the pituitary gland, is considered to be one of the body's most important anti-ageing hormones. It is produced at night during deep (Rapid Eye Movement) sleep, perhaps this is why people who sleep an average of eight hours a night live longer than those who only get six.

When we are young and growing, Hgh levels are high, but after the age of around 20, levels begin to slowly decline. With lower levels of Hgh, your metabolism slows down and you gain weight, you have less muscle and more fat (middle-aged spread), the risk of dehydration increases, wrinkles appear, memory function declines, your eyes don't work as well, in other words – you age.

In young children, this hormone is injected to counteract dwarfism, but in adults it can be used to reverse many signs of ageing. Although growth hormone does not prolong life, it does add quality to it, but there are dangers to taking it long-term.

In a well-known study published in the prestigious *New England Journal of Medicine* in May 1990, Dr Daniel Rudman and his team at the Medical College of Wisconsin, Milwaukee tested the benefits of human growth hormone injections (Hgh) on volunteers in their 60s, 70s and 80s. The results were nothing short of spectacular: six months of injections reversed the ageing process from 10–15 years in patients who received the Hgh, measured in terms of bone density, lean muscle mass, loss of stomach fat, improved cardiovascular risk profile, raised energy levels and a greater sense of health and wellbeing.

These results have been repeated many times. But, Rudman's study concerned men in their 60s, 70s and 80s, so it does not infer that people in a younger age group will also gain back 10–15 years. In fact there is no real support for taking Hgh on a permanent basis, unless you are very old and decrepit.

Also the sceptics warn that growth hormone can trigger a spurt of growth in tumours, though there is no evidence Hgh actually causes tumours in adults. It can cause some degree of bone growth, emerging as thickening of the brows, chin, wrists and other appendages. Also Hgh can cause the major organs to grow, which may pose some health risks.

Hgh can only be given by injection, but there are a number of things you can do to naturally increase Hgh.

Foods to Avoid
■ Reduce the amount of sugar in your diet. This includes cakes, biscuits, pastries, sweets, jams, croissants etc, as sugar makes the pancreas release insulin, and when insulin levels go up, Hgh levels fall.

Friendly Foods
■ See *Diet – The Stay Younger Longer Diet (see page 114)*.

■ Food sources that provide the amino acids that increase Hgh levels are wholewheat, nuts, seeds, organic peanuts, brown rice, soy, and raisins.

■ Short-term fasting helps raise Hgh levels (see *Detoxing p108*).

■ By eating less generally, but making what you eat very high in nutrients, will help raise Hgh levels.

Useful Remedies
■ Daniel Rudman's study has spawned a minor industry on the Internet and pay television, offering compounds that are claimed to stimulate the secretion of Hgh. All quote Rudman for credibility but the Milwaukee study examined only the effects of injected Hgh, nothing else. In fact Hgh can only be administered by injection, if taken by mouth it would be rendered useless by your stomach acid. Therefore, most of the so-called Hgh supplements for sale are "precursors" that naturally help increase levels of Hgh – but they are not Hgh.

■ The term "secretogogue" is used to imply that some substances will enhance the secretion of Hgh, but often proof is lacking. "Hormone precursor" is another common phrase and the claims are large, but again often unproven. Just remember you are being sold herbs, amino acids and minerals, not Hgh itself.

■ One Japanese study showed that gamma hydroxybutyrate increased Hgh by 16-fold. GHB is not approved in the UK. Gamma amino butyric acid (GABA), a derivative compound of GHB, is readily available and offers some value as an Hgh stimulant. It is also a relaxant and can make you drowsy, so take GABA at night. Take 500–1000mgm daily.

■ Other amino acids that work to release Hgh are ornithine, lysine, glysine, arginine and glutamine, the most useful being ornithine. Take 500mgm of each. Some companies now offer these amino acids in one supplement. For details call HB Health on 0207 838 0765. Take on an empty stomach daily for one month, then stop for a month and start again.

■ Symbiotrophin Pro Hgh helps to stimulate the pituitary gland to release more Hgh. It contains the seven peptides that make up natural growth hormone. These peptides are protected in such a way that they are not destroyed by stomach acid. Take 2 tablets (dissolved in water) night and morning for five days. Skip two days and repeat cycle. Not to be taken by children or in pregnancy. For details, call the NutriCentre in London on 0207 436 5122.

■ Minerals such as potassium, magnesium, calcium and zinc are also important for the release of Hgh, therefore take a multimineral daily.

■ Vitamin B3 (niacin) also helps release Hgh, take a high-strength B complex. If you decide to take B3 on its own, beware that it can cause a red flushing of the skin, so ask for No-Flush Niacin.

Helpful Hints

■ An underactive thyroid is linked to low Hgh levels (see *Thyroid in Ageing p313*).

■ Hgh levels decline with obesity (see *Weight Problems in Ageing p330*).

■ Exercise helps to stimulate the pituitary gland to produce more Hgh. Start taking walks, do skipping, swimming, dancing, whatever you enjoy, but get on the move frequently.

■ Proper sleep is very important as most Hgh is released at night. You want deep relaxing REM sleep (random eye movements denote the deepest layers of sleep). Recent research has shown that people who sleep an average of 8 hours per day live distinctly longer than those who get 6 or less. Hgh may be the critical factor in this finding.

■ Hgh injections should never be considered without the help of a fully qualified doctor who works in this field. After a full consultation, and if it is needed, Dr Keith Scott-Mumby, a nutritional physician based in London and Manchester, offers growth hormone injections. He can be reached via his website www.alternative-doctor.com.

■ Hgh injections are also available from HB Health at 59 Beauchamp Place London SW3 1NZ London on Tel: 0207 838 0765, website www.hbHealthOnline.com

■ Read, *Staying Young:Growth Hormone and Other Natural Strategies to Reverse the Ageing Process* by Dr Gilbert Elian and Jim Jamieson, Age Reversal Press. Available to order from The NutriCentre Bookshop (call 0207 323 2382).

■ For more information on Human Growth Hormone log onto www.growyoungandslim.com.

HAIR IN AGEING

(See also *Men's Hormones, Other Vital Hormones* and *Women's Hormones*)

Your hair is made from a protein-like substance called keratin, and research into how to keep our hair as we age is another "Holy Grail" for scientists. Many drugs are claimed to increase hair growth, but some have negative side effects. The most recent drug being Finasteride, marketed as Propecia has helped quite a few men, but the side effect has been an inability to maintain an erection! Before trying these drugs always discuss any implications with your doctor or tricologist.

The average person loses between 70–100 hairs a day and as we age our hair becomes finer, most people find their first grey hair by the age of 30 and by 50 up to 50% of your hairs may have turned grey. Contrary to popular belief, grey hair is not courser, but finer and most hair becomes finer/and or thinner with age.

We tend to associate balding and thinning hair with men and yet just as many women suffer thinning hair as men.

An important factor is the male hormone testosterone, which is also found in women. Although this hormone is responsible for making men hairy during puberty, it also has a large role to play in hair loss in later life, in both men and women. Some woman have too much testosterone, which shows up in excess facial hair and can trigger male-type thinning. In this case the herb vitex agnus castus helps to reduce testosterone levels.

Hereditary factors are also important. The more hair loss there is or was in your father, uncles and grandfather, the more likely you are to lose your own hair, however, dietary supplements and regular daily firm scalp massage can help slow down hair loss. And thinning hair is a growing problem for younger women, even when there is no previous history in the family.

Hair loss in younger female and male executives is also becoming extremely common, showing that stress is definitely a trigger for hair loss. Stress and a toxic bowel prevent production of some of the B vitamins that are necessary for maintaining hair colour and healthy hair.

Hair loss in women is common after childbirth and the menopause, and a lack of protein can trigger thinning hair or even cause it to fall out.

Hair loss is also linked to heavy metal toxicity (see also *Toxic Metal Overload p317*).

The health of your hair depends on the circulation to the scalp and the amount of nutrients present in your blood. It is thought that men lose hair on the top of their heads rather than the back and sides because the blood flow to the top of their scalp is reduced in comparison to the sides. When a person is very stressed, the scalp becomes tight which restricts circulation; the hair follicle becomes malnourished resulting in further hair loss. Adrenal exhaustion, an under-active thyroid and certain prescription drugs are also factors in hair loss.

Naturopath, Steve Langley, adds "If the tissues are too acid then minerals needed for healthy hair, such as iron, magnesium and zinc, are taken from the hair follicles to buffer this acidity" (see also *Acid–Alkaline Balance p18*).

Hair grows faster in summer and a single hair can live for several years. On average human hair grows between 12–15cm (5–6in) a year.

Foods to Avoid

- Reduce caffeine from any source as it increases stress and weakens the adrenal glands.
- Avoid sugar and refined carbohydrates, such as pastries, cakes, desserts, pies etc, all of which deplete nutrients needed for hair growth.
- Reduce the amount of sodium-based salt in your diet.

Friendly Foods

■ Quality protein is the most important food for your hair, especially at breakfast and lunch. So eat some organic lean meats, chicken, game, fish and eggs (egg white).

■ Whey, milk, yogurt and cheese are also rich in protein.

■ Vegetarian-based proteins are found in seeds, nuts, vegetables, wholegrains such as brown rice, barley, spelt, wholewheat and quinoa, plus legumes such as peas, lentils, soya beans, tofu, tempeh, lentils, and peanuts.

■ Eat more iron-rich foods such as egg yolks, green leafy vegetables like spinach, wholegrain breads, cereals, meat and fish.

■ Try adding seaweeds like kombu and arame to meals; you use them as you would a green vegetable as they are a rich source of minerals needed for healthy hair.

■ Essential fats are vital for healthy hair and scalp, therefore eat more oily fish, and use walnut, pumpkin, sunflower or linseeds and their unrefined oils, mixed half and half with olive oil for salad dressings and to drizzle on cooked foods. Essential fats help you to avoid a dry, scaly scalp and nourish the hair follicles.

■ Coriander detoxifies the body of heavy metals and is full of nutrients, especially B vitamins.

■ Muesli, cereals and oats are all high in B vitamins.

Useful Remedies

■ Take a good-quality multivitamin/mineral, most of the companies on pages 13 and 14 supply specific hair nutrient formulas.

■ Romanda Healthcare make an excellent powder (easier-to-absorb) formula that contains all the nutrients needed for healthy hair, plus a growth serum and shampoo, that are really excellent (see *Helpful Hints* in this section for contact details).

■ Steve Langley has formulated a "blood cleanser" that has been shown to help restore hair loss due to stress and mineral depletion. The quality of your scalp depends on the quality of the blood supplying the roots. As we age, the quality of our blood is reduced because of the accumulation of toxins. Once the blood is able to carry more oxygen and nutrients, hair can improve. Take 1 teaspoon in a glass of water three times daily before meals. £11 inc p&p; to order write to Holos Health, PO Box 3063, South Croydon, Surrey CR2 7LZ.

■ Zinc — 30mg daily, is essential for hair and nail growth.

■ The B-group vitamins are vital if you want to keep your hair, and many people who take high-strength B vitamins report that their grey hairs disappear. B5, biotin and folic acid are the anti-greying nutrients and you would need 1000mcg of biotin daily.

■ 50mg of vitamin B6 per day is helpful for women taking the contraceptive pill, which can affect hair loss.

- Find out if you are low in iron. If you are take a liquid easily absorbable formula such as Spatone which is available from health shops worldwide. Don't take iron unless you need it. If you cook in iron pots, you will absorb some of the iron in your food.

- Red meat contains the amino acid lysine, and people who take lysine as a supplement often experience an increase in hair growth. Take 500mg of lysine twice daily on an empty stomach before meals.

- CT241, plus Colleginase, which contain vitamin C, rutin, hesperidin, cellulose, silica, vitamins A and D to strengthen hair and nails. Available from BioCare (see page 13).

- The herb ginkgo biloba helps to increase circulation to the scalp. Kudos make a high-quality one-a-day high-strength capsule (see page 14).

- Herbs that help balance hormones naturally if your hair is thinning because of the menopause, include dong quai, black cohosh, sage and soy isoflavones. All companies on pages 13 and 14 sell these supplements.

- Thinning hair in men caused by excess dihydro-testosterone, can be balanced by taking saw palmetto 500mg daily (under supervision it may need to be higher) and zinc 30mg daily.

Helpful Hints

- There is a myth, saying the more you brush your hair, the thicker and healthier it will grow – it's not true. Too much brushing pulls hair out, breaks it, and scratches the scalp.

- Don't over dry your hair – as this makes it more brittle.

- Take regular aerobic exercise, which will stimulate your heart and circulation, thus increasing oxygen flow, reducing stress and promoting scalp and hair health.

- "Women who lose a lot of hair after giving birth should stop panicking" says London and New York based tricologist, Philip Kingsley, "During pregnancy oestrogen levels are higher and this hormone prolongs the natural life span of a hair. The average person loses 70–100 hairs a day, but during pregnancy hair falls out less, because of the oestrogen. Then 4–6 weeks later the woman gives birth and hormones return to normal levels and all the normal shedding that should have happened during the previous months, occurs all at once. As long as these women eat a healthy diet and take the right supplements the hair should soon get back to normal."

- Philip has formulated various hormone drops for men and women that nourish the follicle and help prevent hair loss. They don't make hair re-grow if the hair loss is permanent, but they help you to keep the hair that you have. For details in the UK call 0207 629 4004. In New York call (212) 753 9600. His website is www.philipkingsley.co.uk. Consult a good tricologist, like Philip, who has numerous trained staff who can help and advise you. He also makes first-class hair products and his sun protection mousse is the best I have ever used.

- For lots more help on hair I strongly suggest you read Philip Kingsley's latest book *The Hair*

Bible, Aurum Press.

■ Some doctors have noticed that smokers tend to lose their hair faster than non-smokers.

■ Shampoo your hair regularly as this helps to re-moisturize the hair. Choose natural-based products such as Aveda, Jurlique, Body Shop and Green People Organic hair products. Use natural hair colours, such as Nature's Dream. Call 0845 6018129.

■ Jojoba oil, mixed with a little essential oil of rosemary and massaged into the scalp, removes dead skin cells and increases circulation. Be firm, you need the skin on your scalp to move so that blood can circulate more freely. Do this before going to bed and leave the oils on overnight.

■ Some yogis say that by doing head and shoulder stands they have kept really thick hair because the circulation to their heads is greatly increased.

■ Chlorine from swimming pools damages your hair and is also linked to asthma and heart disease.

■ Human-growth hormone has been shown to help age related hair loss (see *Growth Hormone* on p156 for specialists who use this hormone).

■ Many readers report that using Romanda lotion and shampoos, along with Romanda hair formula vitamins and minerals, improves hair growth. Call Jan Adams on the Romanda Advice Line on 020 8346 0784, or write to Romanda Healthcare, Romanda House, Ashley Walk, London NW7 1DU e-mail: jan_romanda@hotmail.com, www.romanda-healthcare.co.uk Jan really is incredibly helpful and formed the company after suffering hair loss, she really is a gem.

■ Numerous salons offer hair transplants, which are becoming more sophisticated. Professor Nick Lowe, a dermatologist offers the latest technique called Micro Grafting, which offers a more natural-looking hairline. The surgery is expensive but the results that I have seen are amazing. For details in the UK call 0207 499 3223. In America call (310) 828 8969.

■ Philip Kingsley recommends Dr Patrice Cahuzac in Paris. He says her transplant work is the best he has ever seen. I have met Dr Patrice and was very impressed with her work. She often sees patients for their initial consultation in London – but works in Paris – 16 Rue Clemont-Manot 75008 Paris. Tel: 00 33 15 652 0101.

■ The Hair Clinic at John Bell and Croydon at 50–54 Wigmore Street, London. Tel: 0800 289597 or 0207 224 4640 also offer the Micro Grafting.

■ The Institute of Trichologists can be contacted on 08706 070602, or visit the website at www.trichologists.org.uk, e-mail: admin@trichologists.org.uk.

■ As we go to print, I have seen information about a newly developed battery powered helmet, which pulses an electromagnetic charge into dead or dying hair follicles – which help zap them back into life. Called the BX 3.4, it has been developed by a team of dermatologists in France. The men and women who have tested this helmet have had excellent results. For details call MegaMac (0033) 134 803737, or visit www.BX3-4.com

HAYFLICK LIMIT

(*See Cells in Ageing*)

HEARING LOSS IN AGEING

Hearing loss is one of the most common problems we experience as we age. It often develops gradually over several years, and when you have to keep turning up the volume on the TV and radio until a loved one says, "Are you deaf?", do you even think to have your hearing checked? Alternatively, you may tend to turn one ear towards sounds, suffer inattentiveness, frequently ask for statements to be repeated, respond inappropriately to questions or conversation, or speak louder than necessary. Around one in three of those over 65 have some degree of hearing impairment, with various causes including excessive build-up of earwax, middle-ear infection or inflammation, poor blood supply to the brain or ears, damage to the acoustic nerve from the ear to the brain, or damage to cells in the inner ear called "hair cells" that turn sound vibrations into nerve impulses.

Hearing loss needn't be a natural consequence of ageing and is often a result of accumulated exposure to excessive levels of noise that permanently damage the "hair cells" in your ear. As more of us live in cities and are exposed to more and more noise: traffic, mobile phones, sirens, stereo players, rock concerts and aircraft flight paths; peace and quiet has become a rarity. You can minimize the level of hearing loss you'll experience as you grow older if you reduce your exposure to loud noise throughout your life and it's never too late to protect what hearing you still have.

Earwax is secreted by glands in the external ear to protect the delicate lining of the outer ear and can build up, hindering the travel of sound into the ear. Infections in the middle ear usually follow an upper respiratory tract infection, are often the result of a weakened immune system and are more common in those who eat foods to which they are allergic or intolerant (especially dairy foods and drinks), have a fungal infection (like candida), cancer or diabetes.

Another common hearing problem is tinnitus, characterized by a continuous buzzing or ringing in the ears. This too is commonly triggered by infection, obstruction of the ear canal or noise-induced damage to cells in the ear. Tinnitus can also be triggered by a jaw and neck misalignment and can often be helped by acupuncture and cranial osteopathy, see *Useful Information and Addresses p338*).

Whatever the causes of your hearing loss, you can protect yourself from further deterioration and take more steps to improve your hearing.

Foods to Avoid

■ Avoid saturated fats, as they contribute to excess production of earwax. Take measures to lower your cholesterol level. Studies suggest that people with higher cholesterol levels have greater hearing loss as they age (see also *Cholesterol – High and Low p92*).

- Eliminate foods to which you may be intolerant as they can cause excessive mucus production or a greater risk of recurrent middle-ear infection, hindering hearing. Common culprits are wheat and dairy (see below for alternatives).

Friendly Foods

- Try alternatives to wheat such as rye bread, rice pasta, oat muesli or porridge, rice or oatcakes and wheat-free cookies. A visit to your local health food store can reveal a surprising range of wheat-free products. At least reduce the wheat you eat, as many of us eat wheat three times per day.
- Try alternatives to dairy such as rice, almond or oat milks, soya cheeses (in moderation), tofu ice-cream (definitely in moderation) and non-hydrogenated vegetable margarines.
- Eat fresh pineapple frequently to reduce inflammation.
- Make garlic and fresh root ginger a regular part of your diet. They are anti-inflammatory and anti-bacterial so can reduce the chances of inflammation or infection in your ears.
- Essential fats (EFAs) have been shown to reduce the tendency to produce excessive amounts of earwax. Eat more oily fish plus pumpkin, flax, sunflower and hemp seeds daily and aim for 2–3 portions of oily fish weekly: salmon, fresh tuna, sardines, mackerel or herring (see *Fats for Anti-ageing p139*).
- To lower your cholesterol level, in addition to reducing your consumption of dietary cholesterol, you can help your body eliminate it by increasing the amount of fibre in your diet. Eat plenty of fruits and vegetables, wholegrains, lentils, beans, nuts and seeds.

Useful Remedies

- Appropriate treatment for hearing loss depends on the underlying cause. In addition to a multivitamin/mineral complex providing a balance of all nutrients, try:
- Co-EnzymeQ10, take 30mg per day. CoQ10 is a powerful anti-inflammatory antioxidant involved in the immune system and circulation to the ears.
- A deficiency of the mineral manganese has been linked to ear problems – try 10mg per day.
- Nutrients vital for a healthy nervous system (remember the sound impulse has to get from your ear to your brain along the auditory nerve) are important, especially B vitamins (50-100mg B complex in addition to your multi) and potassium (try 100mg per day).
- Herbs, such as eucalyptus, hyssop, mullein and thyme, have decongestant properties and are useful if congestion, infection or excessive mucus is contributing to your poor hearing.
- If infection is the problem, immune-boosting and anti-inflammatory nutrients and herbs to take include 3 grams per day of vitamin C, vitamin A (especially important for strengthening inner membranes), 15,000iu daily for 2 months (not if you are pregnant) and then reduce to 5000iu daily.

- Zinc (take 50mg per day) plus echinacea, taken in tea or capsule form according to directions.
- Gingko biloba increases circulation to the head. Reduced blood flow to the brain or ears can hinder hearing too and gingko drops or capsules can improve your hearing as well as your memory. Kudos make a one-a-day high-strength capsule, 900mg (see page 14).

Helpful Hints

- Always wear ear protection, such as disposable plugs, when using loud appliances such as power tools or lawn mowers. Do the same if you attend a rock concert.
- If you're prone to ear infections, wear earplugs when swimming. Swimming in water that's overly chlorinated or contains high levels of bacteria can lead to ear infections that can damage your ear and worsen your hearing.
- For earwax build-up try irrigating your ears with a solution of 1-part vinegar to 1-part warm water. Put a few drops in your ear with a dropper, wait a few moments, then drain and do the other ear. Repeat as needed. Many people have reported success in removing excess earwax by using Hopi Ear Candles. Lying on your side, you insert a special wax straw in your ear, you light it, and within several minutes your ear wax is drawn up into the straw. Ask for these "candles" at your local health food store or consult a naturopath.
- If you have experienced permanent hearing loss, ask your family members, friends and co-workers to speak slowly and distinctly and avoid shouting.
- Investigate the suitability of a hearing aid – ask your GP for a referral to a specialist.

HEART IN AGEING

(See also *Chelation in Ageing, Circulation, Cholesterol in Ageing* and *High Blood Pressure*)

Your heart is amazing. A simple pump, it can beat around 70 times a minute non-stop for 100 or more years, pumping more than 10 million litres of blood around your 100,000km of blood vessels every year. While it works we tend to take it for granted, and yet if more people could think of their heart health from their 30s onwards, then heart and arterial disease would not still be the number one killer in the Western world. In 2000, in the UK alone, 125,000 people died from heart disease. The saddest part is that 90% of these deaths are preventable through diet and exercise.

For some there is a genetic predisposition to developing heart disease, but if you eat healthily and change any negative and unhealthy lifestyle patterns practised by your parents and grandparents, then in most cases you can stack the cards in your favour and add decades to your life.

The heart, like any other muscle, needs its own blood supply and receives this via three main vessels called the coronary arteries. Over time, one or more of the arteries can become blocked and if an artery becomes completely blocked, some of the heart muscle may die during a heart attack. Typically, symptoms of a heart attack include a severe pressing band of pain across the chest that can spread up the neck and into the jaw or across the shoulders and down into the left arm. Often termed a "myocardial infarction", this means death of the heart muscle due to an interrupted blood supply. The muscle may simply stop beating or, more commonly, it goes into an irregular pattern, which no longer works like a pump. Sweating, breathlessness and a feeling of nausea can accompany a heart attack which needs urgent medical attention. A heart attack can be fatal, unless someone can apply immediate cardio-pulmonary resuscitation (CPR is something everyone should learn and one day you may save a life with this simple skill). Luckily many people survive their first heart attack. Specialists may recommend drugs and/or by-pass surgery or other operative procedures, but it's important to consider that none of these medical or surgical treatments attempts to solve the cause of the problem, only the result of the problem.

While some heart attacks appear to strike "out of the blue", there are usually warning signs. The most common is angina – a constrictive pain in the chest, provoked by exertion. It's the body's signal that the blood supply to the heart is inadequate, due to narrowed or spasming coronary arteries. If you experience angina, it's time to act. You can still turn the situation around and live another 40 years or more. Some people have gone on to run a marathon after their first heart attack.

If you suffer angina or have had a heart attack, then you need to radically change your diet, increase exercise (gently) and reduce stress.

Other known risk factors for heart disease include smoking, excessive alcohol consumption, high blood pressure, high homocysteine levels (see *High Blood Pressure p170*), high LDL cholesterol levels, being overweight, diabetes, insufficient exercise, eating a high fat, salt, and sugar diet, not eating enough fresh fruit and vegetables and excessive stress

There are also links with heart disease via inflammatory conditions caused by the parasite chlamydia pneumonia and the organism helicobacter pylori, known to cause stomach ulcers. Poor root canal treatment is also linked to heart disease (see *Teeth*).

Foods to Avoid

- Cut down on saturated fats found in meats, cheese, cream and hard margarines. Keep in mind that many low-fat foods are high in sugar which covert to fat in the body if not burned off during exercise.

- You need to have a balance, but if you have a sweet tooth then greatly reduce the amount of concentrated shop-bought fruit juices, fizzy drinks, desserts, cakes and pastries you eat.

- Reduce dairy foods, especially milk. Jeffrey Segall, from London's North Middlesex Hospital, believes the problem may be the lactose, not the fat. Research published in the *Lancet* in 1999 showed how changes in a country's milk consumption pattern, either up or down, accurately predicted changes in coronary deaths four to seven years later.

- Especially avoid any foods containing hydrogenated or trans-fats which are found in most mass-produced biscuits, pies, cakes etc.

■ Don't eat too much fried food, as frying damages fats and turns them into the dangerous fats that heart surgeons find in your arteries!

■ Cut down on sodium-based table salts. Use a low-salt alternative or a little magnesium-and-potassium-rich sea salt, available from all good health stores and most supermarkets.

■ Reduce your intake of mass-produced burgers, pies, sausages, pastries, cakes and desserts.

■ Avoid excessive alcohol consumption. Even though a moderate intake, i.e. one glass a day is slightly protective, large amounts of alcohol over time is a known risk factor for heart disease. Aim for no more than 6 units a week on average.

Friendly Foods

■ Oily fish is rich in omega-3 essential fats: wild salmon, sardines, mackerel, herring, and fresh tuna are good sources, as are linseeds. Try and eat oily fish twice a week.

■ Generally eat more fish of any kind in preference to meats.

■ Unrefined, unsalted seeds such as pumpkin, linseed, sesame and sunflower and their unrefined oils are also a good source of essential fats. Use unrefined organic linseed (flax) oil for salad dressings as people who consume more linseed oil, which contains omega-3 essential fats have a lower risk of developing heart disease.

■ Eat plenty of fruits and vegetables that are high in carotenes and antioxidants such as carrots, asparagus, French beans, broccoli, Brussels sprouts, watercress, cabbage, spinach, cress, sweet potatoes, spring greens, apricots, mangoes and tomatoes.

■ Include brown rice and pastas, beans, wholemeal bread and other grains such as quinoa, amaranth, barley, oats and spelt in your diet.

■ Fibre, derived from fruits and vegetables, is very protective and additional fibre from linseeds, oat or rice bran or psyllium husks all help lower the risk.

■ Eating pistachios, walnuts, Brazil nuts and macadamia nuts on a regular basis has been shown to help lower LDL cholesterol.

■ Wheatgerm and organic soya beans are rich in natural vitamin E, which has been shown to reduce the risk of heart disease.

■ Use non-hydrogenated spreads such as Biona and Vitaquell. There is nothing wrong with a little butter as long as you are eating sufficient omega-3 essential fats.

■ A vegetarian diet using a lot of beans, vegetables and grains dramatically lowers your risk of developing heart disease.

■ Sprinkle 1 dessertspoonful of lecithin granules, to help break down fats, over breakfast cereals and desserts.

■ Olive oil in small amounts helps to raise HDL (the good cholesterol) level, lowers bad LDL cholesterol, as well as containing antioxidants that protect the LDL from damage.

■ Drink more water: at least six glasses daily.

Useful Remedies

■ After the age of 50, unless you have a medical condition that requires iron, do not take extra iron supplements as excessive iron in the body is linked to heart disease.

■ Complete Heart II is a cardiovascular support formula in a powder form, containing garlic, co-Enzyme-Q10, tocotrienols (vitamin E), hawthorn, lipoic acid, bromelain, grape skin extract and amino acids. As a dietary supplement, 1 scoop (20g) daily mixed in a jar or shaker with 60–90ml (2–3fl oz) of juice or other beverages, such as organic rice milk. Drink immediately and follow with several ounces of liquid, if desired. For details call the NutriCentre on 0207 436 5122.

■ Take a high-strength B complex as B6, B12 and folic acid reduce homocysteine levels in the blood.

■ Vitamin C and the amino acid lysine can help to reverse arterial blockages. You would need approximately 3 grams of each per day. (see Higher Nature, page 13)

■ HomoCysteine Metabolite Formula. If you have a high homocysteine level, try this formula which contains vitamin B6 (30mg), folic acid (400mcg), vitamin B12 (400mcg), trimethylglycine (500mg). Take 1 capsule per day with a meal. Available from the NutriCentre as above.

■ Include a good-quality multivitamin/mineral that contains 400iu of natural source vitamin E, 150mcg of selenium, 30mg of zinc, 100mcg of chromium, 400mg of magnesium. Taking 400iu of natural source, full-spectrum vitamin E daily has been shown to reduce the incidence of heart attacks by 40% when taken for two years or more (see Blackmores page 13).

■ Try the herbs hawthorn (100–500mg of standardized extract) and ginkgo biloba (60–120mg of standardized extract daily), either as tea , tincture or capsules. Both are known to improve circulation.

Helpful Hints

■ Stop smoking and avoid places where you will be exposed to passive smoking as both increase the risk for heart disease.

■ If you are overweight – lose weight (see *Weight Problems in Ageing* p330).

■ Gentlemen, unless you are very tall, don't allow your waist to exceed 99cm (39in) and ladies 90cm (35 in) if you want to avoid heart problems.

■ Learn to test your heart health. What's your resting pulse? For 1 minute place your first two fingers on the vein crossing the bony protuberance on the thumb side of your wrist and check your pulse. While your blood pressure tells you about the health of your arteries, your pulse is a measure of your heart health. If your heart is strong and able to pump blood easily around the body, it will pump slowly and rhythmically, around 60–70 beats per minute. If it's weak, and therefore can't pump as much blood as it should with each beat, it will have to beat more often to keep your cells properly oxygenated, so your pulse will be higher. This is why your pulse goes up when you exercise, your cells need more oxygen so the heart pumps more rapidly. In time, this strengthens the heart and it will be able to pump more blood with each beat, so your resting pulse will slow down. A raised pulse is now considered a "normal" result of ageing, though there is no reason you can't have a pulse of 70 when you're over 70.

■ Try chelation, an intravenous therapy which has saved thousands of people from undergoing major heart surgery. It helps to clear clogged arteries, which reduces the likelihood of strokes and heart disease (see *Chelation in Ageing p89*).

■ Reduce stress in your life (see *Stress in Ageing p293*).

■ There is now an easy test to discover your plasma homocysteine levels. Made by York Laboratories and backed by The British Cardiac Patients Association – it's a simple pin prick method that can be done by post. For details call York Labs on 0800 074 6185 or log on to www.yorktest.com

■ Get some exercise. If you have a heart condition, then with your doctor's permission start walking for 30 minutes every day and gradually build up to an hour a day. A little exercise every day is far more effective than a lot of exercise once a week. Even though exercise raises your heart rate while you're doing it, the overall effect is to strengthen the heart and slow your resting heart rate. Research has shown that even moderate exercise after having a heart attack is one very effective way of preventing a second one. If you have had any heart problems only undertake an exercise programme under professional supervision.

■ Stop smoking. The chemicals in cigarette smoke damage your arteries, oxidize the cholesterol that forms plaque in your arteries and increase the likelihood of clotting.

■ Reduce exposure to toxic metals such as lead, cadmium and mercury (see *Toxic Metal Overload*).

■ Homeopathic Arnica 6x, taken twice daily for up to 3 months helps to strengthen the heart.

■ People who are angry and argumentative suffer more heart problems. Millions of people are dying because they don't "get things off their chest". Learn to deal with anger and internal emotions – see a counsellor, your life may depend on it.

■ Contact the British Heart Foundation, 14 Fitzhardinge Street, London W1H 4DH or call the Heart Health Line on 0870 600 6566 website: www.bhf.org.uk

■ Read Patrick Holford's *Say No to Heart Disease*, Piatkus, which is an excellent book explaining the causes of arterial damage and what you can do to prevent or correct high blood pressure and heart disease.

■ See *High Blood Pressure p170* for more on protecting your cardiovascular system.

■ Dr Keith Scott-Mumby, a nutritional physician, recommends that you ask your doctor or specialist about External Counter Pulsation saying, "The name might seem a little intimidating but the principle is simplicity itself. The patient wears five blood pressure cuffs (hence 'External'), one on each calf, one on each thigh and one on the buttocks. A computer arranges that the moment the heart relaxes between beats, these cuffs are thumped in such a way as to send blood backwards (hence 'Counter Pulsation') and so into the heart muscle. It is really like having two hearts: one, which beats properly, and then a second heartbeat, while the muscle organ relaxes. The double blood supply to the heart is terrific and nourishes it when being starved has been the problem. Some 3 dozen or so treatments are needed in all."

HIGH BLOOD PRESSURE

While your pulse is a measure of your heart health, your blood pressure tells you about the health of your arteries. High blood pressure, also known as hypertension, is often considered a "normal" part of ageing, but just because something's common, doesn't mean it's normal. High blood pressure makes you more susceptible to heart disease, strokes and kidney disease. Blood pressure of 150 over 100 or more is classified as high. A normal reading is 120/80, but 140/90 or less is deemed as raised, but acceptable. There is no reason you shouldn't have a blood pressure of 120/80 when you're 80 if you take good care of your arteries.

It's important to remember that high blood pressure is a symptom of a problem, not the problem. The problem is that your arteries are too constricted or "furred up" to properly relax when your heart pumps the blood through. And narrower arteries make you age faster as you have a reduced oxygen supply to tissues, so the heart works harder, which raises your blood pressure even more, exposing arterial walls to damage, which triggers further hardening or furring up, and the problem gets worse.

Think of your arteries as the most amazingly complex system of garden hoses you've ever seen, coming off a single pump – your heart. Every time your heart beats, it's sending oxygen and nutrient-rich blood gushing around your body via your arteries to nourish each of your trillions of cells. These gushes of blood, forced through the arteries with every heartbeat, exert pressure on the walls of your arteries, and this pressure can damage the delicate cells lining your arteries. To reduce the pressure and ensure smooth blood flow, rather than spurts, the arterial walls are flexible, and are surrounded by smooth muscle that is able to expand and contact in response to the pressure being exerted on the arterial walls by the pumped blood.

Over time, many peoples' arteries become gradually harder and narrower, a process called arteriosclerosis (or sometimes atherosclerosis). Arteriosclerosis is a major recognized cause of dementia in the elderly (see *Alzheimer's Disease*). The kidneys, liver and other organs suffer reduced blood flow too and so cannot perform effectively in detoxing the body. Lumps of thickened matter in the artery wall called plaques build up and reduce the diameter of the vessels that the blood flows through. We now know why this happens, and it all starts with damage to the arterial wall. This can occur due to abrasion (from high blood pressure), viral or bacterial infection, or high homocysteine levels (a toxic amino acid formed as a by product of the metabolism of proteins), or free radical damage.

Once the damage is done, the body tries to repair the area, causing scar tissue and this is made worse by high levels of low-density lipoprotein (LDL – "bad cholesterol"), that can pass into the walls of the artery where it is oxidized by free radicals into dangerous rancid forms. This in turn is gobbled up by macrophages (part of your immune system), which become engorged "foam cells". The whole area attracts more and more oxidized cholesterol, more immune responses, more inflammation, and inevitably the arteries become stiffer and narrower.

So now we can understand why LDL cholesterol is bad for us and why levels of unoxidized cholesterol never was the real problem. Total cholesterol, so often touted as the cause of heart and arterial disease, is less a risk marker than high homocysteine levels. Homocysteine, now thought to be one of the key agents involved in damaging the arterial walls, is a damaging compound produced in the body that's normally recycled or broken down by vitamins B6, B12 and folic acid, nutrients often deficient in overly refined foods.

A University of Washington study showed that high homocysteine levels doubled the risk of arterial disease in young women and B vitamins help reduce homocysteine levels (see *Helpful Hints* below to find out how to get these levels tested).

Another key cause of raised blood pressure is a lack of the mineral magnesium. Remember those muscles around the arteries that enable the walls to contract and relax? Magnesium is needed for muscles to relax after they've contracted (muscle cramps or eye ticks are a symptom of magnesium deficiency) and research has shown that arteries are considerably narrower in those who are deficient in magnesium. In Japan, paramedics inject magnesium directly into the heart of heart-attack victims to relax the muscle and the blocked arteries supplying it. Many heart attacks and strokes are now thought to be due to arterial spasms blocking blood supply to the heart or brain, rather than a clot.

Stress and excessive exercise are known to deplete magnesium that may be deficient in your diet if you don't eat enough dark green leafy vegetables, wholegrains and seeds. This may explain why fit, apparently healthy people sometimes die suddenly of a heart attack or stroke.

A dangerous side effect of arteriosclerosis is an increased tendency towards (and greater dangers from) blood clotting. Turbulence in the blood caused by rough areas in the normally very smooth arterial walls can increase clotting. Also the plaques can break off and travel along the artery until they get stuck in a narrower blood vessel, commonly known as thrombosis. If these clots reach an area sufficiently narrowed by arterial plaques, they can block the vessel completely and starve the tissues "down stream" of blood, oxygen and nutrients. If this happens in the vessels supplying the heart or brain, a heart attack or stroke can occur. But there is plenty you can do to help yourself.

Eighty-five per cent of all cases of high blood pressure can be treated without drugs if the person is willing to change their lifestyle and diet. For example in societies where salt is virtually absent, hypertension is equally absent. Too much caffeine, alcohol and smoking when combined with high blood pressure greatly increases your chances of suffering heart disease or stroke. Stress is a major factor in high blood pressure, because adrenaline is released into the bloodstream and increases your heart rate, breathing and blood pressure.

In short, your arteries are literally a lifeline to a longer life. So if longevity's your goal, you need to look after your arteries – from today onwards.

Foods to Avoid

■ Salt. There is a clear link between the use of sodium-based salt and high blood pressure because sodium causes more water to be retained by your kidneys, so keep the sodium level in your diet low. More water means more blood volume, and therefore higher blood pressure. There are plenty of magnesium and potassium-based salts, such as Solo Salt, available from health shops. Use sparingly on the food that's on your plate.

■ Reduce stimulants. Blood pressure has been shown to drop as much as 20 points when all caffeine is eliminated, because caffeine causes arteries to constrict. Some decaffeinated drinks contain formaldehyde, so look for decaffeinated drinks and coffee that has been decaffeinated using the more natural water method.

■ Sugar is also a problem as sugar coverts into fat in the body if not used up during exercise and be aware that many low-fat foods are high in sugar. Always check the labels.

■ Replace refined grains, for example white bread, pasta and rice, with wholegrains such as brown rice, breads and pastas, to increase your intake of the B vitamins: B6, B12 and folic acid, which are involved in breaking down homocysteine.

■ If you have eliminated all of the above and still have a tendency towards high blood pressure, consult a nutritionist who can check for food intolerances, particularly if you are a migraine sufferer (see *Useful Information and Addresses p338*).

Friendly Foods

■ Green vegetables, fresh fruit, unprocessed and unsalted nuts, seafood, soya, roast potatoes, butterbeans, currants, dried figs, apricots, almonds, black treacle and sunflower seeds are all rich in minerals such as magnesium and potassium.

■ Potassium can help lower blood pressure because it balances sodium. Two bananas a day (rich in potassium) have been shown to help lower blood pressure.

■ Another useful salt is organic Herb Seasoning Salt by Bioforce. Made from organic sea salt, dried celery, leeks, cress, parsley, kelp, garlic and basil. Sold globally in health stores and supermarkets. www.bioforce.co.uk

■ If you are not a fan of eating fresh fruit and vegetables, at least drink a couple of glasses of freshly made fruit or vegetable juices, so although you miss out on the fibre, you still get much of the nutrient content.

■ Try switching to a more vegetarian-based diet as the more fruit, vegetables, beans and lentils you eat, the greater your potassium intake and, generally speaking, the lower your sodium intake. And vegetarians tend to have much lower blood pressure.

■ Eat more garlic, onions, broccoli (which are antioxidant, anti-viral and anti-bacterial) and celery (which is diuretic).

■ Use unrefined organic virgin olive, walnut, pumpkin, flax or sunflower oils for your salad dressings and eat oily fish three times a week (see *Fats for Anti-ageing p139*).

■ As high levels of toxic metals, such as lead, can contribute to high blood pressure, buy a good-quality water filter. The fibre in apples (pectin) and seaweed (alginates) helps to detoxify metals from the body (see also *Water in Ageing p325*).

■ Natural-source vitamin E helps to thin blood naturally, therefore eat more soya beans, wheatgerm, alfalfa sprouts, dark green vegetables, hazel nuts, almonds and avocados.

■ See also *Friendly Foods* under *Elimination*, as constipation can aggravate blood pressure.

Useful Remedies

■ If you are on blood pressure medication tell your doctor about any supplements you are taking, as in time your prescription drugs may be able to be reduced, and these supplements help to lower blood pressure naturally and you don't want your blood pressure to go too low.

■ Take 500mg of magnesium with 500mg of calcium daily. Both of these minerals have been shown to help lower blood pressure.

■ Essential fats thin the blood (to protect you from clots) and reduce inflammation (in your arterial walls). Take a 1gram fish oil daily or 1gram of linseed oil, both omega-3 fats (see *Fats for Anti-ageing p139*)

■ Take 900mg garlic a day. When used long-term, garlic can help gently lower blood pressure and thin the blood. Kudos make a high-strength 1000mg capsule (see page 14 for details).

■ Hawthorn, either as tincture or as tablets, is a gentle way of bringing blood pressure back down to normal. Take 1–3mls of tincture or 1–2grams of the tablets.

■ Begin taking 100iu of natural source, full-spectrum vitamin E and gradually increase to 500iu a day. Vitamin E thins the blood, protecting you from clotting, and is also a powerful antioxidant that protects fats (such as cholesterol) from free radical damage.

■ Include a high-strength multi-vitamin/mineral in your programme, as the B vitamins help to support your nerves, controlling muscle contraction and improving your tolerance to stress.

■ If your homocysteine level is high, take an extra 10–50mg of vitamin B6, 400–1000mcg of folic acid plus 10mg of B12.

Helpful Hints

■ High blood pressure can occur in pregnancy – and will need medical attention.

- Toxic metals in the body are also linked to high blood pressure. So if you have tried all the dietary guidelines, have levels checked (see *Toxic Metal Overload p317*).

- Cigarettes, plus the chemicals in cigarette smoke, damage your arteries and make the blood more likely to clot, raising your risk of developing heart disease.

- Reduce stress. Try to find a method of relaxation that you enjoy whether it's meditation, t'ai chi, yoga, exercising, walking or swimming (see also *Stress in Ageing p293*).

- Have a regular aromatherapy massage using relaxing essential oils such as rosewood, ylang ylang, clary, sage and marjoram.

- Get a pet. Researchers from the State University of New York have shown how having a pet can protect against the effects of stress better than drugs designed to lower blood pressure.

- Exercise is vital for reducing blood pressure. With your doctor's permission start walking briskly for 30 minutes daily. People who are overweight and don't get much exercise are much more likely to suffer high blood pressure.

- Have a nutrition consultant conduct a hair mineral analysis for you. This inexpensive test determines your level of calcium, magnesium and other important minerals, identifies any raised heavy metals in your system, plus gives you an indication of your glucose tolerance, adrenal and thyroid functions. For further information call Sarah Stelling of ARL (UK) on 01313 127454 or write to ARL (UK), 44 Park Crescent, Edinburgh EH4 7RP.

- Have your doctor obtain an ordinary cardiac risk blood profile. This will check your total cholesterol, HDL (good cholesterol), LDL (bad cholesterol) and triglycerides. There is no doubt statistically that raised triglycerides put you in the high-risk category, though this does not mean triglycerides are necessarily to blame. If you're prescribed cholesterol-lowering drugs get a second opinion. Cholesterol is made in the body naturally, and as explained above, oxidized cholesterol is the problem. So increase your intake of antioxidants and eat more fibre, to support your body's own method of reducing cholesterol (via the bowels) (see also *Cholesterol, High and Low p92*).

- Additionally, have your homocysteine levels checked. It should be below 8; above 10 is poor; above 12 is definitely dangerous. But the good news is that homocysteine can be brought down by supplementing just 3 vitamins: B6, B12 and folic acid. If yours is high, you need higher levels of these vitamins than you can get in your diet alone (see *Useful Remedies,* above).

- There is now an easy test to discover your plasma homocysteine levels. Made by York Laboratories and backed by The British Cardiac Patients Association – it's a simple pin prick method that can be done by post. For details call York Labs on 0800 074 6185 or log on to www.yorktest.com

- If you need to check for food intolerances, see either a kinesiologist or to take a more scientifically accepted blood test from York Test Laboratories, call 01904 410410.

- Many men who suffer arteriosclerosis have low levels of testosterone (*see Men's Hormones*).

- Patrick Holford's *Say No to Heart Disease*, Piatkus, is an excellent book explaining what you can do to prevent or correct high blood pressure.

HOMOCYSTEINE

(See *Cholesterol – High and Low, High Blood Pressure* and *Heart in Ageing*)

IMMUNE FUNCTION IN AGEING

Our immune system is made up of a network of cells, organs and fluids that help defend us against the millions of bacteria, viruses and fungi that bombard us in our daily lives. And one of the most important things you can do to hold back ageing, is to keep your immune system in good shape. For instance, when I was younger and did not realize how diet and lifestyle affected my ability to fight off illnesses, when I was under pressure, not getting sufficient sleep and eating the wrong foods, I was always ill. At times, when I felt ghastly, I would turn to a sugary snack to keep me going and I could literally feel my immune system going "over the edge".

These days I recognize my limits, I know when to stop, get more sleep, eat a clean diet, detox and de-stress. You need to get in touch with your body, listen to it and take notice!

Meanwhile, most people don't think of their skin as being part of the immune system, but it forms a physical barrier against attack and the immune system is in charge of cell regencration within your skin. The more efficient your immune system – the younger your skin will be.

Then comes your stomach acid, which also helps to destroy harmful organisms but as we age, stomach acid levels fall and more bacteria can get through (see *Low Stomach Acid*). And within a child's bone marrow are "stem cells" which, as we grow, develop into various types of immune cells some of which mature in the thymus gland – known as T cells.

The spleen also contains immune cells that manufacture antibodies and the lymphatic system, often called the master drain, is also a major player in immune function. The lymph system removes toxins and microbes from the body's tissue and along with bone marrow manufactures lymphocytes (a specific kind of white blood cell that come in three types – B cells, T cells and natural killer cells that keep your immune system in good shape). Lymph nodes are found all over the body but the ones most people are aware of are situated in the neck, groin and arm pits. During an infection the lymph glands can swell as they produce more white blood cells, and this is very common in throat conditions for instance. If the lymphatic system becomes congested, the fluid thickens and becomes more gel-like, which inhibits proper drainage and detoxification and puts more pressure on the liver and kidneys (see *Detoxing p108*).

Hence why a fully functioning lymph system helps you to fight off invading bacteria and viruses. The liver and thymus gland also play a huge role in immune function (see *Liver in Ageing p189*).

Unfortunately, as we age, our immune system becomes less effective at protecting us and more viruses and bacteria get through our defences. Conversely our immune system can also over-react, which produces chronic inflammation when we eat certain foods, or are exposed to pollen, pollutants etc, or even begins attacking the body's own tissue, called an autoimmune response, in conditions such as lupus and rheumatoid arthritis.

The secretion of hormones, including growth hormone and melatonin, also decline in old age and may also be related to a compromised immune system.

High cholesterol levels are also linked to a lowered immune response, because cells containing high levels of cholesterol can disrupt our cells' ability to communicate with each other, which is vital for proper immune responses (see *Cholesterol, High and Low*).

Lowered immune function is also linked to chronic fatigue, allergies, parasite infections, and some forms of heart disease.

Prostaglandins, which are hormone-like substances, become more out of balance as we age. This has an effect of suppressing the immune system and affecting important processes such as body temperature and metabolism. Essential fatty acids, such as EPA (from fish oil) and GLA (from evening primrose, blackcurrant, and borage oils) help to restore the proper prostaglandin ratios, thereby supporting the immune system (see *Fats for Anti-ageing p139*).

Aging of the immune system is also characterized by increased levels of a protein called tumour necrosis factor alpha (TNF-a) in the bloodstream. TNF-a is involved in increased inflammation and reduced immunological responses. Nettle leaf has been shown to reduce the levels of TNF-a.

Foods to Avoid

■ I'm afraid it's our old friend sugar, which greatly compromises your immune system. Use a little fructose if you need sugar, but generally cut down on pies, biscuits, sweets and shop-bought sugary snacks and drinks (see *Sugar in Ageing p302*).

■ Reduce your intake of caffeine and alcohol, which place an extra burden on the immune system.

■ Avoid foods containing lots of preservatives, additives and especially the artificial sweetener aspartame.

■ Avoid all smoked foods and cheeses.Reduce your intake of saturated fats found in red meat and full-fat dairy produce and hydrogenated and trans-fats (see *Fats for Anti-ageing*).

Friendly Foods

■ Eat organic food as much as possible. Make sure your diet is high in all fresh fruits and vegetables, which are high in immune-boosting nutrients.

■ Eat more fresh fish, chicken, broccoli, cabbage, cauliflower, parsley, green beans, apples, green salads, buckwheat, soya beans and millet.

■ Sprouts such as alfalfa and brown rice, and algaes, such as spirulina and chlorella.

■ Eat more purple, red and orange foods: blueberries, bilberries and blackberries are high in immune boosting nutrients, plus sweet potatoes, apricots, papaya and red peppers.

■ Nuts and seeds are packed with essential fats and minerals like zinc and selenium (see *Fats for Anti-ageing p139*).

■ See *Diet – The Stay Younger Longer Diet (see page 114)*.

Useful Remedies

■ Take a good-quality multivitamin/mineral and an antioxidant formula daily. For information on the most effective anti-oxidants (see *Antioxidants in Ageing p38*).

■ See details of Kudos 24, the multi-active age management complex that contains a full spectrum of vitamins, minerals, brain nutrients, essential fats, antioxidants and more. An ideal once-a-day supplement to keep your immune system in better shape – see page 348.

■ I believe that an important supplement for boosting immunity is essential sugars – these are a new food group fairly recently discovered that are essential to life, see *Essential Sugars* on page 126.

■ Plant sterols derived from the wild South African potato have been shown to boost immune function. Usually sold as Moducare. Take 3 capsules daily on an empty stomach. Call 01782 56/100 for stockists.

■ Use organic spirulina, especially while detoxing. It is an easily digestible food that helps protect the immune system. One heaped teaspoon in juice, or 8 tablets per day in-between meals. Blackmores make an organic formula (see page 13 for details).

■ Include organic chlorella and garlic as these foods contain germanium, a trace element beneficial for the immune system. Chlorella, a single-celled algae, helps to build up the immune factors. It is one of the most efficient foods on earth with its high chlorophyll content–a natural, pure, wholefood. Up to 15 tablets daily.

■ Colostrum, which is the pre-milk fluid produced by all mothers after giving birth. It arrives before breast milk and contains 37 natural immune boosting factors and 8 growth factors that support the immune system and regeneration of cells. Dose: 2000–4000mg per day. For details, call The NutriCentre or Sloane Health Shop (see page 14).

■ Whey protein powder helps to boost immune function, thus inhibiting cancer cell proliferation. It protects against free radicals and boosts cellular antioxidant levels. Take 20grams per day.

■ Echinacea is known for its ability to stimulate the body's immune system. Several trials have shown echinacea to be effective, especially if taken with vitamin A, zinc and selenium at the first signs of an illness. Blackmores stock it (see page 13).

- Take 250mg–500mg of echinacea per day, 14 days on, then 7 days off, to improve overall immune function.
- Astragalus is a traditional Chinese herb used to strengthen the immune system. It boosts T-cell levels close to normal in some cancer patients, suggesting the possibility of a synergistic effect of astragalus with chemotherapy. Take two 250mg tablets per day.

Helpful Hints

- Stress alone can suppress immune function by up to 60%. Stress during a lifetime, causes the over-production of the hormone cortisol, which is thought to shrink the thymus gland (which is where T cells mature – situated in your upper chest area, just below the hollow in your neck). Therefore keep your stress levels in check (see also *Stress in Ageing p293*).
- Greatly reduce your exposure to external pollutants such as cigarette smoke, car fumes, chemical-based sprays and heavy metals (see *Toxic Metal Overload p317*).
- Make sure you get sufficient sleep, which helps boost immune function.
- If possible take regular holidays in the sunshine, which really helps to boost your immune system.
- Laugh a lot, watch films that make you laugh. Make friends with people who make you laugh. Laughter and having some *fun* strengthen immune function.
- Think positively – people who are cheerful and who look on the bright side have stronger immune systems.
- Take regular exercise but not to excess. Don't over exercise if you are truly exhausted.
- See *General Anti-ageing Health Hints p147* for more help.

INCONTINENCE

(See *Bladder Problems* and *Prostate in Ageing*)

INSOMNIA

(See *Sleep*)

INSULIN RESISTANCE

(See also *Carbohydrate Control, Diabetes – Late Onset,* and *Low Blood Sugar*)

If blood sugar imbalance (discussed in *Carbohydrate Control* and *Low Blood Sugar*) is not addressed, over time it can develop further into insulin resistance or Syndrome X and finally diabetes (see *Diabetes – Late Onset*). Anti-ageing doctors are increasingly concerned about the problem of insulin resistance as a causative factor in degenerative diseases associated with ageing.

As explained in *Carbohydrate Control*, carbohydrates of all types are digested as simple sugars, such as glucose, when they enter the gut. Eating large amounts of carbohydrates such as cakes and biscuits, can result in a "sugar rush", which has to be dealt with safely. One of the key hormones that regulates your levels of blood sugar is insulin. Basically, insulin makes cells more receptive to glucose, so they can either metabolize it, or store it for future use as glycogen or fat. This takes glucose out of your blood and into your cells, lowering your blood sugar levels.

"However", says nutritional physician Dr Keith Scott-Mumby, "When this process has been abused for many decades, it's liable to break down. Eventually the body ceases to respond to glucose as it should and despite ever increasing levels of insulin, glucose in the blood begins to rise. The cells can no longer utilize it properly. Insulin receptors on the surface of cells seem to have switched off and stopped listening to the signal from insulin, hence the term for this condition.

Insulin resistance is dangerous. Apart from the obvious risk of progression into Syndrome X and eventually diabetes, high insulin levels result in excess sympathetic nervous system activity, which keeps the individual tense and prone to fatigue. What's more, because insulin is usually only released when there's an excess of blood sugar, conversion of fat back to sugar for use as fuel is blocked by the hormone, so weight loss becomes increasingly difficult."

Syndrome X

In 1988, our understanding of disordered blood sugar control was advanced considerably by Dr Gerald Reaven of Stanford University, who published a paper describing what he called "Syndrome X". A "syndrome" simply means a group of symptoms that appear together in a characteristic pattern. In this case, the syndrome consists of 5 features that are common among the elderly (and becoming more common in the young too), obesity, insulin resistance, high blood pressure, high LDL (the bad) cholesterol and low HDL (good cholesterol). Because Dr Reaven had no idea what caused this group of symptoms to occur together, he named it "Syndrome X". Doesn't sound so frightening now does it? As we age, all the manifestations of Syndrome X are more frequently seen, but even elderly people without these problems tend to have increasing insulin resistance.

Patients with Syndrome X do not have the dangerously raised glucose levels of diabetes. But they do have insulin resistance and higher than normal levels of circulating glucose. The high level of insulin stimulates the kidneys to re-absorb sodium, which in turn results in a tendency to high blood pressure. Dr Reaven believes that half of all people with high blood pressure have insulin resistance (see *High Blood Pressure p170*).

Unfortunately, high levels of insulin also reduce blood enzymes that prevent or dissolve blood clots. Thus, along with the undesirable changes in blood fats comes a possible increase in the likelihood of blood clotting, making the risk of heart attack or stroke far greater than for healthy individuals.

Abnormal glucose and insulin metabolism are also associated with increased free radical formation. And the more free radicals you have in your body, the faster you will age (see *Antioxidants in Ageing p38*).

Foods to Avoid

- See *Carbohydrate Control p80*.

Friendly Foods

- Follow the *Friendly Foods* guidelines in *Carbohydrate Control* as closely as possible, plus, eat more lentils and beans. Dr Jeffrey Bland and fellow researchers at the Functional Medicine Research Centre in Gig Harbour, Washington, have found that legumes create a very low insulin response and that increased intake of lentils, chickpeas, beans and peas is desirable in the management of Syndrome X.

- In general, vegetables have a beneficial effect on blood sugar and insulin, but certain vegetables appear to be even better at maintaining blood sugar and insulin levels, including members of the brassica family (cabbage, cauliflower, broccoli) and other green leafy vegetables.

- Fermented soya products – such as tempeh and miso – are also very desirable as they help to balance blood sugar levels. Soya helps improve glucose transport as well as containing soluble fibre that slows the absorption of glucose from the gut, thereby reducing insulin response.

- See also the dietary guidelines in *Diabetes – Late Onset p110*.

Useful Remedies

- A high-strength multivitamin/mineral complex taken every day provides a baseline of nutrients. In addition to the useful remedies listed in *Carbohydrate Control*, especially the 200mcg of chromium daily, for glucose tolerance factor.

- Fish oil supplementation has been found to not only improve insulin sensitivity in diabetic animals, but also to prevent diabetes-induced nerve damage. Take 1gram daily.

- Antioxidant nutrients have also been found to improve insulin sensitivity. Take a good-quality antioxidant formula containing 100–400mg of vitamin E and 20–50mg of alpha-lipoic acid, both known to improve insulin response (see *Antioxidants in Ageing p38*).

- UltraGlycemX is a specially fortified, vegetarian, powdered beverage mix designed for the nutritional support of glucose metabolism and insulin regulation. Contact NutriCentre on 020 7436 5122 for more information.

Helpful Hints

- One of the best ways to improve glucose control and insulin sensitivity is through regular aerobic activity. This doesn't have to be intense exercise and can be as moderate as a regular walking programme. Twenty minutes per day of walking on level ground has been shown to improve insulin sensitivity and glucose management.

- Moderate alcohol consumption is OK. A recent study by Dr Reaven and colleagues indicated that light-to-moderate alcohol intake was associated with improved insulin sensitivity, while more than two drinks per day worsened it.

■ See the other *Helpful Hints* in *Carbohydrate Control p80*.

JOINTS IN AGEING

(See also *Acid-Alkaline Balance, Exercise, Muscles in Ageing* and *Osteoporosis*)

As we age, the cartilage "cushioning" between the joints, which is made up of dense connective tissue, tends to degenerate over time. Cartilage also begins to thin and eventually it cannot replenish itself as quickly as it is worn down.

Normal wear and tear on our joints can thin or disintegrate the cartilage to the point where the edges of our bones touch each other, which degenerates our bones even faster. At this point bones can become misshapen as in arthritis (see *Arthritis*).

This is why long-distance runners and sports people, who regularly play impact sports such as football, rugby, squash etc, tend to end up with rather painful knees, ankles, spines and hips. It's usually the weight-bearing joints that experience the worst symptoms.

Our joints, depending on their degree of movement, can be divided roughly into three categories: fixed joints such as the skull, slightly moveable such as the spine and freely moveable as in the knees, shoulder, wrists, ankles and elbow.

In free-moving joints, the joint cavity or the space between the ends of the bone, is filled with a small amount of slippery, synovial fluid which supplies nutrients and fluid to the cartilage. This fluid is produced by the synovial membrane which lines the joint capsule and is well supplied with blood. The capsule is reinforced by slightly elastic ligaments, which act like straps to prevent excessive movement of the bones.

As we age, our spine loses mobility, and you can greatly help your spine by keeping your abdominal muscles, which stabilize the spine and pelvis, in good shape. We also tend to become more round-shouldered, therefore make the effort to stand, walk and sit straighter. So if you want your joints to be healthy in later life, you need to begin practising prevention in your thirties, but at any age you can help your joints to become more supple and healthier.

Foods to Avoid

■ The nightshade family include tomatoes, potatoes, peppers and aubergines, which many arthritics find difficult to digest, and they often have a sensitivity to this food group. Recent research has shown that arthritics who consumed devil's claw tablets were much better able to digest the nightshades and their arthritis improved as well.

■ Acid-forming foods deplete the body of vital minerals that support healthy bones and tissue (see *Diet* under *Acid–Alkaline Balance p18*).

Friendly Foods

■ Oily fish, calves' liver, cod liver oil, sweet potatoes and pumpkin are good sources of vitamin A, which aids tissue repair.

■ Pineapple contains bromelain, an enzyme that helps reduce pain and inflammation.

■ Adding ginger and turmeric to foods can provide pain relief and improve circulation.

■ Linseeds, sunflower seeds, pumpkin seeds, walnuts, Brazil nuts and their unrefined oils, are rich in omega-3 and 6 fats which help keep joints supple (see *Fats for Anti-ageing p139*).

■ Black cherries increase elimination of uric acid, which can deposit in the joints – as in gout.

■ Dark blue fruits, such as blackberries, blueberries and plums are acid forming in the body but they help to mobilize uric acid out of the joints, reduce joint inflammation and aid collagen production.

Useful Remedies

■ For healthy cartilage formation you need vitamins A, B5, B6, zinc, copper and boron, which are all available in good-quality, organic green-based powders, such as chlorella, wheat grass, barley grass, alfalfa-type powders. Dr Gillian McKeith makes a Living Food Energy Powder which is available from all health shops, or try Alkalife powder available from www.bestcare-uk.com. Tel: 01342 410303. Take 2 teaspoons daily.

■ Take a high-strength antioxidant formula which contains vitamin C, natural source vitamin E and 25–30mg of zinc such as Kudos 24 Multi-active Age Management complex (see page 348).

■ A daily multimineral in a colloidal or chelated form is easier for the body to absorb.

■ CT241 contains chondroitin sulphate, aecerola concentrate, kelp, silica, boron and digestive enzymes, plus Ligazyme, made by BioCare which all help to prevent cartilage damage (see page 13).

■ The amino sugar glucosamine (usually now blended with chondroitin) helps to re-hydrate cartilage, which helps to thicken the cartilage, if taken regularly for at least 6 months. If your joints and spine are in pain 500mg can be taken three times daily. Otherwise 500mg can be taken daily as a preventative and maintenance dose after the age of 35 – especially for those keen on exercise. Note: this supplement is derived from crab shells, therefore if you have a severe allergy to shellfish don't take this supplement.

■ Joints need essential fats to keep them supple (see *Fats for Anti-ageing p139*).

■ Cat's claw, 1000mg, is very useful, especially if you feel the need to use conventional pain killers or anti-inflammatories, as it benefits the arthritis.

■ Niacinamide, vitamin B3, is a great alternative to glucosamine. But this vitamin can cause a tremendous red flushing of the skin, so ask for a **no-flush** variety. Begin with 500mg daily and increase to 500mg three times a day. It should begin working after three to four weeks.

■ Sodiphos, sodium phosphate, helps to reduce lactic acid (and uric acid) build-up in the joints and re-alkalizes an over-acid system. Take 600mg daily for three months (Blackmores page 13).

■ Joints need water, so make sure you drink at least six glasses of water daily.

Helpful Hints

■ Exercise in a warm swimming pool, which supports the joints, bringing nutrient-rich blood flow to the area and helps keep joints supple.

■ If you are overweight, this places extra strain on your joints, which can wear the cartilage down more quickly.

■ Wobble boards improve balance which helps to strengthen the muscles around the joints, especially ankles and knees, which gives more protection to the joints. Available from all good sports shops.

■ Don't over-exercise and never practise impact sports without at least wearing proper cushioning footwear.

■ Whenever you exercise for an hour or more, always stretch for at least 5 minutes before working out.

■ In Chinese medicine, heated moxa (herbs) are used in conjunction with acupuncture to warm painful, stiff joints and encourage blood flow to the area.

■ Sometimes a crusting of mineral salts, known as crepitations, can form around the joints and cause extreme pain. Joints begin clicking, sometimes noisily. If you have these types of symptoms, firstly consult an osteopath or chiropractor and if they cannot help, have the affected joint X-rayed, as the build up of crystals can be removed using keyhole surgery.

■ Topically apply oil of wintergreen to help reduce pain and inflammation in the joints.

■ When you keep your muscles working, this helps to support the joints and holds them in their correct position.

■ If your joints become swollen or painful, practise the standard therapy of rest, ice packs (apply for 20 minutes as needed), compression and elevation.

■ Apply magnets to the affected joints, which increase, circulation and reduces pain. For further details call Homedics UK Ltd on 0161 798 5876 or write to them at Parkgates, Bury New Road, Prestwich, Manchester M25 0JW or log on to homedics.co.uk

■ Acupuncture is excellent for reducing swelling and painful joints (see *Useful Information and Addresses p338*).

■ If you have suffered from any joint injury or are in pain that stops you from exercising, I strongly recommend that you try Pilates. It is a way of exercising that is totally brilliant if your injury prevents you from working out properly. I ruptured two discs in my back a couple of years ago and after trying many treatments, Pilates truly reduced the pain and has given me the confidence to start exercising properly again. For your nearest practitioner send an SAE to The Pilates Foundation UK Ltd, PO Box 36052, London SW16 1XQ. Tel: 07071 781859 website: www.pilatesfoundation.com Anoushka Boone is my teacher and if you live near London, she is a miracle worker. Tel: 0208 746 1199.

■ To keep your spine healthier, use a back board for 10 minutes a day – or buy a Swiss Ball. These inexpensive balls are available from all sports shops. Simply sit on the ball and carefully slide your feet forward so that your body and back are lying on the back of the ball – and just hang there for a few minutes every day. This really helps to keep your spine supple, as does yoga and t'ai chi.

KIDNEYS IN AGEING

By the age of 70, the average person's kidney function can be reduced by up to two-thirds, which greatly reduces its ability to aid in the detoxification process.

Your kidneys filter the plasma of your blood and extract all the waste and unwanted toxins, which are excreted in the urine, which is a sterile liquid. Also, antibiotic, prescription drug and hormone residues, vitamins and minerals are excreted in the urine.

The kidneys maintain the acid–alkaline balance of your blood within very narrow limits; and if the blood becomes too acid or alkaline, life is not possible. General body acidity is one of the factors which accelerates ageing (see also *Acid–Alkaline Balance*). Without functioning kidneys you cannot live for very long.

These remarkable organs weigh just a few ounces each and yet, if they cease to function (kidney failure), they must be replaced with a huge dialysis machine.

Two of the main threats to our kidneys are blood pressure and toxins. If you tend to have a poor diet or take little or no exercise, it's likely that you may develop hypertension, which, sooner or later, plays havoc with the kidneys (see also *High Blood Pressure p170*).

Other toxins that affect the kidneys are in our air, water, food and other pollutants: cadmium, from cigarettes, is a major kidney poison and accumulation of this metal in the kidneys is one of the reasons why smokers tend to succumb sooner than average. Smokers simply cannot clear their bloodstream of the harmful waste products as efficiently. Similarly, mercury, arsenic, pesticides and a huge amount of chemical pollutants all pose potential problems to the kidneys, which have to work harder and may weaken under the strain (see also *Toxic Metal Overload p317*).

Over time, if we eat a poor diet, kidney stones can start to form as miniscule crystals that look like gravel, which can damage the delicate tubules in the kidneys and impede proper urine flow. Kidney stone episodes are more common in the summer when urine becomes more concentrated when we tend to sweat more.

Kidney stones are generally made from minerals such as calcium and uric acid deposits, the most common component being calcium oxalate. Kidney stones can cause excruciating pain as they try to move out of the kidneys and into the bladder. Passing a kidney stone is one of the worst pains in all of medicine. So, try and make sure this never happens to you.

Vegetarians have a 40–60% less chance of developing stones. Whereas high meat eaters tend to suffer more stones.

Foods to Avoid

- If you tend to eat a lot of foods high in oxalic acid such as chocolate, cocoa, tea, spinach, rhubarb, chard – don't eat these foods too regularly.

- Beetroot, instant coffee, grapefruit, oranges, gooseberries, peanuts and strawberries also contain oxalic acid, so reduce your intake of these if you suffer from kidney stones.

- Reduce or avoid high-acid-forming foods such as red meat, full-fat dairy products, sugar and sweet foods.

- Sugar is the worst food for your kidneys, it stimulates the release of insulin from the pancreas, which in turn stimulates calcium excretion through the urine that can over time increase the risk of kidney stones.

- Cut down on all fizzy canned drinks and reduce alcohol and caffeinated drinks.

- Antacids, excess milk, bicarbonated drinks such as soda water and fizzy water can all add to the problem.

- Avoid sodium-based salts, ask at your health shop for magnesium-and-potassium based sea salts – use sparingly.

Friendly Foods

- The three keys to healthier kidneys are to increase fluids, fibre and green vegetables.

- Drink plenty of plain pure water and increase to 8 glasses daily in summer.

- Add cranberry juice, parsley tea, dandelion leaf tea, mullein tea and barley water which all help to break down any stone formation.

- Black cherries help to remove uric acid crystals out of the body.

- Use carrot, celery and parsley juice, or make "smoothies" with these ingredients. Celery does contain a little oxalic acid, but makes a great kidney cleanser as it is rich in potassium.

- Garlic, horseradish, asparagus, parsley, watermelon, apples, cucumber, kale, parsnips, turnip greens and mango are all great kidney foods.

- All magnesium and calcium-rich foods help you to avoid kidney stones and encourage healthier kidneys. Green leafy vegetables, plus apricots, blackstrap molasses, honey, curried vegetables, watercress, yoghurt, muesli and sesame seeds. Raw wheatgerm is also high in magnesium and vitamin E.

- Try rice or oat milk as non-dairy alternatives to cows' milk.

- Use organic, unrefined olive, walnut or linseed oils over salad dressings.

- Sprinkle lecithin granules which help emulsify saturated fats that can contribute to stone formation. Lecithin also contains choline and helps to protect the kidneys from the damage of arteriosclerosis and hypertension. Take 2 tablespoons a day.

■ Kelp and all seaweeds are a great source of calcium, magnesium and trace minerals.

Useful Remedies

■ A good B complex – especially if you are under stress.

■ Vitamin C – 2grams taken daily with food is a good detoxifier.

■ Vitamin D3 – contained in a cod liver oil capsule; take daily.

■ Choline also protects the kidneys from inflammation. It is available as the amino acids methionine and s-adenosyl methionine (SAMe), which is super-strength methionine. Take 500mgms a day of methionine or 50mgms of SAMe.

■ Alka herb tea helps to re-alkalize the system and is delicious with a little added molasses or honey. To order call 01342 410303 or www.bestcare-uk.com

■ The tissue salts silica and calcium fluoride help to break down kidney stones. Take four of each daily.

■ The herb horsetail acts as a diuretic which promotes kidney function. It can be taken either as capsules or a tincture to help reduce stones, but should not to be used if your kidneys are already damaged.

■ 1 cup of nettle tea taken three times daily is useful.

■ Or try Parsley Piert, available from health stores – 1 teaspoon per cup of boiling water can be taken morning and evening. Parsley Piert is also a diuretic which helps to dissolve stones in the urinary tract.

■ Include either a liquid multimineral, such as Concentrace, available from Higher Nature (see page 13) or a multimineral tablet in your regimen.

Helpful Hints

■ Taking 1 teaspoonful of neat lemon juice every half hour during the day for two days may help to smooth the kidney stones.

■ If you have reflexology, massage, manual lymph drainage and other therapies which help remove toxins out of the tissues, this can temporarily overload the kidneys. Warn your therapist to be gentle if you have a kidney problem. Drink plenty of water afterwards.

■ Skin brushing and lymphatic drainage massage also help remove toxins.

■ If you need painkillers, avoid paracetamol, which has a negative effect on the kidneys. If you are taking a diuretic medicine, be sure to get enough potassium. We need potassium to shed the more toxic sodium. Excess sodium leads directly to hypertension (high blood pressure) and kidney damage. You can take a potassium supplement (maximum 800 mgms per day). Or use a potassium chloride table salt, available from most pharmacies and health stores.

■ Some homeopathic remedies are excellent for strengthening kidney function. Populus and Solidago are well-known kidney remedies. HEEL also make Mucosa compositum, which helps the healing process. Available from Bio Pathica on 01233 636678.

- Avoid excess sweating. Do not consume strong (concentrated) drinks, which means no sodas, carbonated pops or alco-pops. If you have alcohol, make sure that you swallow plenty of water between each drink. Remember that salty food is also proportionately deficient in water; take less salt. Avoid dehydration at all costs!

LEAKY GUT IN AGEING

(See also *Absorption* and *Elimination*)

As we age, the small villi (small finger-like protrusions) in the small intestine can become irritated or eroded, which allows larger, undigested food molecules and toxins to pass through our gut wall into the bloodstream, which affects both the liver and the lymphatic system and places a greater strain on our immune system.

These undigested food molecules are treated as foreign invaders and provoke an immune reaction. Our bodies then begin reacting to food as though it were an infection entering our system and sends out antibodies to fight it. This is one of the possible mechanisms that trigger rheumatoid arthritis, and is now recognized as a major trigger for most food intolerances, allergies, and, for some people migraines.

Various toxins accumulate in our body, especially in the small intestine and large bowel. It tends to be a combination of undigested food, impacted faeces, bacteria, fungi, parasites and dead cells. As the toxins accumulate, the gut wall can become irritated and damaged which enables partly digested food molecules to cross the gut (small intestine) wall into the bloodstream. And the more toxins in the body – the faster you will age.

Also if you have a leaky gut you are unlikely to absorb or utilize as effectively the beneficial nutrients from your food, which will also accelerate the ageing process.

Leaky Gut Syndrome has now reached epidemic proportions, thanks mostly to stress, eating too many of the wrong foods, eating in a hurry and so on. People with irritable bowel tend to always have a leaky gut. Generally, if you suffer bloating, constipation and/or diarrhoea, crave sugary, refined foods, feel tired all the time and notice that your food sometimes comes out the other end looking much the same as it went in, you may well have a leaky gut. Candida, a yeast fungal overgrowth, is also a common cause or results from a leaky gut. Most people with a leaky gut also tend to have low stomach acid (see *Low Stomach Acid p199*).

Foods to Avoid

- Grains from wheat, rye, oats and barley if not properly assimilated will continue on into the bowel and feed the bad bacteria, which can increase constipation. Eliminating grains for even a week will help reduce a leaky gut.

- Sugar encourages fermentation and growth of unfriendly bacteria in the bowel, so keep sugary foods and drinks to a minimum.

- If you tend to bloat a lot after meals, don't eat large amounts of fruit directly after a large protein meal, as fruit likes a quick passage through the gut. If it gets stuck behind proteins, such as meat, the fruit will ferment which adds to the problem.

- Alcohol, vinegar and most pickled foods contribute to fermentation.

- Any foods to which you have an intolerance will only aggravate the problem, the most common being wheat, citrus fruits and sometimes cows' milk.

- Particularly bad is melon, this should only ever be eaten on its own.

- Avoid heavy, fatty, large meals which place a strain on the digestive system and the liver.

- Cut down on low-fibre foods such as jellies, ice cream, burgers, biscuits, cakes, pies, pastries etc.

Friendly Foods

- If you are desperate for sugar, use a little fructose or blackstrap molasses.

- Include more natural low-fat, live yoghurt containing the friendly bacteria acidophilus and bifidus.

- Pineapple and papaya are rich in enzymes, which improve protein digestion making it less likely that undigested proteins end up in the bowel.

- Beetroots, artichokes, radishes, celeriac and dandelion are all good liver cleansers, which also improves digestion. They contain inulin which helps encourage the growth of bifidus within the large bowel. This helps to reduce the load on the liver in the long-term (see *Liver in Ageing p189*).

- Unsalted sunflower, pumpkin, sesame seeds, linseeds and nuts are all rich sources of fibre. A great way to get more nuts and seeds into your diet is to place 1 tablespoon each of sunflower, pumpkin, sesame seeds and walnuts, hazel or Brazil nuts and place them in a coffee grinder or food mixer and pulse for a few seconds. Then keep them in a screw-top jar in the fridge and sprinkle over cereals, salads, desserts, fruit, yoghurts etc.

- Drink plenty of water, at least six glasses a day.

- Garlic and onions help fight infections and encourage growth of friendly bacteria in the bowel.

- Organic source chlorella is a great way to detoxify the system. You do need to use liberal amounts and it is better in powder form than taking tablets.

- Use fresh root ginger in your cooking which soothes and heals the gut.

- Green cabbage is rich in the amino acid L-glutamine which helps heal a leaky gut. Eat more cabbage, raw and steamed, and use the liquid from the cooking to make gravy and sauces.

- Eat plenty of fresh vegetables, and if you eat fruit, eat it between meals.

- Figs, apricots, apples and bananas all help to reduce constipation.

- Try quinoa, buckwheat or millet and plenty of brown rice.

- Most health shops sell pastas made from corn, millet, spelt or rice flour.
- Sprinkle rice bran over cereals.

Useful Remedies

- Take two acidophilus and bifidus bacteria capsules after main meals to replenish healthy bacteria which aids digestion and elimination.
- Take a digestive enzyme capsule with meals, such as Polyzyme Forte, available from BioCare (see page 13).
- L-glutamine, the amino acid, helps to heal a leaky gut. Take 1–4grams a day, on an empty stomach for the first month and then reduce to 1gram daily.
- Take a high-strength multivitamin/mineral supplement daily.
- Sprinkle Alkalife greenfood, rich in wheatgerm and green foods that re-alkalize your system over cereals and desserts. To order call Best Care Products on 01342 410303, www.bestcare-uk.com
- Add 1–3 dessertspoons of raw, ready-cracked linseeds (such as Linusit Gold) to your cereals or yoghurts every day.
- After taking these supplements for three months, your gut should be in better shape and you could then reduce this regimen to a good multi-vitamin/mineral, plus a digestive enzyme.

Helpful Hints

- It is vital that you chew food thoroughly and more slowly, which helps break down the food more effectively. Many people with a leaky gut swallow large food particles in a hurry, which places a great strain on an already labouring digestive tract.
- Smoking increases the toxic load on the body and can make the situation worse.
- At least try to sit down to eat, and in between, make sure you get plenty of regular exercise and always walk for at least 15 minutes after a meal to aid digestion.
- Lower your stress levels (see *Stress in Ageing* p293). Never eat a heavy meal when stressed.
- For further help, read a brilliant book called *The Good Gut Guide* by Stephanie Zinser, Thorsons, £10.99.

LIVER IN AGEING

It is no coincidence that the word "liver" contains the word "live" and if you want to stay younger longer, you really need to look after this vital organ. When it's working properly the liver can clean up to 99% of bacteria and toxins from the blood, around four pints of blood pass through the liver every minute for detoxification, and every day the liver manufactures about two pints of bile that help carry away toxins via the bowel.

Your liver, in essence, is the chemical factory of your body that builds or recycles substances you need and breaks down those you don't. If your liver isn't functioning properly, toxins that would normally be filtered by the liver accumulate in the body and certain nutrients are not processed and stored as they should be, resulting in a more rapid degeneration of your whole body, which is obviously ageing.

Typical symptoms of a sluggish liver are, feeling constantly tired even though you have slept, nausea, skin disorders such as acne, eczema and psoriasis, muscle and joint pain, age spots on the skin and regular infections. Also, most people don't associate being constipated with poor liver function, but blood from the bowel goes first to the liver, via the portal venous system, hence why a bowel loaded with rubbish is going to overwork the liver.

Other symptoms of poor liver function can include yellowing whites of the eyes, yellow-looking skin, fever, nausea, difficulty digesting fatty foods, and an increased sensitivity to cigarette smoke, strong perfume, petrol and other chemicals.

And because the brain is unable to disarm a wide range of toxins it relies on the liver to clean the blood before it gets there. So an under-performing liver can have dire consequences for the brain and nervous system over the long-term, including memory loss, Parkinson's and Alzheimer's.

While detoxification is the key function of the liver, it also produces bile to eliminate toxins and aid fat digestion, manufactures and balances hormones, stores various vitamins and minerals, assembles amino acids, makes cholesterol, controls glucose and fat supplies and plays a key role in immunity.

Your digestive system (see also *Digestion*) is closely involved in the health of your liver, as the blood from your digestive system, where nutrients are absorbed from your food, goes directly to the liver for filtering before it goes anywhere else in the body. If your diet is good and your digestion and absorption are working well, then the nutrients needed for good health will make it to the liver and then on into the body.

However, if your digestive system is generally toxic thanks to a poor low-nutrient, high-fat diet, constipation, poor gut flora and so on, these toxins, and any others you ingest, will similarly be delivered directly to your liver which adds to the liver's work load and accelerates ageing.

As we age, it's common for liver function to decline, however, the liver is capable of regenerating itself, so with a good diet, lifestyle and the right supplements there's no reason you can't maintain liver function at an optimal level at any age. And when you look after your liver, your skin literally glows with health.

To aid this regeneration process, you need to reduce your toxic load. Begin by eliminating as many unnatural chemicals as possible from your home and environment. The American Chemical Society has now registered the 10 millionth artificial (man-made) chemical compound, of which around 100,000 are in production at any one time. Millions of tons of these potential poisons find their way every year into our food, water and air. A worrying aspect of these foreign chemicals is that many act like hormones. The incidence of hormone-related cancers (including breast, ovarian, testicular and prostate) are all increasing. Average sperm counts of men around the world have fallen steadily in the last five decades, and it's thought that these man-made oestrogens, particularly plastics and pesticides, are to blame.

Researchers worry that unchecked, this may lead to widespread fertility problems (one in four couples in the UK now have fertility problems). These chemicals are present throughout the world, detectable even in the remotest places on Earth, but you needn't look far to find them in your immediate surrounds: plastic food packaging, non-organic food, plastics and laminates, synthetic fabrics (clothes, carpets, furniture), dry cleaning chemicals, air-fresheners (a misnomer, most of them poison the air), cosmetics, paints, glues, food additives, medicines, household cleaning products, wallpaper, the list is virtually endless, and they are all around us.

You could drive yourself crazy trying to avoid all these things, but you would be surprised at how many healthier, safer alternatives to all the above are available if you are willing to seek them out.

Foods to Avoid

- Avoid excess alcohol, which is a liver toxin. Drinking 1–2 units per day is generally not considered to be harmful, although the best gauge is how you feel afterwards or the next day. If you feel worse than you should, your liver is probably struggling to detoxify the alcohol.

- Reduce your consumption of non-organic food as much as possible, as certain foods like lettuces are often sprayed up to 11 times with pesticides and/or fungicides.

- When you can't avoid non-organic fresh produce, wash it thoroughly, or use specialist vegetable cleaning solution (e.g. Vegi-wash), or a weak vinegar/water solution to remove the majority of the pesticide residues, which are designed to resist being washed off easily by water (i.e. rain). Until very recently even the UK government advised peeling fruit for young children to reduce the risk.

- If you're trying to detox or suspect your liver is under functioning, avoid eating or drinking grapefruit. It contains narningenin, a compound known to slow liver detoxification (a glass of grapefruit juice can significantly affect the action of some medications, which explains why some very expensive medications are prescribed with grapefruit juice, it slows down the body's ability to remove the drug, thus increasing it's efficacy).

- Avoid eating excessive protein, as protein metabolism gives the liver a lot of work to do. Generally, reduce your animal protein (meat, chicken, dairy) intake, and increase the amount of vegetable protein in your diet from beans, lentils, nuts, seeds, soya and wholegrains, such as brown rice.

- Reduce your intake of saturated fats, especially hydrogenated or trans-fats, fried and highly processed foods. Your liver needs nutrients not junk. Essential fats from oily fish and seeds are vital for proper liver function (see *Fats for Anti-ageing* and *Detoxing*).

■ Caffeine, paracetamol, aspirin and most other medications place a strain on the liver. A good alternative to coffee is dandelion coffee, available in health food stores.

Friendly Foods

■ Increase your intake of all fruit and vegetables, especially those rich in antioxidants such as organic carrots, tomatoes, alfalfa sprouts, peppers and watercress.

■ Eat more berries, beetroot, celeriac, grapes, cabbage, broccoli, Brussels sprouts and kale. Aim for 40 % of your diet to be raw in summer.

■ Eat artichokes, this Mediterranean staple is not only delicious, it helps protect the liver.

■ Eat more beetroot, raw or cooked it's one of the best vegetables for the liver. Beetroot aids digestion, improves liver function and reduces constipation.

■ Eat organically produced food as much as possible, the Food Standards Agency in the UK acknowledges that pesticide residues are likely to be considerably lower than in conventional produce. You are also likely to encounter far fewer food additives and unnecessary artificial colourings or flavourings.

■ Sprinkle a dessertspoon of lecithin granules over breakfast cereals, fruits and yoghurts, as lecithin helps the body to digest fats which eases the burden on the liver.

■ If you know that your liver is a problem, then eat lighter meals regularly and don't eat heavy, rich meals. If you eat too much in one sitting, especially fatty or fried foods and alcohol then you place an enormous burden on the digestion and liver, which could make you nauseous.

Useful Remedies

■ As always, start with a good-quality multivitamin, which provides a baseline of nutrients you can then add to, such as Kudos 24 (see page 348).

■ Add 1 gram of vitamin C daily.

■ Take a 1 gram fish oil or linseed oil capsule daily. Try BioCare, Higher Nature, FSC and Seven Seas One A Day fish oils which are all free of toxins such as PCBs and dioxins (see page 13).

■ Magnesium is required by literally hundreds of enzymes throughout the body, many of which have a detoxifying function. Take at least 350mgms daily. Twice that if you have backache, twitching and/or can't sleep.

■ The best-known remedy for the liver is the herb milk thistle which contains the bioflavonoid silymarin, which promotes cell regeneration in the liver, increases levels of glutathione (see below), and has been shown to repair liver damage from alcohol. For optimum effects you need 600mg of standardized extract daily. Kudos make a high-strength milk thistle, which means you would only need 1 capsule a day. For details see page 14.

■ The most powerful antioxidant and detoxifying compound in the liver is glutathione, a naturally occurring amino acid combination. Both alpha-lipoic acid (50–100mg per day) and N-acetyl cysteine (500–600mg per day taken away from food) increase production of glutathione in the liver, as well as protecting the liver and being first-rate antioxidants in their own right.

■ Another key nutrient needed by the liver is sulphur. It can be supplemented as MSM or the amino acids cysteine and methionine. Take 500mgms of all three daily. Also include sulphur-rich foods in your diet, including garlic, asparagus, cabbage and broccoli.

■ The nutrients choline, inositol and L-methionine, prevent the accumulation of fat in the liver, thereby enhancing general liver function (take 300–400mg of each one to three times per day). Methionine also aids liver detoxification.

■ The herb dandelion is also known to be highly beneficial for the liver, mostly due to its ability to enhance the production and flow of bile (where the liver expels the toxins). It can be taken as capsules (500–1000mg daily), the leaves can be drunk as tea, and the roasted root is a common coffee substitute.

Helpful Hints

■ Standard tests for liver function involve measuring levels of key enzymes. If they're raised, it means your liver is struggling. This indicates a chronic problem and while it's useful in indicating a problem exists, it doesn't tell you the best way to help recovery. A better test, non-invasive and available through nutritionists, is a comprehensive Liver Detoxification Profile. This urine test tells you exactly which detox phases and pathways in the liver are under-performing and you can then be advised which nutrients are needed to restore normal function (to find a qualified nutritionist see *Useful Information and Addresses p338*)

■ Stop smoking and reduce the amount of time you spend in traffic there can be more pollution inside your car than outside! If you are walking or cycling avoid busy roads where possible.

■ The intravenous therapy chelation is marvellous for delivering large amounts of nutrients, especially glutiathione into the body (see *Chelation in Ageing p89*).

■ We tend to think of pollution as being solely an outdoor problem, though the home and office may be more of a concern. Indoor air pollution is now recognized as a real problem, and the availability of more natural household cleaning products, paints and fibres has improved dramatically in recent years. Visit your local health food store for natural cleaning products and see health, environmental, and organic magazines for details of more natural products.

■ Use a water filter to remove unwanted chemicals from your drinking supply. Reverse osmosis filters remove 99.999% of all known chemicals, they also remove minerals and will even filter anthrax spores. For details of reverse osmosis water filters, contact The Pure H2O Company on 01784 21188, or www.pureH20.co.uk. Or the Fresh Water Filter Company on 0870 442 3633, or www.freshwaterfilter.com (see also *Water in Ageing p325*).

■ Another good option is to drink bottled still, natural mineral water such as Volvic or Belgian SPA Water. A filter jug containing a simple carbon filter is the bare minimum but don't forget to change the cartridges regularly.

- Plants also do a remarkable job of filtering indoor air, though make sure the soil doesn't become mouldy, as this is a common source of indoor air pollutants.

- Because the liver is responsible for balancing hormones, if it's not working efficiently, hormones can accumulate inappropriately or become unbalanced, triggering problems such as facial hair. Also many women who take the Pill and orthodox HRT have put on weight, which could be because these hormones place a greater strain on the liver.

- According to traditional Chinese medicine, the liver does most work between 1 and 3am in the morning, liver dysfunction will often wake a person up at these times.

- The liver detoxes more efficiently when we are lying down and relaxed, so make sure you are getting sufficient sleep.

- Don't eat large meals late at night or drink alcohol after 11pm if you know your liver is in trouble.

- Repressed anger and resentments affect liver function, so deal with any stress-type issues.

- Dr Keith Scott-Mumby suggests this liver cleanse, **which should only be attempted with your doctor's consent** It could be considered if you wake up feeling hung-over but haven't been drinking, you are constantly tired and don't know why, you are slow getting started in the morning or have a very low tolerance to alcohol.

RECIPE
6 tablespoons of lemon juice
3 tablespoons of organic extra-virgin olive oil
1 small garlic clove, crushed
pinch of grated ginger
pinch of cayenne pepper
Whisk in a blender and drink immediately. Do not eat for at least 1 hour afterwards.

- Coffee enemas have long been known to stimulate liver function. Its use is largely retained in the natural (biological) treatment of cancers.

- A great book to read is *Tired or Toxic?* by Sherry Rogers, Prestige Publishing, New York.

LOW BLOOD SUGAR (HYPOGLYCAEMIA)
(See also *Carbohydrate Control, Essential Sugars, Insulin Resistance* and *Sugars in Ageing*)

Do you tend to miss breakfast and then crave sugary snacks by 11am? Do you suffer a brain "fog" in mid-afternoon and ease it with another coffee and a biscuit? Are you Type A – a generally stressed, rushed and/or exhausted person? If the answer is "Yes" to any of these questions, you may well have blood sugar problems. One major reason to avoid eating sugar is to slow down the ageing process. If you want to stay younger longer, you definitely need to limit your sugar intake. Sugar is the most significant physical factor that accelerates ageing. It does this by two mechanisms.

Firstly it attaches itself to proteins in the body forming sugar-protein substances called advanced glycation end-products (AGEs). The higher the AGE levels, the faster your skin will wrinkle and the AGEs also trigger inflammation, especially in the brain, which can cause mental "fogginess", and in the long-term degenerative conditions of the brain. Also, sugar increases free radicals in the body, which accelerates ageing, and the average person in the West consumes around 14kg (30lb) of sugar annually!

Eating foods with a high sugar content causes a rapid rise in your blood sugar levels. In response, the pancreas over-reacts by secreting too much insulin to remove the excess sugar from the bloodstream. This results in a drop in blood sugar, and the adrenal glands then begin secreting cortisol to balance the pancreas, which prevents glucose levels from dropping too far or too quickly. If this situation continues, over-production of insulin not only places an additional burden on the pancreas (that can lead to diabetes), but also the adrenal glands. And if the adrenal glands become exhausted, then production of cortisol is greatly reduced. If this happens, because cortisol is needed to help regulate blood sugar levels, they can eventually drop too low, which triggers headaches, brain fog and in extreme cases blackouts.

While all this is going on in your body, you will most probably crave even more sugary foods and drinks as your body strives to achieve a proper glucose/insulin balance.

Nutritionist, Kathryn Marsden, once explained this brilliantly in one of her lectures. Imagine you are setting fire to a piece of paper. Initially it bursts into bright flames which last for a few minutes, but then quickly subsides into ashes, and if you want bright flames again, you need more paper. This simple analogy is perfect to explain blood sugar problems. You eat sugar, you get the quick energy burst and then thirty minutes or so later you need more to keep the flames bright. It's an addictive vicious cycle that needs a fair amount of discipline to overcome.

Fluctuations in blood sugar can trigger feelings of depression, anxiety, mood swings, fatigue and even aggressive behaviour. Proper sugar balance is also needed for muscle contractions, the digestive system and nerve health. Additional symptoms range from restlessness, insomnia, dizziness, general shakiness and trembling, ravenous hunger and craving for sweets, plus heart problems, nausea, blurry vision, and frequent headaches or migraines.

The fluctuation in blood sugar levels is particularly harmful to the brain, which is highly sensitive to blood sugar levels. The brain uses glucose, as a source of fuel to think and function clearly, and when you become hungry then the hypothalamus area within the brain simply demands more sugar. But at this point you need to eat more foods that release their natural sugars more slowly into the bloodstream such as wholemeal bread and pastas, brown rice, etc while avoiding high sugar foods.

Sugar depletes the body of vital minerals, especially chromium, manganese, cobalt, copper, zinc, and magnesium, which are all needed to process sugar.

During my 10 years as a health writer, I have heard some dreadful stories about blood sugar problems. I have heard of dozens of cases of young women who skip breakfast, live on colas and snacks and then have fainting and blackout episodes. Such symptoms can usually be avoided by just watching your diet.

Foods to Avoid

■ The most important thing is to remove all refined and most processed foods, sugar, soft drinks, caffeine, pre-packaged fruit juices and alcohol. Alcohol severely stresses blood sugar control, particularly if you drink on an empty stomach. I'm afraid all those wonderful chocolate croissants, sugary cakes, biscuits, white rice and bread – generally "white" foods need to go. Not forever, just keep things in balance. You can have treats, but don't live on them.

■ The average can of a fizzy drink contains 8 to 9 teaspoons of sugar. When a person drinks it, the blood is hit with a hefty dose of sugar eight to nine times more than normal.

■ All these foods are low in fibre and minerals, the very things that you need to help control blood sugar.

■ Limit the foods with a high glycaemic index (see opposite).

Friendly Foods

■ Begin the day with breakfast – you are literally breaking a fast – and to keep your blood sugar on an even keel try porridge oats, sweetened with chopped fruit and a few prunes or raisins. Otherwise a low-sugar cereal, beans on toast or an egg is fine. If you cannot face breakfast, at least take with you a couple of bananas, a yoghurt and a packet of raisins and pumpkin seeds.

■ Fibre helps to slow down the release of sugars, so if you have porridge or cereal add extra rice or oat bran to increase fibre, or eat a piece of fruit before the porridge.

■ Eat sugar in the form of complex carbohydrates, high in fibre, like brown rice and pasta, barley, lentils, spelt, amaranth, millet and vegetables. The body slowly breaks these down into simple sugars, which are steadily released into the bloodstream giving sustained energy.

■ Eat a little protein with each meal. Good proteins are fish, unrefined nuts, seeds, tempeh, skinless turkey or chicken, low-fat yoghurt (preferably sheep or goats').

■ Reduce saturated fats found in meats and dairy foods, but include more good-quality oils, such as olive oil, unrefined flaxseed or fish oil, walnut or sunflower oil. (Do not use these for cooking, apart from olive oil.) The presence of some fat in the diet helps to slow the uptake of glucose into the blood (for more details see *Fats for Anti-ageing p139*).

■ To keep the blood sugar at a relatively constant level, eat little and often, about 4–6 small meals/snacks a day. Do not allow yourself to become really hungry. Some people with chronic hypoglycaemia find it helpful to eat a small snack such as a banana with a few seeds at bedtime.

■ During a hypoglycaemic reaction, a good snack would be a couple of oatcakes with nut butter (almond, hazelnut, cashew or peanut), or oat or rice cakes with goats' cheese or avocado. However, in acute cases, such as fainting, extreme weakness, trembling and giddiness, it is vital to restore blood sugar balance as quickly as possible. Although it's not the long-term solution, give the person a sugary drink such as Lucozade, or a sugary biscuit, which should alleviate their symptoms fairly quickly.

■ The glycaemic index is a measure of how a given food affects blood-glucose levels, with each food assigned a numbered rating. The lower the rating, the slower the digestion and absorption process. Conversely, a high rating means blood-glucose levels are increased quickly.

■ Eat foods which are low on the glycaemic index. The lower the number the better, although you can take a small portion of food which is high on the glycaemic index if you mix it with a protein food.

Glycaemic Index Table

Biscuits	70
Fruit preserve (without sugar)	25
Fructose (fruit sugar) (Fructose is many times sweeter than ordinary sugar – use for baking etc.)	20
Glucose	100
Honey	87
Jam	55
Maltose	100
Sugar (sucrose)	59
White bread	70
Brown bread	65
Wholemeal bread or bread with bran	46
Wholemeal rye bread	41
100% stoneground wholemeal bread	35
Refined cereals with sugar	73
Wholegrain cereals without sugar	66
Oat flakes	49
Cornflakes	80
Popcorn	85
Chocolate bars	68

Dark chocolate (over 60% cocoa)	22
Milk products	36
White rice	72
Wholegrain rice	66
Non-wholewheat pasta	55
Wholewheat pasta	42
100% stoneground wholewheat pasta	30
Fresh fruit juice (without sugar)	37
Fresh fruit	30
Bananas	62
Lemons	15
Red kidney beans	29
Dried peas	35
Dried beans	31
Lentils	29
Corn (maize)	70
Chickpeas	36
Soya	15
Peas	51
Carrots	49
Beetroot	64
Mashed potatoes	90
Baked jacket potatoes	85
Boiled potatoes	70 New potatoes 50
Green vegetables, tomatoes, mushrooms	Less than 15

Useful Remedies for Hypoglycaemia

■ Chromium in the form of chromium picolinate, chromium polynicotinate, or GTF chromium, helps control blood sugar levels by assisting insulin to carry glucose into cells to be burned for energy. American research has found that taking just 200mcg daily can reduce the likelihood of late-onset diabetes by as much as 50%.

- You also need a multimineral formula that contains 200–400mg of magnesium, which helps to keep you calm and balances blood sugar.

- A high-strength vitamin B-complex helps support the adrenal glands and plays a major part in carbohydrate metabolism.

- Carnosine is a naturally occurring antioxidant made within the body and as we age the levels fall. High concentrations of carnosine are present in long-lived cells such as in nerve tissues and people who live longer have higher levels of this nutrient. Carnosine has been shown to help reverse age-related damage caused by advanced glycation end-products (AGEs) especially in the skin. It's also found in lean red meat and chicken. Take 100mg daily on an empty stomach. Available from The NutriCentre and Sloane Health Foods (see page 14) or order from the Life Extension Foundation on www.lef.org

- Vitamin C helps support the adrenal glands, which help to regulate blood sugar levels. Take 1gram daily.

- Glucobalance is specially formulated for hypoglycaemia, and contains chromium polynicotinate and vitamins C and B5 which support the adrenal glands. Other ingredients include vanadium and L carnitine. It also contains vitamins B1, B3 and B3 which are needed for energy production. For details contact The NutriCentre (see page14 for details).

Helpful Hints

- If you are an adrenaline junkie, live on your nerves, snacking on junk foods, you need to take a long hard look at your life, and change your diet.

- Living on adrenaline is an alternative way to produce energy as this causes blood sugar to be released from the cells. In time, the adrenal glands become exhausted due to overuse and low blood sugar problems worsen. Make efforts to reduce or eliminate stress.

- In some people low blood pressure is linked to low blood sugar.

- Regular exercise is very important as it improves insulin sensitivity, glucose tolerance and increases tissue chromium concentrations.

- Read *The Low Blood Sugar Cookbook* by Patricia and Edward Krimmel, Franklin Publishers.

- Read *The X Factor Diet* by Leslie Kenton, Vermilion.

LOW STOMACH ACID

(See also *Digestion* and *Leaky Gut in Ageing*)

As we age, stomach acid levels tend to fall, which means that we no longer absorb sufficient nutrients for good health. This is especially true of protein foods such as meat, which are harder to digest and this accelerates with age.

When we eat, our stomachs should produce a lot of gastric juice in response. This juice is a combination of mucous, which protects the stomach lining, and a very strong acid, hydrochloric acid – HCl. High levels of hydrochloric acid are needed for proper digestion before the food moves on to the small intestine and the nutrients can be absorbed. Thanks to our modern lifestyle of eating in a hurry, eating too many fried foods that are hard to digest, stress and not chewing properly, the amount of acid we produce over time tends to decline.

Conditions linked with low stomach acid levels are asthma, candida and allergies. Many people feel they make too much stomach acid, whereas in reality they usually make too little. A simple test is featured under *Helpful Hints* in this section.

For instance, when we eat a cheese sandwich, hopefully we chew it thoroughly and it moves down to the stomach, which begins the digestion process. If, however, the stomach doesn't produce enough acid, the valve that shuts off the oesophagus from the stomach doesn't close properly, because it will only close in response to a high level of hydrochloric acid. If it doesn't close properly then a little acid can leak up and trigger a burning feeling in the chest, known as acid reflux. At this point most people take an antacid, which neutralizes what little acid was there, making digestion even harder.

Undigested foods can end up leaking into the bloodstream triggering food intolerances. Also undigested food can rot in the bowel causing wind, bloating, and overgrowth of unhealthy organisms such as candida. Low stomach acid also allows bacteria such as helicobacter pylori, known to cause stomach ulcers, to thrive.

Foods to Avoid

- Cut down on alcohol, sugar, caffeinated foods and drinks, cows' milk and dairy produce, which can all cause an acid reflux.
- Don't eat in a rush and keep heavy, rich meals containing red meat and creamy sauces to a minimum.
- Avoid all fried foods, and especially melted cheese, which are hard to digest.
- Avoid eating proteins like fish and meat with potatoes or pasta. This is the basis for food combining (see *Useful Information and Addresses* p338).
- Avoid drinking too much liquid with meals.
- Stop chewing gum, this makes the stomach think that food is about to arrive and so it begins producing stomach acid.
- Don't eat a large amount of fruit directly after a heavy meal, as it can get stuck behind the meal and ferment, which makes the problem even worse.

Friendly Foods

- 2 teaspoons of apple cider vinegar and 1 teaspoon of honey in a glass of warm water taken before each meal is a superb way of improving low stomach acid.
- A natural way to discover if you have low stomach acid, it to eat some beetroot and if your urine turns pink, this denotes lack of stomach acid.

■ Chew your food thoroughly and eat more slowly, you would be amazed how this simple practise can hugely improve your digestion.

■ Eat fruit generally in-between meals, or have a little papaya or pineapple before meals as these fruits are packed with digestive enzymes.

■ Bitter vegetables are great for stimulating digestion, such as celeriac, artichoke and celery. These foods stimulate gastric juices in anticipation of the arrival of food.

■ Ginger aids digestion.

■ Manuka honey can help heal the stomach and discourage helicobacter.

■ Drink mint or peppermint herbal teas to aid digestion.

Useful Remedies

■ Levels of stomach acid tend to drop as we age, or when we are under stress. Take 1 betaine hydrochloride (stomach acid) capsule with main meals. If you have active stomach ulcers, use a good-quality digestive enzyme supplement instead.

■ Take 10–20 drops peppermint formula before a meal. If you suffer with symptoms of feeling bloated and uncomfortable take 10–20 drops after a meal.

■ Acidophilus/bifidus are the healthy bacteria that help to regulate digestion. Take 1–2 capsules at the end of the meal. If the gut flora is in good shape the body's ability to manufacture hydrochloric acid is improved.

■ Chloride Compound helps to encourage the body to produce more stomach acid. Available from Blackmores (see page 13). Take 3 tablets daily, 1 with each meal.

Helpful Hints

■ Some people have found separating proteins and carbohydrates at one meal greatly improves digestion.

■ Avoid eating when you are stressed, on the move, or when you are distracted from eating as this makes digestion very difficult.

■ Eat small meals regularly rather than large rich meals, especially at night. Become a grazer.

■ Dr John Briffa suggests this home test for low stomach acid in his book *Body Wise* (Cima Books). Take a level teaspoon of bicarbonate of soda and dissolve in some water. Drink this mixture on an empty stomach. If sufficient quantities of acid are present in the stomach, the bicarb mixture is converted into gas, producing significant bloating and belching within 5 to 10 minutes of drinking the mix. Little or no belching denotes low stomach acid.

■ If you have pronounced longitudinal ridges in your nails, this is a common sign of low stomach acid.

■ Walking for 30 minutes each day aids digestion.

LUNGS IN AGEING

(See also *Breathing* and *Oxygen in Ageing*)

Your ability to take a really lung-filling deep breath can decline by up to 40% by the time you reach 70. That is, unless you exercise regularly and learn how to breathe properly. Over time, it becomes harder to completely fill the lungs on the inhalation or to empty them on exhalation, which leaves more stale air in the lungs.

This leads us onto another important biomarker of ageing which is called Aerobic Capacity. Your aerobic capacity is your ability to sustain exercise over time, it is one of the most important measures of your fitness level and greatly affects how well you will age. The greater your aerobic capacity the healthier your lungs will be, you have more energy and will stay younger longer.

Normal ageing brings about a decline in aerobic capacity as the lungs take in less oxygen and the heart pumps less forcefully during exertion. Therefore, the more optimally you can fill and empty your lungs, the more oxygen exchange takes place, which gives every cell more energy. People with healthy lungs also tend to have healthier hearts and circulation, more muscles and less fat.

Unfortunately, long-term exposure to pollution, pesticides, air-borne chemicals, cigarettes, dust and so on, can cause the lungs to become congested and the more congestion, the less oxygen gets through to our blood and we tire more easily, we experience memory problems, tired-looking skin and so on. And if even light amounts of exercise cause breathlessness, you need to take urgent steps to improve your lung function.

Avoidance of smoking is the most important way to minimize the affect of ageing on the lungs. And regular exercise will improve aerobic capacity.

Stress and sitting around all day, can cause you to shallow breathe and lungs lose their elasticity, which leaves you more likely to suffer conditions like bronchitis (see also *Breathing* p67 to learn how to breathe more deeply).

Foods to Avoid

- Avoid foods that contain hydrogenated/trans-fats and oils. These types of fats are linked to asthma (see *Fats for Anti-ageing p139*).

- Wheat and cows' milk can trigger coughing. To find out if these foods are a problem eliminate them from your diet for one week and see if your breathing eases. Try rye and amaranth crackers, spelt or rye breads and organic rice or goats' milk as a substitute. Keep a food diary and note when your breathing becomes more laboured.

- Avoid mucus-producing foods such as full-fat dairy products, processed foods, desserts, croissants, chocolate, cheese and "white" doughy foods.

- Too much sugar places an extra burden on your immune system and if you already have poor lung function and you eat too much mucus-producing foods and then become run down, don't be surprised if you end up with a cold or worse (see *Immune Function in Ageing*).

■ Some people also find soya milk produces a lot of mucus.

Friendly Foods

■ Make the effort to eat more fresh fruits and vegetables, make sure they are organic as much as possible. Fruits like apples. which are great for lung health, can be covered in up to six pesticides – you need the apples but not the chemicals!

■ Eat vine-ripened tomatoes which are rich in the carotene lycopene, which helps support the lungs. When the tomatoes are cooked with a little oil then the lycopene is released.

■ Eat more broccoli, cauliflower, cabbage, Brussels sprouts and turnips, which are rich in beta-carotene and protect mucous membranes, especially in the lungs.

■ Quercetins – flavonoids found in apples, pears, cherries, grapes, onions, kale, broccoli, garlic, green tea and red wine – help protect the lungs from the harmful effects of pollutants and cigarette smoke.

■ Eat more oily fish, pumpkin and sweet potatoes, which are rich in vitamin A, to support your immune system. Make fresh soups, which are a healthy way to ingest lots of nutrients.

■ Limonene may help to protect the lungs and is found in the rinds and the edible white membranes of citrus fruits such as oranges, grapefruit, tangerines, lemons and limes.

■ Vitamin B1 (thiamine) is essential for maintaining health in the lungs so eat foods such as peas, wholegrain rice, and pistachio nuts.

■ Brown rice, avocados, spinach, haddock, oatmeal, baked potatoes, navy beans, lima beans, broccoli, yoghurt, bananas, and unrefined nuts are all rich in magnesium, which is vital for healthy lungs.

■ Eat more garlic and onions, which help to fend off infection and clear the lungs.

Useful Remedies

■ As a good base, take a multivitamin/mineral daily.

■ Bromelain, extracted from pineapples, is great for bronchial conditions, which helps to loosen mucus. If symptoms are acute take 1000mcu daily.

■ Drink fenugreek or liquorice teas to soothe the lungs.

■ Antioxidants protect the lungs, especially from pollution (see *Pollution Protection* and *Antioxidants in Ageing*).

■ Vitamin C and magnesium. *The American Journal of Respiratory and Critical Care Medicine* reported on a study which confirmed that people who consume high levels of vitamin C and magnesium tend to have healthier lungs and experience less decline in lung function over time. Take 1gram of vitamin C daily along with 400mg of magnesium. Magnesium is also often lacking in those who suffer asthma-type conditions.

■ N-acetyl cysteine is a great amino acid that not only helps to break up excess mucus, but also reduces the bacterial count for anyone suffering from bronchitis. Take 500mg twice daily, 30 minutes before food.

■ Expectorant herbs that will help clear any "gunk" in your lungs are garlic, white horehound and euphorbia, which can be found in tablets and tinctures.

■ The herb mullein helps to support and strengthen the lungs. Take 2mls twice daily in water.

Helpful Hints

■ Ask your doctor, or a local health clinic, for an aerobic capacity lung function test. This usually consists of simply blowing into a tube for as long as you can and the results can be monitored instantly.

■ Regular exercise at any age can help strengthen the heart and lungs. It gets the blood circulating, delivers more oxygen into the lungs and boosts metabolism. If you have not exercised for a long time, begin by walking for 15–20 minutes a day and gradually increase to one hour daily. As much as possible, exercise away from busy, polluted main roads and go on holiday to destinations with cleaner air – and *breathe*.

■ Many mass-produced household cleaning fluids, perfumes, paint sprays and gardening products contain chemicals that you definitely don't want to inhale into your lungs. Use environmentally friendly products such as Ecover available in health stores and supermarkets.

■ Practise taking deeper breaths (see *Breathing p67*). You can increase the efficiency of your lungs a thousandfold by increasing your air intake by a mere 5% on each breath. Sing, when you are home alone – as singing really helps increase lung capacity. But please, don't drive your neighbours crazy!

■ Use an Ultra Breathe, a small inexpensive device that really does a great job of exercising the lungs. For details call 0870 608 9019 or visit: www.ultrabreathe.com

■ Inhaling steam is a great way to open up the lungs, either use the steam room at your local health club or, if you become congested, place some boiling water in a bowl, add a few drops of Olbas or eucalyptus oil, and place your head over the bowl, cover your head with a dry towel and inhale the steam for 5 minutes twice daily.

■ If you end up with a lung infection and take antibiotics, then make sure you take a course of acidophilus/bifidus, healthy bacteria that will have been killed by the antibiotics. And remember by taking more antioxidants all year round, you boost immunity, which helps prevent many illnesses from taking hold.

MACULAR DEGENERATION

(See also *Cataracts* and *Eyes in Ageing*)

Macular degeneration (AMD – aged-related macular degeneration) is the slow deterioration of cells in the macula, a tiny yellowish area in the central part of the retina which is responsible for visual sharpness. This deterioration affects your ability to read, write, drive and so on. Macular degeneration is now the leading cause of blindness in people over the age of 55, and 25% of people in the West over the age of 65 have symptoms of AMD, which increase with age.

There are two types of macular degeneration, wet and dry. Ninety per cent of people with macular degeneration have the dry type, in which small, yellow spots called drusens form underneath the macular. Drusens are waste products that accumulate because of lack of antioxidants to clear them from the eyes. The drusens slowly break down the cells in the macular, causing distorted vision. In the wet type, abnormal blood vessels begin to grow toward the macular, causing rapid and severe vision loss.

Scientists now believe that AMD is triggered by oxidative stress, caused by free radical reactions in the body, especially in the retina because of its high consumption of oxygen (see *Antioxidants in Ageing p38*). Free radical reactions occur as the normal by-products of living, eating and breathing, but also from over-exposure to ultraviolet radiation, smoking, a poor diet and a compromised immune system.

It is also linked to hardening of the arteries and poor circulation (see *High Blood Pressure p170* and *Circulation p100*).

Some people believe that macular degeneration is inherited, but diet is a far more important factor. However, women with light coloured irises are more at risk from AMD.

Foods to Avoid

■ Avoid full-fat dairy foods, plus meats, hamburgers, mass-produced pies, sausages, cheeses, chocolates and sugary, fatty foods. All the usual suspects.

■ Definitely avoid too many fried foods and hydrogenated/trans-fats found in most margarines and mass-produced vegetable oils (see *Fats for Anti-ageing p139*).

■ Cut down or eliminate sodium-based salt, use a natural mineral sea salt available from all good health stores.

■ Avoid monosodium glutamate (MSG), which is a potential retinal toxin.

■ Excessive alcohol, but the occasional glass of wine is fine. Too much alcohol interferes with liver function, and reduces protective glutathione levels in the eyes.

■ At all costs avoid foods and drinks containing aspartame.

Friendly Foods

■ The most important foods for reducing and preventing AMD are carotenes (especially lutein and zeaxanthin). Lutein is found in all dark green leafy vegetables such as spinach, kale, broccoli, spring greens, cabbage and so on. Zeaxanthin is found in yellow and orange fruits and vegetables such as carrots, yams, peaches, persimmons, pumpkin, sweet potatoes, mangoes, apricots and cantaloupe melons.

- Other great eye foods are onions, apples, green tea, cherries, pears, grapes, cranberries, red onions, garlic, mustard greens, alfalfa sprouts, asparagus and butternut squash.
- Generally eat more wholefoods such as brown bread, rice and pastas.
- Eat oily fish and other fish in preference to meats.
- Eat more blueberries, bilberries and blackcurrants.
- In addition, green drinks of organic grasses, blue-green and sea algae, herbs and other nutrients are very helpful.
- Vitamin E-rich foods help reduce the risk of developing AMD. These include hazel nuts, almonds, cod liver oil, raw wheatgerm and tomato purée.

Useful Remedies

- Take a high-strength multivitamin/mineral daily as a base. Make sure your multi contains 200mcg of selenium and 50mg of zinc.
- Bilberry has been called the vision herb for its powerful effect on all types visual disorders. British Royal Air Force pilots during World War II reported improved night-time vision after consuming bilberry. Bilberry supports the structural integrity of the tiny capillaries that deliver oxygen and nutrients to the eyes, take 200-300mg daily.
- Bioflavonoids, such as quercetin and rutin, are neither vitamins nor minerals but plant pigments rich in antioxidants that protect the eyes from sunlight damage. Take 1,000mg daily of a mixed bioflavonoid supplement daily.
- Glutathione is essential for vision. It is an antioxidant found in large concentrations in the eye. Diminished levels of glutathione occur during aging which makes the lens nucleus susceptible to oxidative stress induced clouding, take 500mg daily.
- Cysteine is important for a healthy retina. Taken as N-acetyl-cysteine (NAC), it increases production of glutathione, one of the most important antioxidants in the eye. Take 500mg daily.
- Taurine is another potent antioxidant that is highly concentrated within the eye. A deficiency of this amino acid alters the structure and function of the retina. Taurine also helps prevent cataracts. Take 500mg daily.
- If you don't eat plenty of carotene-rich foods, you definitely need to take a high-strength natural source carotene complex.
- Vitamin C helps make collagen, which strengthens the capillaries that nourish the retina, and protects against UV light. The eye contains the second highest concentration of vitamin C in the body next to the adrenal glands. Take 1gram daily in an ascorbate form.
- Most of the companies listed on pages 13 and 14 make all-in-one eye formulas that contain most of the above.

M.E. (MYALGIC ENCEPHALOMYELITIS)
(See *Chronic Fatigue*)

MEDITATION
(See also *Mind Power*)

In the past, meditation was usually associated with the hippy, New Age culture. But these days science has validated its numerous benefits.

Dr Serena Roney-Dougal, a parapsychologist based at the PSI Research Center in Glastonbury in the UK, says "Regular meditation slows the ageing process because it decreases the amount of thyroxin produced by the thyroid gland, which acts as the metabolic regulator – or body clock. High levels of thyroxin means that all body processes speed up (see *Thyroid in Ageing*), lower levels of thyroxin allow the body to slow down to an optimal level. Regular, meditation helps to keep the thyroid balanced.

Meditation also stimulates the pineal gland situated in the centre of the brain, traditionally known as the third eye or the Ajna Chakra, which acts as the off switch for many of the hormones that contribute to ageing."

Dr Serena adds, "It has been my experience in 23 years of yoga and meditation that when one attains total stillness and no thoughts, that linear time, as we know it, stands still and I consider from that experience that whilst one is experiencing time as being stopped, the body stops ageing." Dr Deepak Chopra makes similar statements in his book, *Grow Younger, Live Younger*.

Meditation reduces the release of the stress hormones adrenalin and cortisol which are major contributing factors in heart disease, strokes and ulcers and it helps you to better tolerate stressful situations. Researchers have also found that people who meditate regularly sleep more easily, as they produce more of the hormone melatonin .

Naturopath, Steve Langley, who studied meditation in a Zen monastery in Kyoto, Japan says, "Being in the alpha state has been proven to increase our immune system and even deeper states can help raise levels of the anti-ageing hormone DHEA" (see *Other Vital Hormones p237*).

Meditation costs nothing, you can practise it daily on your own or with friends and it has proven health benefits. Studies show that the positive effects can be greater than those gained from sleep – so that's a pretty profound reason to begin today. People who meditate regularly look younger, enjoy better mental clarity, more peace of mind, feel more contented with their lives, have a reduced heart rate and lower blood pressure; they breathe more easily and if they become ill, recover more quickly. Under pressure they remain calm and are generally less anxious.

The single biggest reason people don't meditate is because they do not have the time. Well, it seems if we could make time, the benefits would far outweigh the loss of 15–20 minutes per day.

The basis of meditation is to switch your brain waves from their normal busy "beta" state to a more relaxed "alpha" state. This allows your right, intuitive, psychic brain to click in. Many spiritual masters are almost permanently in a theta state, which most doctors say would require you to be comatose!

Chronic insomniacs soon learn to shut off their "brain chatter", which allows deeper more refreshing sleep. Researchers have also found that regular meditation is as powerful as some drugs for lowering blood pressure, and meditation does not have the negative side effects. In some areas learning meditation is available on the NHS.

Foods to Avoid

■ Meditation is best done in the morning before you begin the rush of the day, or at dusk. Even if you just sit quietly for 10 minutes daily on an empty stomach, this will help.

■ Generally don't meditate on a full stomach which may make you uncomfortable and reduce your concentration.

Friendly Foods

■ If you like to meditate before going to bed, make sure you eat a light meal early, have a walk and then settle for your meditation.

Useful Remedies

■ The herb sceletium, from South Africa, has been used for centuries to reduce anxiety, improve mood and increase one's sense of connection and perception. Take 100–200mg one hour before meditating. Nutritionist, Patrick Holford, has formulated a Connect Formula containing this herb and others that aid meditation. For details call Higher Nature (see page 13).

■ Isopogan is an Australian Bush Flower Essence that helps to integrate left and right brain activity. Available from The NutriCentre and Sloane Health (see page 14).

■ Bach Flower Remedies – white chestnut and walnut – taken in water will help still the mind.

Helpful Hints

■ There are now hundreds of books teaching you how to practise this age-old art, one of my favourites is *The Meditation Plan* by Dr Richard Lawrence. Piatkus.

■ Meanwhile, find a straight-backed comfortable chair and sit with your back straight and your feet firmly on the ground. Take a few deep breaths – breathe in – close your eyes and *relax*, say the word "relax" to yourself and as you see the word in your mind's eye, allow the feeling of calm to flood from the top of your head right down to your toes. Then simply invite a golden light to come from the Heavens and imagine it flowing, like a liquid, through the top of your head, down to your toes and into the ground. Then visualize your mind as a bowl of clear white light that is totally empty and enjoy the peace. Many people have a mantra such as Om or "I am", which they repeat silently over and over to help reduce their "brain chatter". It takes a while but with practice you will get better. There are thousands of meditations, it is just a question of finding which one really suits you.

- Frankincense oil placed in a burner helps the mind to relax, or use incense sticks, or dab a small amount of the oil on the third eye area to help induce a calmer state.
- Light a candle or, even better, several to create the right atmosphere.
- Chanting induces similar results to meditation. Again find a chant that suits you best. I discovered a tape called *The Sounds of Creation – How To Set Your Spirit Free*, by healer Kim Hutchison. She uses powerful sounds for each chakra, that over time alter your DNA structure, which encourages the body to release its own healing power. The sounds are quite unusual, but since I have been using the tape, my psychic abilities have improved considerably. If you find it really hard to still your mind, then try this tape 3 times a week and then meditate quietly on alternate days. For further details, you can call Kim on 01844 217772.

MEMORY

(See also *Alzheimer's Disease, Brain in Ageing, Circulation and Oxygen in Ageing*)

At the age of 53, I regularly forget people's names and where I placed my car keys, but just because you forget a few things, it doesn't automatically mean that you have Alzheimer's or dementia, so don't panic. Most people think that once a brain cell dies, it's gone forever, but scientists in America have now proven that brain cells can be regenerated (see *Brain in Ageing p59*).

Like any other muscle in the body, the brain needs regular use and if you don't use it you lose it. The secret to improving your memory is to keep your brain active, eat less junk food but more brain foods. There really is no need for your memory or brain function to decline with age – my mother-in-law is 88 and her brain is as sharp as a razor as she has spent 30 years regularly completing crosswords.

Temporary memory loss is not uncommon after drinking alcohol, if your blood sugar level is low, after a high fever, surgery, an epileptic fit, or when under stress. Depression and acute anxiety can also cause temporary memory loss.

More serious memory loss can occur after an accident, brain injury or stroke. Senile dementia involves progressive loss of short-term memory until the individual is unable to remember what they did or saw only a few moments before. Many prescription drugs also affect memory.

External influences such as poor eyesight and hearing can inhibit our ability to learn – thus affecting memory.

However, the vast majority of cases of poor memory are caused by a lifetime of eating too many of the wrong foods, especially saturated fats which clog the arteries until the small capillaries are affected, and if insufficient fresh blood reaches the brain, it is deprived of oxygen. Most of us forget to breathe deeply on a regular basis, so make sure you take really deep breaths at least every 20 minutes.

Lead is well known to affect memory, hence why lead free petrol was introduced on both environmental and health grounds. Mercury fillings are also linked to memory loss (see *Toxic Metal Overload p317*).

Foods to Avoid

- If you want to retain a good memory, you need to cut down on high-fat foods such as meat and full-fat dairy foods. This includes mass-produced pies, cakes, biscuits, white bread, pizzas, burgers etc which not only deplete nutrients but also contribute to clogging your arteries as most of these foods are usually high in fat, sugar and salt. Research shows that people who eat high-fat, nutrient-poor foods, such as burgers and chips are less intelligent and have poorer memories than those who eat a low-fat nutrient dense diet.

- Stimulants like tea, coffee and alcohol all deplete the body of vital nutrients.

- Avoid excess sodium-based table salt and don't add salt to food once cooked.

- In some people excess wheat triggers "brain fog".

- Avoid too much sugar, which ages your brain (see *Sugar in Ageing p302*).

- Also see *Foods to Avoid* under *Brain in Ageing p59*.

- Avoid aspartame and monosodium glutamate (MSG).

Friendly Foods

- Low blood sugar levels can trigger "foggy brain" symptoms like memory loss. Therefore eat small meals regularly to balance blood sugar (see *Low Blood Sugar p194*).

- Always eat breakfast, a low-sugar cereal, such as muesli or porridge is great, as they are rich in B vitamins that are often lacking in dementia patients, especially B12.

- Omega-3 essential fats rich in EPA and DHA, are vital brain nutrients found in oily fish: tuna, salmon, sardines, herrings, and mackerel.

- Use unrefined, preferably organic, olive oil, sunflower, walnut and sesame oils for salad dressings and drizzle over cooked foods (see *Fats for Anti-ageing p139*).

- Fresh coffee is often criticized, but in terms of memory function it seems to help it, particularly in the elderly. Two cups a day is fine.

- Green leafy vegetables, particularly spinach, cabbage, pak choy, celery, broccoli, spring greens, plus red and purple fruits like strawberries, blueberries, blackberries and cherries are rich in antioxidants, which help to slow age-related memory decline.

- Apples, peaches, lychees, pineapple, grapes, prunes and raisins are all great memory foods.

- Eat more brown pasta and rice, wholemeal bread and flour, barley and buckwheat.

- For those with a sweet tooth, use a little brown rice syrup or fructose.

- Phosphatidyl choline is a vital brain nutrient found in egg yolks (ask for Columbus eggs, which are free-range eggs from chickens that are fed on healthy essential fats), fish (especially sardines), plus lecithin granules, which also reduce the amounts of LDL, the "bad" cholesterol in your body. Taking this brain nutrient during pregnancy can result in brainier children. Sprinkle a tablespoon of lecithin over your breakfast cereal, into salads or yoghurts. Make sure the brand you buy is a GM-free product with at least 30% phosphatidyl choline content, such as cytoplan. Available from health stores, or call The NutriCentre (see page 14).

- Eat more ginger and live, low-fat yoghurt to aid digestion.

- Add freshly chopped sage to your salads and meals as it has been shown to improve memory and brain function – but not if you are pregnant.

Useful Remedies

- As some of the detailed supplements thin the blood naturally, if you are on blood thinning drugs, speak to your doctor before trying those marked * below, as in time your prescription drugs dose could be lowered.

- Firstly, take a good all-round combination formula that contains vitamins, minerals, antioxidants, brain nutrients and essential fats all-in-one powder, such as Kudos 24 – for details see page 348.

- The Siberian herb, rhodiola, has been shown to greatly improve concentration and memory. In Siberia where rhodiola tea is drunk regularly, many people live until well past 100. It also reduces the negative effects that stress hormones have on our body and mind. Kudos make a high-strength one-a-day capsule. Call 0208 392 6524.

- The herb *gingko biloba is proven to increase memory as it improves blood flow to the brain. Take 1 dose three times a day either as tincture or tablets, around 60–300mg of standardized extract. Kudos, as above, also make a high-strength one-a-day capsule.

- An extract of the periwinkle plant called *Vinpocetine, like ginkgo, is another herb that helps improve circulation. It is especially useful when blood flow to the brain is diminished, as in hardening of the arteries or minor strokes, and it also helps some people with tinnitus (ringing in the ears). Take 20–40mg daily. Available from the NutriCentre (see page 14).

- Phosphatidyl serine, taking 100mg up to three times a day has been shown to improve mental function. Take early in the day, as at night this can increase dreaming and delay you getting to sleep.

- Co-enzyme Q10, taking 100mg a day can improve energy production within the brain.

- Include a daily vitamin B-complex, as B vitamins are essential for normal brain function.

- The amino acid, glutamine, also makes a great brain food as it is the most abundant amino acid in the fluid that surrounds the brain. Take 250mg daily.

Helpful Hints

■ Regular exercise is vital for aiding memory, the more oxygen you get to the brain, the less likely you are to lose your memory.

■ Common sage contains considerable amounts of thujone (a naturally occurring substance that gives sage its flavour) which, if used as an essential oil of sage, can trigger fits in sensitive individuals. However, Spanish sage contains almost no thujone. All sage is great and safe for cooking – but if using sage essential oil, make sure it is derived from Spanish sage, as regular head massage with this oil (diluted in a base oil) has been shown by Dr John Wilkinson at Middlesex University to increase memory functioning. For details of Spanish sage oil contact Essentially Oils Ltd, Chipping Norton, Oxfordshire. Tel: 01608 659544, or visist: www.essentiallyoils.com.

■ Chelation therapy helps to unclog your arteries, which increases the amount of blood and oxygen that reach the brain (see *Chelation in Ageing p89*).

■ Keeping the brain active is a crucial aspect for improving memory. Studies have shown that people who do not retire, but work and stay active into their late 60s or 70s have a better memory. Play more word games, do crosswords. During car journeys or when on a train or queuing in a supermarket add or multiply varying numbers in your head.

■ Minimize aluminum exposure, this includes many deodorants, cooking pans, some cheeses etc (see *Alzheimer's Disease p33*).

■ Minimize exposure to mercury (see *Toxic Metal Overload p317*).

■ Avoid using a mobile phone for more than 10 minutes at a time, and avoid using them in cars and trains which amplifies the negative effects, not only for you, but for those sitting around you (see *Radiation in Ageing p265*).

■ If, after trying these remedies for three months you are still experiencing memory problems, consult a nutritionist who is also a doctor (see the *Hints* section under *Alzheimer's Disease*).

■ Rubbing essential oil of basil and/or rosemary, in a base of almond oil, into the scalp will help to increase circulation to the scalp and clear your mind, thus aiding concentration. .

■ For further help read *Optimum Nutrition for the Mind* by Patrick Holford, Piatkus.

MENOPAUSE

(See also *Osteoporosis, Other Vital Hormones* and *Women's Hormones*)

The menopause is not an illness for which you need a drug (orthodox HRT). It is part of the normal cycle of a woman's hormonal life when the menstrual cycles cease. Menopause generally occurs between the ages of 45 and 55, though it can occur as early as 35 or as late as 65 years of age.

Dr Marilyn Glenville, an expert on the menopause, says, "At the time of menopause, a women still produces oestrogen but not sufficient to prepare her womb for pregnancy. Levels of progesterone plummet or disappear completely. The ovaries continue to produce small quantities of oestrogen for at least 12 years after the onset of the menopause."

For most women the menopause happens in three phases. Firstly comes peri-menopause when you still have periods but they may become heavier or lighter, and symptoms such as hot flushes can appear. Then comes menopause when ovarian function decline, and periods stop. The last phase is called post-menopause, which begins 12 months after your last period.

Throughout this time, many signs associated with ageing can appear as the hormonal balance alters with the drop in oestrogen and progesterone levels. Skin is more likely to wrinkle, there can be growth of facial hair and a thinning of hair in the temple region. Muscles lose some strength and tone, and many women suffer hot flushes and insomnia. Your joints may begin to ache and bones can become more brittle, increasing the risk of osteoporosis.

Vaginal dryness often results from these hormonal changes. The vaginal wall also becomes thinner and blood flow is restricted. Dryness can make sexual intercourse painful or uncomfortable and can lead to irritation and increased risk for infection. You will be happy to note that having regular sexual intercourse increases blood flow into the vagina.

Loss of bladder tone, which can result in stress incontinence (leaking urine when you cough, sneeze, laugh or exercise), can also result (see *Bladder Problems in Ageing*).

You may also experience a whole host of emotional ups and downs, one minute feeling on top of the world and the next in the pits of despair. The good news is that by eating the right diet, taking the right supplements, doing some exercise and using natural hormone replacements – virtually all these symptoms can be alleviated.

I do not advocate taking orthodox hormone replacement therapy (HRT) because of the increased risk of high blood pressure, weight gain, gall bladder and liver problems, not to mention breast and endometrial (uterine) cancers. The increased health risks of orthodox HRT have now been shown to far out-weigh the benefits. Yes, it slows the rate of bone loss, but only while you are taking it. Also, if you are under a lot of stress at this time, adrenal function is greatly affected. Healthy adrenal glands continue to supply post-menopausal women with oestrogen. But if you are stressed, then your adrenal glands are kept busy pumping the stress hormone cortisol and less oestrogen is made.

On the subject of oestrogen, most women are also becoming aware of the condition known as oestrogen dominance. This occurs when the amount of oestrogen in the body is not balanced by the proper amount of progesterone. This can occur from failed ovulations, or by over-exposure to environmental chemicals found in herbicides, pesticides and plastics, called xenoestrogens, which have an oestrogen-like effect on the body. These chemicals accumulate in our fatty tissue and greatly increase the risk of cancers.

When you have too much oestrogen activity compared to progesterone, you can suffer symptoms such as water retention, bloating, and menstrual irregularities. Globally we are living in a dangerous ocean of hormone-disrupting chemicals, which are triggering lowered sperm counts, animals and fish are changing sex, and we too are seeing sexual mutations.

One problem with conventional HRT is that they do not use progesterone but synthetic hormone-like substances called progestins, which are artificial hormones. These have side-effects such as irritability, liver dysfunction, vaginal bleeding, blood clots etc and they reverse the positive effects of oestrogens on the heart. Conventional HRT also uses much higher levels of oestrogen than natural HRT. Hence why I prefer to use natural HRT (see *Useful Remedies* opposite).

If you have had a partial hysterectomy (ovaries remaining) before menopause you will still have hormonal changes similar to the normal menstrual cycle. If you need supplemental hormones and are told that you only need oestrogen because you do not have a uterus, you should also take real (natural) progesterone with any oestrogen supplementation. If you have had a total hysterectomy and need hormone replacement therapy, use the lowest dose of oestrogen possible for you and always use real (natural) progesterone with it (see *Useful Remedies*).

Some women go through early menopause, which can happen for many reasons, ranging from oestrogen-like chemicals in the environment or smoking, drinking heavily, or being severely malnourished. Whatever the cause, it is important to make sure that the bones remain healthy, therefore have a bone scan periodically and a urine – deoxypyrodinoline test to measure bone breakdown. If bone loss is occurring then you need to take the appropriate measures (see *Osteoporosis p233*).

Foods to Avoid

- In general, the typical Western diet of white flour, and full-fat dairy and meat is not only unhealthy but also contributes to hot flushes.

- Avoid chemicals that mimic oestrogens (xenoestrogens) found in pesticides or herbicides by eating organic foods.

- Intensively reared animals have often been treated with antibiotics and hormones, another reason to eat organic meat and chicken.

- Minimize your exposure to foods stored in plastic containers and never heat or microwave food in plastic containers – as they will leach xenoestrogens,

- Cut down on all caffeine, fizzy cola-type drinks, sugar, chocolate and too much alcohol, which all act as stimulants and trigger blood sugar problems.

Friendly Foods

- See also *Diet – The Stay Younger Longer Diet (see page 114).*

- Increase your intake of fresh, locally grown and preferably organic fruits and vegetables.

- Fermented soya-based foods are truly one of the best foods for managing the symptoms associated with the menopause. Soya contains isoflavones (phyto-oestrogens), which have oestrogen-like effects on the body and block the harmful effects of oestrogens and xenoestrogens. There has been much misinformation written about about soya and Dr Glenville says, "Soya foods in their traditional forms of miso, soya sauce and tempeh (a fermented form of soya) are all rich in isoflavones which have been proven to reduce the risk of developing cancers. But they are best eaten cooked. "

- Eat more organic miso, tempe or tamari soy sauce.
- Isoflavones are also found in chickpeas, lentils, alfalfa, fennel, kidney beans, sunflower, pumpkin and sesame seeds, Brazil nuts, walnuts and linseeds. All seeds and their unrefined oils are rich in essential fatty acids which also help reduce joint pain, risk of heart disease and help lubricate the vagina (see *Fats for Anti-ageing p139*).
- Foods from the brassica vegetable family also help protect against oestrogen-sensitive cancers, including breast cancer and cervix cancer, and help to balance hormones. These include cabbage, broccoli, pak choi, Brussels sprouts, cauliflower, kale, kohlrabi, mustard, rutabaga and turnips.
- Brazil nuts and sesame seeds are a better source of calcium than cows' milk.
- Live, low-fat yoghurt increases healthy bacteria in the gut, which aids absorption of nutrients from your diet.
- Vitamin B12 has been shown to reduce irritability, bloating and headaches associated with the menopause and is found in oily fish, eggs and meats.
- Potassium and pantothenic acid (vitamin B5) help support adrenal function. They are found in wholegrains such as brown rice, amaranth, barley, quinoa, salmon, tomatoes, broccoli, cauliflower, avocado, dried apricots, banana, cantaloupe melon, oranges and fish.
- Use dried seaweeds such as kombu in your cooking and stir-fries, as seaweed is rich in iodine (which supports the thyroid) and calcium (see also *Thyroid p313*).
- Eat organic foods including meat, chicken, vegetables and fruits to avoid ingesting too many toxins from herbicides and pesticides.
- Folic acid found in wheatgerm, eggs, leafy greens, calves' and chicken liver, dried yeast and boiled beetroot is very important during the menopause to protect the bones.
- Include garlic in your diet, which helps to keep cholesterol levels in check.
- Drink more spring water which helps to regulate body temperature.
- Avoid very hot drinks and hot spicy foods.
- If you have trouble sleeping, try valerian and passionflower teas.

Useful Remedies
- If you dislike the taste of soya foods, then take soya isoflavone capsules. Most of the health companies on pages 13 and 14 make them. Take 30–40mg daily.

- Natural hormone replacement therapy can reduce many of the symptoms of menopause. Natural hormone replacement therapy consists of natural progesterone extracted from wild yam and/or natural oestrogens from soya. The natural progesterone most often comes as a cream that you rub on the skin called Natural Progesterone Cream. Natural oestrogens are mostly available in a combination formula with the three types of oestrogens found in a woman's body mixed with natural progesterone. This is called phyto-estrogen with Progesterone Cream, both of which contains bio-identical hormones (meaning the exact same molecule that is found in the human body). Phyto-estrogen with Progesterone supplementation can be used in place of HRT under the direction of a gynaecologist. Phyto-estrogen and progesterone creams are available on prescription in the UK, but you can order them for your own use from PharmWest in USA (see page 14). Use the natural progesterone for 2–3 months but if there is not sufficient improvement then switch to the phyto-estrogen cream. For an information sheet on these creams Tel: freephone with in the UK 0 800 8923 8923, website: www.pharmwest.com

- If you are suffering low-level hot flushes, insomnia, vaginal dryness or mood swings you may only need natural progesterone.

- Don't use hormones unless you have been tested by your doctor and if you have no hormonal symptoms and good bone density there is no need for extra hormones.

- Take a good-quality woman's multivitamin/mineral such as Biocare's Femforte or Lambert's Gynovite. Any women's multi that you choose should contain boron, vitamin K, selenium, folic acid, vitamin D, vitamin E, calcium and magnesium to support you through the menopause.

- A very interesting remedy extracted from a Peruvian cruciferous root vegetable called Maca has been used for centuries as a natural remedy for hormonal-type symptoms. The root is rich in protein, minerals, vitamins, fibre and essential fats. Dr Gloria Chacon de Popivici, a biologist in Lima Peru, says her research shows that Maca helps to stimulate the pituitary gland into producing hormone precursors, which eventually raises oestrogen and progesterone levels naturally, as well as balancing the adrenal glands, the thyroid, and the pancreas. Taken regularly, this root has been shown to reduce hot flushes, depression and palpitations associated with the menopause. Take 1 capsule daily. For details call Kudos on 0800 389 5476.

- Take 400iu of full-spectrum, natural-source vitamin E per day to help reduce hot flushes and if your vagina is very dry you can insert a capsule into it nightly for six weeks.

- Indolplex, by Enzymatic Therapy, is a nutritional supplement made from extracts of the brassica vegetables that contain indole 3 carbinole and diindolymethane, which increase what scientists now believe to be the "good" oestrogen (2-hydroxyestrone) and decreasing the "bad" oestrogen (16-a-hydroxyestrone). Take 2 tablets per day. To order call The Society for Complementary Medicine on 0207 487 4334.

- Vitamin K, 10mg per day, can reduce the heavy menstrual bleeding that is common in the peri-menopausal years. Vitamin K is also needed to keep minerals such as calcium in the bones and out of the arteries.

- Vitamin B-complex, 100mg per day, helps to relieve stress, depression and mood disorders and is needed for energy production.

- Black cohosh can effectively relieve hot flushes and other menopausal symptoms after four weeks of use. Additional herbs that are great for reducing menopausal symptoms include agnus castus, hops, liquorice root, dong quai and wild yam. These herbs can be taken individually or in combination formulas. Dr Glenville has an excellent formula containing all these herbs. One teaspoonful can be taken twice daily. Call 01892 750511 for details.

Helpful Hints

- If you are suffering heavy bleeding you must have this checked by your doctor or gynaecologist.

- Regular weight-bearing exercise not only helps raise levels of DHEA, a vital anti-ageing hormone (see *Other Vital Hormones p227*), but also reduces stress, which makes symptoms and hormone imbalances worse. Also in mid-life our waistlines tend to expand! Exercise keeps you trim and increases bone density. It also makes you feel more positive and cheerful about life and women who exercise regularly tend to suffer fewer hot flushes.

- Use relaxation techniques such as meditation or yoga (see *Meditation p207*).

- Add essential oils of geranium, camomile and jasmine to your bath to further aid relaxation.

- If you suffer from night sweats, wear loose-fitting cotton nightwear and have a change of nightwear ready. Use cotton blankets and keep the room cool.

- Homeopathic Sepia 30c, taking 1 daily for a week, has been found to reduce hot flushes.

- To further help prevent vaginal dryness and painful intercourse, avoid deodorant soaps or scented products in the vaginal area.

- Use a water-soluble lubricant to facilitate penetration during intercourse.

- An acidophilus pessary can be vaginally inserted to help produce copious amounts of lubrication. There are many creams containing wild yam available in health food stores that can be used topically as a vaginal lubricant. Contact The Perfect Woman range for wild Mexican yam on 0117 968 7744, www.wildmexicanyam.co.uk

- Read *Natural Alternatives to HRT* and *Eat Your Way Through The Menopause*, both by Dr Marilyn Glenville, published by Kyle Cathie. Marilyn's website, www.marilynglenville.com, offers postal consultations and is packed with useful information.

- If you require further information on natural progesterone and a list of doctors who use it, send a 1st class stamp to Natural Progesterone Information Service (NPIS), PO Box 24, Buxton SK17 9FB.

- Some women find the menopause a thoroughly depressing time, perhaps because children have left home and a few women say they feel empty and useless. But the menopause heralds new freedom and a whole new chapter. I did not become a writer until the age of

43. It's never too late to begin a new career or a new hobby. Find things to feel passionate about and know that you can make a huge difference to your friends, family – and the world – if you just decide to take the first step.

MEN'S HORMONES

(See also *Mid-Life Crisis, Other Vital Hormones, Prostate* and *Sex in Ageing*)

Testosterone, produced within the testicles, is a critical hormone for men and is intimately tied to sexuality as well as generating strength, stamina, increasing lean body tissue, lowering cholesterol, stimulating red blood cell production, reducing blood sugar levels, and fortifying bone density. Women also have traces of testosterone in their bodies.

From the age of 30 onwards, free testosterone levels (the biologically active part of the testosterone) decrease at around 1.5% per year. Half of all men over 80 have low testosterone levels. While the total testosterone of a male does not drop drastically with ageing, the free testosterone does. The effects of this decrease have been called andropause (see *Helpful Hints*) or the male menopause (see also *Mid-life Crisis p221*).

In addition to testosterone, men also make oestrogen. As men age, oestrogen levels increase, which has been linked to prostate enlargement and prostate cancer. Regular supplementation with zinc helps to block the enzyme that converts testosterone to oestrogen for men.

Oestrogen levels can also be raised by environmental toxins that act like oestrogens within the body. These hormone-altering substances are found in plastics, pesticides and chemical residues from industry, such as dioxins from incinerators. These chemicals cause increased oestrogen activity which is linked to prostate enlargement, cancers and a reduced sperm count.

Impotence is another alarming symptom for men, which is also linked to low testosterone levels. This hormone has often been given a bad press saying that excess testosterone increases risk for heart disease – in fact recent research has found that testosterone levels in cardiovascular patients was low and that testosterone offers some protection against heart disease. This is also true for women.

A note of caution. Some testosterone is converted into an unwanted oestrogen form, by an enzyme called aromatase. More so in later life. It is this male oestrogen that leads to prostatic enlargement and *not* testosterone itself, as you may have been led to believe. Male oestrogen adds to the risk of heart disease. Therefore, never self-medicate with any hormones – have a blood test and find out if you need them first.

Foods to Avoid
■ High saturated fat foods such as red meat, full-fat dairy products, hamburgers, sausage

rolls, meat pies, hydrogenated or trans-fats tend to accumulate environmental toxins which can affect testosterone and the prostate gland.

- Refined carbohydrates, such as croissants, refined cakes, white bread, rice and pasta plus biscuits etc, cause insulin resistance, which affects free testosterone levels.

- Cows' milk may be bad for the prostate. Overall, countries that consume the most milk have the highest incidence of prostate cancer. The culprit appears to be milk's calcium. Excessive calcium intake, regardless of source, suppresses the synthesis of a form of vitamin D that inhibits prostate cancer.

Friendly Foods

- Cabbage, kale, broccoli, Brussels sprouts all contain a powerful plant substance called indole 3 carbinole which blocks the bad effects of oestrogen and has also been shown to be very helpful against women's hormone dependent cancers, such as breast and cervical cancers. Men can benefit from the same breakthrough. Details: www.lef.org

- Eat foods high in natural carotenes, such as carrots, pumpkin, tomatoes, apricots and all orange and yellow foods.

- Oats are also said to increase free testosterone, therefore make organic porridge your breakfast cereal of choice, which also helps balance blood sugar.

- Lean beef, turkey, shellfish (especially oysters), cereals and beans are good sources of zinc.

- Selenium is found in whole cereals, seafood, meat, eggs and brewer's yeast.

- A little alcohol is fine – but as always everything in moderation. Excess alcohol increases oestrogen and decreases testosterone.

- An ailing prostate can reduce your ability to have erections, putting a severe damper on your sex life. Prostatitis, a deep, sometimes painful and debilitating inflammation of the gland, can be eased by foods such as unrefined nuts, seeds and wholegrains, especially rye products. They contain plant hormones, oils and other agents that decrease swelling, congestion and inflammation of the prostate. Pumpkin seeds in particular contain oils that ease the discomfort and pelvic pressure associated with enlargement of the prostate (benign prostatic hyperplasia-BPH). Soy products, rice and Chinese cabbage can help to reduce BPH.

Useful Remedies

- A good-quality multivitamin/ mineral for men.

- Taking 50mg per day of zinc helps to block the conversion of testosterone to oestrogen. Zinc is also linked to fertility, potency, sex drive and long-term sexual health. Zinc is critical to sperm production, and low zinc levels have been blamed for decreases in semen volume and testosterone levels.

- Indole 3 carbinole, is also available in capsules, and taking 200mg per day protects the prostate from oestrogens.

- Testosterone hormone replacement therapy for men is available in the form of creams that are put on the skin, patches, capsules and implants. The testosterone used should be a natural form of testosterone and not a synthetic form, such as methyl testosterone, which is linked to cancer. Extra caution needs to be used when testosterone supplementation is used to prevent an excess of the male oestrogen being formed. This can be accomplished by taking the herb saw palmetto as well as zinc.
- But *do not* use testosterone supplementation if you have an elevated PSA or known prostate cancer.
- Saw palmetto – taking 160mg 2 tablets per day helps to block the formation of the very strong testosterone, DHT, in the prostate that can cause prostate swelling.
- Lycopene, a carotene found in tomatoes and carrots, is one of the best antioxidants for the prostate. Take 15mg daily.

Helpful Hints

- Andropause – Dr Keith Scott-Mumby, a nutritional physician who specializes in hormonal problems in ageing, says, "It is not widely known that men undergo a hormonal transformation in middle age, much like the menopause of women. The event tends to be more gradual than for women and so often goes unnoticed, but it can be a time of great unhappiness for a man: there can be fatigue, depression, aches and pains, sweating and flushing and reduced libido, exactly the same as for women. Loss of erectile function is particularly poignant, since most men continue to judge themselves by sexual prowess, even when it's inappropriate. Many men are reluctant to discuss their sexual symptoms at this time, which is why the andropause continues to be little regarded, even by some doctors. The andropause must be distinguished from the mid-life crisis, which is a totally separate phenomenon. The distinction is important, because the andropause will respond to supplementation of testosterone, whereas this hormone has little or no effect on the mid-life crisis, since the latter is not caused by testosterone deficiency."
- Regular exercise, try and walk for at least 30 minutes daily and get to a gym twice to three times a week. Exercise helps to increase production of another vital anti-ageing hormone – DHEA (see *Other Vital Hormones p237*).
- Stress causes the adrenal glands to produce the stress hormone cortisol instead of DHEA, so watch your stress levels (see *Stress in Ageing p293*).
- Heavy metals such as lead, mercury and cadmium also inhibit testosterone production (see *Toxic Metal Overload p317*).
- Smoking can have an adverse effect on hormone production.
- For more help read *The Testosterone Revolution* by Dr Malcolm Carruthers and Jed Diamond, Harper Collins.

MID-LIFE CRISIS IN AGEING

(See also *Men's Hormones, Diet – The Stay Younger Longer Diet (see page 114)* and *General Anti-ageing Health Hints*).

As a woman, this is as much a mystery to me as most other women, so I asked my friend, Dr Keith Scott-Mumby, a nutritional physician who specializes in Ageing and Allergy Medicine to write this section for me. Over to you Keith...

The menopause is a well-known event for women. What is much less known is that men have to endure a similar biological and emotional experience. It is mostly obscured by the usual male inability to come to terms with personal issues, their lack of communication skills and the fact that it is perceived as less than masculine to even admit to such feelings.

Matters are made more complicated by the fact that there are really two phenomena rolled into one and these easily become confused. It is vital that women appreciate what is happening to their loved one and that more doctors get to grips with this important aspect of growing older. Although men like to believe they are tough and immune from care, the truth is they are often desperately insecure, and failing to understand what is happening to one's self can be a major cause of anxiety and suffering.

There is a male hormonal shutdown, akin to the menopause, which is therefore named the "andropause" (see also *Men's Hormones*). But this is quite distinct from the mid-life crisis, as we shall see. The trouble is that both happen at a similar time, though the mid-life crisis tends to occur somewhat earlier. How can we tell these two apart?

Let us consider first the true andropause. When a man is in his 50s, testosterone levels fall, resulting in true biological changes, which can be measured in a laboratory. The resulting symptoms are not unlike those experienced by women at the menopause: fatigue, depression, aches and pains, sweating and flushes, and reduced libido. Loss of erectile function can also become a problem. This is particularly disturbing to a man and difficulty in talking about this problem is one of the reasons why the male menopause isn't discussed much.

The true mid-life crisis often falls earlier than the andropause, often in a man's 40s. Typically, it occurs in response to life events: marriage breakdown, career failure, bankruptcy, death of a peer or loved parent, redundancy and so on. Essentially, it is an emotional crisis and not a hormonal one. Deep introspection often results in the feeling that life is passing by and precious years have been wasted with so little achieved. Dreams that were once so important seem to have faded or gone forever beyond reach. It can be a time of great anguish, despair, inadequacy and feelings of guilt or futility.

Whereas anyone, sooner or later, will experience a sharp fall in hormones, the man who suffers the mid-life crisis is typically one who has been challenged and cannot come to terms with his life. There has been a shock which brings him face to face with his self and he doesn't like what he sees. In trying to rationalize the unhappy feelings he may begin to see his life partner in negative terms, or blame his bosses and work dissatisfaction. Therefore he seeks change: a new partner (times of infidelity and experiment), a new career, new home territory and so on.

Unfortunately, alcohol and drugs are often seen as the answer. They shut out the pain temporarily but of course solve nothing. This may be the start of a slippery slope to abuse, addiction and early demise.

Far from the libido shut-down characteristic of the andropause, a man in a mid-life crisis wants to boast of sexual prowess and seeks new thrills and adventure. This is the man likely to start buying younger-generation fashions and have an affair with his secretary! But it is a kind of denial, an admission that things are not as they were, underscored by a great desire to prove everything is OK.

Whereas, the andropause man lacks energy or drive and cannot be bothered with sex or adventure. He feels it is already is too late.

While less common, the mid-life crisis can occur for women. Almost all of what is said here applies equally. Even the search for new loves, thrills and adventure can lead to women also becoming unfaithful or seeking divorce. Obviously, it needs to be distinguished from the onset of the menopause.

What You Can Do

The most important first step is to have blood tests to check up on the man's hormones. If this reveals there is a problem, testosterone supplements – hormone replacement therapy (HRT) for men – can bring about a satisfying and sometimes dramatic change. Fatigue and depression lift, life becomes worthwhile, energy levels and zest return to former levels, potency problems recede. What's more, testosterone improves circulation, protects against heart disease, aids weight loss, improves skin condition, increases muscle strength and works in a host of healthy ways to rejuvenate the man (see *Men's Hormones p218*).

Testosterone supplementation does need some care. Generally, though, one can say that the dangers of *not* supplementing testosterone well into old age are far greater than any theoretical risks to prescribing it. Be clear about it: testosterone saves lives, hearts and minds!

On the other hand, what if the tests show that testosterone deficiency is not significant? Clearly supplements will not help. This is an emotional or life-events crisis and needs handling as such, at whatever age it occurs.

The man concerned has to be brought to confronting his situation. The pretence that there is nothing wrong and everyone else is to blame does not help. Dr Malcolm Carruthers, a male hormone and lifestyle specialist and author of *The Testosterone*

Revolution makes the point that the kind of man likely to suffer a mid-life crisis is one with an unhappy childhood, maybe abusive or with cold and unloving parents. Such early formative experiences often engender a feeling of unworthiness which emerges later in life, at a time of crisis. This is fruitful ground for counselling or other therapy.

Even without a therapist, a man can sit down with pen and paper and start to write down what matters. Nothing changes the meaning of life more than working out what one's values truly are. Often we aspire to false goals, imposed by others, which have little meaning to ourselves. Society at large, and the media in particular, often impose ridiculous standards of goodness and value. There is a cult of greed, materialism and celebrity worship in vogue, which is very dangerous and tends to create envy, desire, inadequacy and misery in those who do not have all the trappings of a luxurious film-star lifestyle.

The irony is, you only have to look at the stories in that same press to realize that the people we are supposed to envy sometimes have disastrous, miserable or even tragically short sick lives.

The mid-life crisis is a challenge for all concerned, make no mistake. Maintaining strong personal relationships, especially with stable marriage, is a key feature in the longest-lived people around the world. Remember this throughout life and especially at times of crisis. Another attribute of successful agers is the ability to turn difficult or uncomfortable situations into positive experiences or outcomes. The mid-life crisis certainly gives you an opportunity to practise this valuable skill.

Foods to Avoid
■ See under *Men's Hormones p218 and Depression in Ageing p104*.

Friendly Foods
■ See under *Men's Hormones* and *Depression in Ageing*.

Useful Remedies
■ See under *Men's Hormones* and *Depression in Ageing*.

Helpful Hints
■ Find a good doctor that you trust and to whom you can talk about how you feel. There are now many clinics that specialise in sexual disfunction. They will be able to check all of your hormone levels and so on. There is also a fountain of knowledge on the internet, but it is always advisable to seek professional help.

■ Dr Keith Scott-Mumby can be reached via his website: www.alternative-doctor.com

■ Read *The Andropause Mystery: Unravelling Truths About The Male Menopause* by Robert S. Tan, Amred Consulting, or, *A Woman's Guide to Male Menopause* by Marc C Rose, Keates.

MIND POWER

(See also *Meditation*)

Scientists have shown that people who have a positive outlook on life and who are adaptable – regardless of their diet and lifestyle – live on average seven years longer than anyone else. And if you want to also look and feel younger than your actual chronological age, you can re-program your mind to help turn back the clock.

Your mind has the power to determine whether you are healthy or sick and the power to help you slow down, and in some cases, greatly reverse the ageing process. For some, this may seem like a nebulous, totally unrealistic possibility – but I have seen it happen with my own eyes.

During April 1998, I underwent an incredible near-death experience and for several months following this experience, I truly began to understand just how much our minds can affect our health and the length of our lives.

I was in such a heightened state of awareness, that through the power of my thoughts I could appear older or younger at will, which was witnessed by others. It was fantastic and my story, plus scientific explanations as to how this is possible, are documented in my book *Divine Intervention* (Cico Books, November 2002).

The average person has 40,000 thoughts a day, and scientists have proven that if you have a clear intention for a specific result, you can re-programme your computer – your brain – to bring your dreams into reality.

Back in 1994 in the American magazine, *Science of Mind*, I found an interview with biophysicist Beverley Rubik PhD, who at that time was Director at the Centre for Frontier Sciences at Temple University in Philadelphia. Her experiments showed that there is a definite interaction between consciousness and matter. In other words – what you think about becomes your reality. In Dr Rubik's words, "The research has shown a significant relationship between what we intend in consciousness and what we experience. Of course, if our intention is not clear, the results we get will be muddled by deeper, unconscious inclinations that may even work in the opposite direction. But when we do have a clear intention for something to occur and it is not blocked by contrary subconscious thinking, or a feeling that we don't deserve it, our thought does tend to create the results we desire. Our thoughts matter. Thought matters, thought materializes. A clear intention will create a reality."

Hence why I suggest you start thinking young and *know* that it can happen.

Havard psychologist, Ellen Langer, tried this a few years ago. She brought together a group of men in their 70s and 80s. They were asked to dress, behave and think as they had 20 years earlier. Within just five days their biomarkers of ageing (blood pressure, hearing, vision, mobility, heart rate, aerobic capacity etc) showed changes associated with age reversal.

It *can* happen. But, you have to be realistic. Start by knocking 10 years off your actual age and begin believing and thinking 100% that you are that age. It takes time to re-program a lifetimes mind set, but over several months it can happen. Total belief can trigger positive results.

During a recent lecture, a renowned American doctor told us about a patient with terminal liver cancer. The patient had approximately one month to live and his family and doctors decided it would be best if he could go home. *But*, they didn't tell the patient that he was dying. His doctor joked with him saying there was nothing more that needed doing and he was free to go home. The patient *presumed* that this was because he was now cured. He believed 100% with his conscious and subconscious mind that he was well. And he became well. The cancer disappeared and he lived until his natural death some 22 years later.

Cancer sufferers who show a "fighting spirit" and positive attitude are 60% more likely to still be alive 13 years after their initial diagnosis.

This is the power of the mind. You can be hypnotized and told that a lighted cigarette is being placed your skin and when you "awake" you may have burns on your skin, but no cigarettes have been used.

A senior medically trained nurse, Bernadine Coady aged 62, in Northern England, has hypnotized herself twice in the past three years to enable doctors to operate and cut through bones in her feet. In a study at Imperial College in London, patients with severe cases of chronic genital herpes that were not responding to medication, were taught self hypnosis and the doctors were astonished that the recurrence rate dropped by 50%. We are capable of anything we can imagine and truly believe.

Dervishes, a Sufi religious sect in Muslim countries, regularly pierce their skin and skull with swords, spikes, knives and so on, without any pain or any blood. They are neither in trance nor hypnotized. I don't suggest you try this at home, but again it demonstrates the mind's incredible power. Monks in the Far East can move huge objects using mind power and my co-author Steve Langley has witnessed this phenomenon in his travels. Mind over matter is a reality.

Dr Serena Roney-Dougal a parapsychologist based in the UK says, "In the experience of practitioners of human psychotherapy, if a person begins repeating positive self statements regularly, such as "I always have sufficient time" instead of "I never have enough time" that person can reprogramme their mind to believing that they always have sufficient time – and time appears to expand." Serena says changing one's attitude is the most important action you can take.

How many times have you said to yourself, "I'm too fat, too old, too unfit" or whatever – and then were you surprised when your constant affirmations came true? Now you know why. So let's re-direct our minds to staying younger longer.

Foods to Avoid and Friendly Foods

■ See *Brain in Ageing* and *Diet - The Stay Younger Longer Diet (see page 114)*.

■ Eating more of the right foods and taking the right supplements will help this process.

■ See also *General Anti-ageing Health Hints*, plus the supplements in that section.

Useful Remedies

■ The placebo affect also has a great effect on the mind. 35% of patients given dummy medication that they are told will heal them – get better.

■ When it came to testing Prozac, the paperwork submitted to the federal authorities in America, showed that the placebo pills were 80% as effective as the active drug! This proves that in many cases we can think ourselves well.

■ See *Ageing p25, Antioxidants in Ageing p38*, and *Meditation p207*.

Helpful Hints

■ Begin by setting your new age – it is realistic to reduce your chronological age by 10 years.

■ Then change your attitude and begin thinking that age. Place a note of it on the fridge, by your bedside, on your bathroom mirror – and at least three times a day look at your words and say something like "It's great to be only..., I feel healthier, happier and have more energy than I have had in years!" And even if it's not completely true in that moment, just keep on saying it – and feeling it – and acting as if it is true.

■ Remember, repetition over several months is the key to success.

■ Then once a day, five days a week (or as often as you can) begin practising the Stay Younger Longer Meditation:

Find a quiet space, turn off the phone, and sit somewhere in an upright but comfortable chair, where you won't be disturbed for 10 to 15 minutes.

Light a candle and place it in front of you. Breathe deeply in and out a couple of times and then just become aware of your natural breathing. Let your chest rise and fall and stare at the candle and begin to feel more relaxed.

In your own time – allow your eyes to gently close. Then imagine a beautiful, healing, calming, anti-ageing, white light is flowing in through the top of your head and all around your body – feel it slowly flow down through every part of your body. Feel it repairing your cells and as it reaches each major organ – imagine that organ having a huge smile on it's "face". And if, for instance you want thicker hair, visualize your hair as looking thicker and so on.

Allow the light to travel down through your feet and into the ground. As it moves downwards, feel every part of yourself becoming younger – see yourself looking and feeling younger and feel how that feels.

Remember your mind cannot tell the difference between a real or an imaginary event and if you practise regularly, certain physical changes will take place.

■ Begin dressing in a younger way – I'm not saying it has to be "mutton dressed as lamb"! – just dress younger so that you feel younger.

■ Become more spontaneous and adaptable – do things that you haven't done – or thought you should do – for years. Do something that you really enjoyed doing when you were younger.

- If you find it hard to "get started" try hypnotherapy or Neuro Linguistic Programming – both brilliant ways to begin training your mind, see *Useful Information and Addresses*.

- Lisha Spar distributes a powerful CD and cassette tape programme called InnerTalk developed by Dr Eldon Taylor. You can choose *InnerTalk* tapes on practically every subject from inner desires and inner doubts to inner hopes and inner health. For details log on to www.innertalk.co.uk, or call 0207 610 9221

- A brilliant book clarifying and explaining this concept is *Grow Younger, Live Longer* by Dr Deepak Chopra, Rider/Random House.

- Read *The Human Effect in Medicine*, a brilliant book about how our minds can heal, by Michael Dixon and Kieran Sweeney, Radcliffe Publishing.

MUSCLES IN AGEING

(See also *Exercise in Ageing, Joints* and *Oxygen in Ageing*)

One of the most important biomarkers of ageing is your Lean Body Mass – which is how much of your body is lean muscle compared to fat. As we age we tend to replace muscle with fat. In a gym recently my instructor asked me to grip a small hand-held device into which he programmed my height 5'9" and my weight 8 and a half stone. Now that's thin. But, the result was that I was carrying 5% too much body fat and insufficient muscle. In other words I don't need to lose weight, I need to exchange the excess fat for muscle. If you are worried that by building muscles you will start looking like a weight lifter, you won't if you follow professional guidance, and you will greatly help to slow the ageing process.

When you exercise and use weights, you increase bone density and as muscle is more dense than fat, you may actually weigh more, but you will look trimmer, younger and fitter! The more muscle you make, the more efficient is your metabolic rate, which means that you burn more calories even when you are resting. And as soon as I finish typing this book (I have been here for 8 months) I'll be returning for more regular workouts to the gym.

As we enter our 30s, we tend to lose an average of 300g (10 oz) of lean body mass a year, mostly in the form of muscle tissue. Most adults gain about 454grams (1lb) a year, nearly all in the form of fat, which masks the loss of lean body mass.

Over time, muscles become less flexible and, unless you stretch regularly and keep muscles supple, they will shorten, which not only makes you look and feel "stiffer" but also increases the risk for injuring your ligaments, tendons and bones. Muscles work in pairs, so if you work a particular muscle, then you should also work its opposite. For instance, if you do lots of stomach exercises, you would also then need to work on your lower back muscles.

Regular exercise (especially resistance and weight-bearing exercises) can prevent or reverse much of the muscle loss normally associated with ageing.

Women are usually more flexible than men, but it's the same old song, "Use it or lose it", hence why exercises such as yoga, Pilates and t'ai chi will all help you to stay supple for longer (see *Useful Information and Addresses p338*).

Inactivity is associated with many age-related medical conditions, such as high blood pressure, heart disease, diabetes, obesity, and osteoporosis. Research shows that if you do exercise, you benefit, if you don't, you increase your risk of disease. And some people use their illness as an excuse as to why they cannot exercise, when in the majority of cases it would make them healthier!

Muscle cramps, or twitching muscles, denote a build up of toxic waste products such as lactic acid and carbon dioxide in the muscles. Cramp is also triggered by a poor blood supply to the muscles. You are also likely to be lacking in the minerals potassium, calcium or magnesium.

Muscle wasting in later years is triggered by reduced levels of glutamine (a naturally occurring amino acid which is high in muscles) from the muscles. Stress, repeated illnesses, injuries and so on all add to glutamine depletion and thus muscle loss. Less muscle means less burning of calories, more storage of food as fat and less strength and stamina, which is the number one complaint heard from older patients by their doctors. Supplementing with glutamine in times of stress, and daily for older people, will go a long way towards preventing these complaints.

Muscles improve your ability to utilize oxygen, which aids circulation and reduces the risk for heart disease. They also help to protect you against Syndrome X (see under *Insulin Resistance p178*), which will also help slow the ageing process.

Foods to Avoid

- Avoid foods loaded with calories: cakes, pies, desserts, sausage rolls, pizzas, mass-produced hamburgers and high-sugar foods and drinks, which all deplete vital minerals from the body.

- Sugar converts to fat and lives on your hips if not burned off during exercise. So, if you're working out regularly, some sugar is fine, but not to excess.

- You need some salt, but use organic sea salt such as Celtra (available in supermarkets) rather than sodium table salt.

Friendly Foods

- Protein foods are vital for building muscle and help to keep you energized and alert.

- Unless you are a professional athlete whose requirements will be different, then men should eat around 175–225 g (6–8 oz) of organic meat, poultry or fish daily and ladies around 100–175 g (4–6 oz) would be fine.

- Eggs, whey, milk, yoghurt or cheese are also rich in protein.

- Vegetarian-based proteins are found in seeds, nuts, vegetables, wholegrains such as brown rice, barley, spelt, wholewheat and quinoa, plus legumes such as peas, lentils, soya beans, tofu, tempeh, lentils and peanuts.

■ Make sure you eat plenty of essential fats (see *Fats for Anti-ageing p139*).

■ Bananas, raw cauliflower, jacket potatoes, fresh fruits and juices, dried apricots and dates, leafy greens, avocado, mackerel, and beans (dried beans) are all great sources of magnesium and potassium which are needed for healthy muscles.

■ Almonds, sesame seeds, Brazil nuts, dried skimmed milk, sardines, muesli and Parmesan cheese are rich in calcium.

■ Drink plenty of water to avoid dehydrated muscles.

Useful Remedies

■ Glutamine – an amino acid needed to prevent muscle wasting and build lean body mass. Take 500mg twice daily before meals.

■ Carnitine is a vitamin-like nutrient that is found in the heart, brain, and skeletal muscles. Its job is to transport fatty acids across the cell wall to the mitochondria, providing the heart and muscle cells with energy. It enhances athletic performance and strength and promotes weight loss. Carnitine is found in meat and animal products. Red meat is the best source, or take 500–1,000mg per day.

■ Pycnogenol is an antioxidant found in pine bark and grape seed extract. It helps increase elasticity and flexibility in muscles, tendons and ligaments, relaxes smooth muscles in blood vessels and inhibits allergic reactions. Take 30–60mg per day.

■ Include a liquid, easily absorbed multimineral in your regimen for healthier muscles, this will also help reduce cramps. From Higher Nature (see page 13).

■ See also details of Kudos 24 – a multimineral, vitamin, essential fats, antioxidant formula that also contains carnosine (see below). For full details of Kudos 24, see page 348.

■ Leg cramps, especially at night should benefit from taking extra magnesium. Take up to 800mg in a chelated form daily before bed.

■ Sodiphos contains sodium phosphate which helps to reduce lactic acid (and uric acid) build up. Take 600mg daily for three months (See Blackmores, see page 13).

■ Carnosine is an excellent supplement for better muscle tone in ageing (for full details see under *Useful Remedies* in *Cells in Ageing p88*).

■ If you are under stress, then good-quality whey protein powder, is an excellent way to take in more protein, as it is easier to digest and helps retain muscle tone. Solgar make a great formula (see page 14).

Helpful Hints

■ Begin walking, stationary cycling or swimming, for at least 20 minutes, three or more times a week.

■ Always stretch and warm up your muscles before working out to reduce the risk for injury.

■ If you suffer from cramp rest for a few moments to allow more oxygen into the muscles. Gently massage the muscle and if the cramp starts in your calves at night, stand up for a few minutes to aid blood flow and reduce the discomfort.

■ Treat yourself to a regular massage which helps to reduce the amount of lactic acid in your muscles. Use essential oils of lavender, ginger, rosemary, black pepper or camomile in a base of almond oil to reduce aches and pains in your muscles.

■ Weight training and resistance exercises are the best way to build healthy muscles. Buy yourself a couple of dumb-bells or join a local gym. Have your Lean Body Mass tested (virtually all gyms will offer this service) and then ask the in-house instructor to help you with a suitable exercise programme.

■ Since no one can force you to train, it's imperative that you engage in activities that are fun. Choose something active that you truly enjoy doing, and vary your routine so that you work all the muscle groups and you don't get bored.

■ Always try to eat meals about two hours before your workout. Don't try to fit in a quick meal just before you go to the gym. Eating a lot of carbohydrates within 45 minutes of your workout could make your body over-produce insulin, the hormone that helps convert blood sugar into fat. But if I am hungry then a banana usually gets me through a one-hour session – but I eat it at least 45 minutes before working out.

■ Deep, quality sleep promotes your body's release of growth hormone, which helps to melt fat and aids muscle development. Steady exercise will also increase your levels of DHEA, an anti-ageing hormone and human growth hormone.

■ If you suffer an injury which prevents you from exercising, to help keep muscles toned and aid rehabilitation, try the Ultra Tone System. You place small pads on the muscle groups and an electrical impulse stimulates the muscles' motor points, which causes them to contract and relax. This brings more blood to the muscle and surrounding tissues, which aids drainage of toxins and tones the muscles. They also make small hand held units for lifting facial muscles. For details call 0207 935 0631, www.ultratone.co.uk

NAIL PROBLEMS IN AGEING

(See also *Low Stomach Acid* and *Absorption*)

Your nails are a great barometer for your health. For instance as we age, and stomach acid levels often fall, you may experience longitudinal ridges, which denotes low stomach acid.

Nails are made up mostly from keratin, a protein-like substance, with fat and water molecules in-between the keratin, that help to keep nails healthy and supple.

White spots can denote that you are either ingesting too much sugar, alcohol and junk foods or have insufficient zinc.

Brittle, transparent and flat looking nails that curl up at the edges, are a common problem with ageing associated with low iron levels, but as too much iron after the age of 50 is linked to heart disease, don't take too much iron unless a blood test shows you need it.

Brittle, splitting nails are a sign of silica deficiency while soft peeling nails indicate a calcium deficiency. Excessively curved nails (like an upside down spoon) can indicate a potassium deficiency.

Anyone who has their hands in water for long periods usually has weaker nails. Biting the nails is an obvious cause for poor nails.

Fungal infections turn the nails white or at the very least they cause a discolouration and deformity in the nails. Nails can thicken if you eat too much protein or when the immune system is at a low ebb.

Horizontal ridges across the nails can denote a lack of calcium and/or magnesium, and stress.

If your nail beds are red, your liver may be congested from too much fat and alcohol and you should have your cholesterol levels checked.

Foods to Avoid

- Junk foods, fizzy drinks, white bread, biscuits and pastries – all these foods deplete the body of nutrients, especially B vitamins.

- Reduce your intake of caffeine and alcohol.

- Keep sugar to a minimum.

- Avoid hydrogenated or trans-fats and avoid too much fat from animal sources – full-fat milk, cheeses, chocolates, pies, desserts and so on as hard, thick nails can denote that you are eating too much fat and excess protein.

Friendly Foods

- Make sure you eat good-quality protein at least once a day. Either chicken, fish, tempeh, or a little organic red meat. But don't overeat protein which can make the nails hard and thick, 175g (6oz) daily is fine.

- Eggs, blackstrap molasses, almonds, red meats and spinach are rich in iron.

- Oily fish, unrefined nuts, seeds, especially hazel nuts, Brazil nuts, walnuts plus sunflower, pumpkin, sesame and linseeds are rich in zinc and essential fats. Use their unrefined oils over salads and cooked foods to nourish your nails.

- Drink six glasses of water daily.

- Eat more pumpkin, apricots, green leafy vegetables, cantaloupe melons and sweet potatoes for their vitamin A content.

- Cereals, brown rice, oats, organ meats, eggs, lentils, peas, nuts and leafy green organic vegetables are all rich in B vitamins, which are vital for healthy nails.

- Eat a small amount of pineapple and papaya before meals to aid digestion.

- Eat one avocado a week and sprinkle organic wheatgerm over cereals and desserts, as they are rich in vitamin E.
- Silica-rich foods are lettuce and all high fibre foods, vegetables and wholegrains.

Useful Remedies

- A comprehensive multi-nutrient powder that includes essential fats (see *p348*).
- Take a B-complex plus 2.5mg of biotin, a lack of which is linked to brittle nails. Vegetarians and vegans often also have low levels of B12 found in meat, fish and eggs, therefore make sure your B-complex contains at least 50mcg B12.
- The mineral silica is important for healthy nails, take 75mg daily.
- If you have fungal infections, as well as following a low-sugar diet, take 2 x 500mg capsules twice daily of both herbs pau d'arco and cat's claw to reduce fungus in the body and nails.
- Tissue Salt Combination K help reduce brittle nails and Combination L helps reduce fungal problems.
- MSM, a sulphur-based supplement helps to strengthen nails. Take 250mg daily.
- White blobs (more than tiny spots) on the nails can denote a lack of selenium. Take 200mcg daily.

Helpful Hints

- Nail polish remover contains solvents that are notorious for drying nails out and making them more brittle. Most nail salons and beauty counters sell oils specifically for the nails that can be used after polishing. Always use a base coat.
- To remove yellow stains from nails, soak them in a cup of warm water that contains the juice of one lemon for 15 minutes daily.
- Massage your nails regularly with jojoba, olive or almond oil.
- If you have a fungal infection, soak nails in white distilled vinegar for at least 10 minutes twice a day. You can also use diluted tee tree oil or neem oil on the nails.
- Bacteria and viruses can breed under the nails and being in close contact with someone who has dirty nails is a great way to pass them on. Also if you shake hands with someone who has a cold, this too will spread the virus. Keep your nails clean.
- If your nails are constantly in water, then wear surgical or rubber gloves. Wear gloves when gardening.
- Only use nail salons that keep their instruments scrupulously clean.

OBESITY IN AGEING

(See also *Carbohydrate Control* and *Weight Problems in Ageing*)

OSTEOPOROSIS

(See also *Acid-Alkaline Balance, Exercise, Joints in Ageing*)

Osteoporosis is not inevitable. The ageing process causes a gradual reduction in bone density but fractures should be a rare occurrence. When osteoporosis develops, there is a greater than normal decrease in bone mineral density that leads to the bone fragility which results in fractures, especially in the hips, wrists and spine. One in 3 women and one in 12 men will develop osteoporosis during their lifetime. It is estimated that 3 million people in the UK alone suffer this condition, but many cases go undiagnosed. The occurrence increases with age, especially after 50 and women are at greater risk of developing osteoporosis after menopause, when the reduction of hormonal protection causes accelerated bone loss, which increases to 3–5% per year for 3 to 5 years and then continues at the rate of 1–1.5% per year.

Although osteoporosis is thought of as a disease of old age, recent research suggests that its roots lie in adolescence. A poor diet lacking in vitamins and minerals such as calcium, magnesium and boron, during the teens can sow the seeds for brittle bones. Phosphorous is a vital mineral, but high levels in the diet can deplete bone. Unfortunately, high levels of this element are found in fizzy, canned drinks, which is undoubtedly contributing to the growing numbers of young people with brittle bones. Junk foods, alcohol, too much caffeine and sugar also deplete minerals.

Osteoporosis is also associated with a lack of weight-bearing exercise, excess animal protein in the diet, low body weight and lack of skin exposure to sunshine, which increases vitamin D levels in the body. My mother suffered with osteoporosis, in part due to her poor diet, but also, she never exposed her skin to the sun. When she died at 78, her skin was amazingly wrinkle-free, but her bones were in a dreadful state. Hence why I firmly believe that women who are fanatical about staying out of the sun, would definitely benefit from exposing their skin regularly to 15 minutes of early morning or late afternoon sun to boost their vitamin D levels. A family history of osteoporosis, premature menopause, some cancers and long-term use of certain drugs, such as tranquillizers and steroids, can also increase the risk for osteoporosis.

Other risk factors are a thin body frame and smoking. Women who suffered anorexia when they were younger are also at risk. Women who exercise to the point where their periods stop are at risk because of low hormone level.

The hormones adrenalin and cortisol, when produced to excess, such as in long-term stressful situations and lifestyles, can thin bone, hence why keeping yourself stress-free encourages healthier bones (see *Stress in Ageing p293*).

Lack of absorption of nutrients within the gut is another contributing factor to thinning bones (see *Absorption p16*).

Traditionally, osteoporosis is prevented and treated by hormone replacement therapy (HRT). But naturopath, Bob Jacobs, says "Women who have taken HRT for 10 years or more may have a greater bone density than those who have not taken it, but they lose increased density rapidly when the HRT is stopped and end up with only 3.2% higher bone density than women who took nothing. HRT can only prevent osteoporosis if women take it for the rest of their lives. When women exercise regularly, eat a healthy diet and take the right vitamins and minerals, bone density can be maintained and even increased, without having to endure the potential side effects of conventional HRT, which are increased risk of breast and endometrial (womb) cancers, thrombosis and strokes. Far better to use natural hormone therapy." (See *Useful Remedies* in this section).

Foods to Avoid

- Generally cut down on caffeine-based foods and drinks. More than 3 cups of strong coffee a day can increase your risk of developing osteoporosis by as much as 80%.

- Our Western diets tend to be very high in acid-forming foods, which cause more calcium to be excreted in urine. These include all the usual suspects of "white" foods: breads, cakes, croissants, biscuits, white pasta and rice etc (see *Acid–Alkaline Balance p18*).

- Reduce sodium-based table salt, which increases calcium loss.

- On average we eat 50% too much animal protein, which increases acidity of the blood and can promote calcium loss from the bones. Therefore, eat quality protein such as fresh fish, chicken, tofu, eggs or beans which are less acid-forming than red meat.

- Avoid fizzy drinks, because the artificial carbonation creates carbonic acid that dissolves bone and the excess phosphates force more calcium to be excreted.

- Avoid excess alcohol. Consuming more than 2 alcoholic drinks daily decreases calcium absorption from your diet. It also interferes with the synthesis of vitamin D, which helps the bones absorb calcium.

Friendly Foods

- Vegetarians tend to suffer less osteoporosis as their diet usually contains far more vegetables, grains and fruits.

- Ideal foods for strong bones which are high in calcium and reduce calcium losses are green leafy vegetables like kale, alfalfa, kelp, cabbage and spring greens. Dairy is not as good a source for calcium as green vegetables and 100g (3½oz) of kale, or spring greens will have at least as much beneficial effect on calcium balance as 200g (7oz) of milk or 100g (3½oz) of Cheddar cheese.

- Eat fermented soya-based foods, which are high in phyto-oestrogens (see *Menopause p212*).

- Calcium is found in green leafy vegetables, fish – and sesame seeds contain more calcium than milk.

- Magnesium is found in brown rice, buckwheat, lentils, peas, corn, almonds, cashew and Brazil nuts, sunflower, sesame and pumpkin seeds, wheatgerm and wholegrain cereals.

- Vitamin D is found in egg yolks, oily fish, organ meats and milk. It allows the body to absorb calcium and phosphorous needed for healthy bones.

- Vitamin K is vital for healthy bones, as it keeps calcium in the bones and out of the arteries where calcium deposits add to arterial plaque. Vitamin K is found in broccoli, green cabbage, lettuce and especially kale.

- As low stomach acid is often a factor in osteoporosis, eat more pineapple or papaya before meals to aid absorption of nutrients from your diet.

- Silica is another vital mineral for healthy bones, found in lettuce, celery, millet, oats and parsnips.

- Boron is a trace mineral needed for healthy bones and is found in raisins, prunes, nuts, non-citrus fruits and vegetables.

- Add 1 tablespoon of organic cider vinegar and honey to a glass of warm water daily, and sip throughout the day. This helps the body to assimilate more calcium.

- Drink mineral waters in preference to tap water.

Useful Remedies

- Natural plant phyto-oestrogens and soya-based isoflaone supplements promote a positive calcium balance, they help make bone more resistant to releasing calcium and reduce urinary calcium loss. Oestrogen levels decline with age in both men and women, with a particularly dramatic drop in women at menopause. Take approximately 40 mg daily.

- Natural phyto-estrogen cream contains natural (meaning the exact molecule that is found in the human body) progesterone from wild yam and oestrogen from soya beans, which helps to prevent osteoporosis and can, with proper nutrition, help increase bone density.

- To find out if you are at risk of osteoporosis, have a bone density scan via your doctor and also ask for a urine DPD test to show if you are currently losing bone. If the bone scan is OK and the urine test shows no bone loss then you don't need extra hormones. But if your density is low and the urine test shows excessive bone breakdown, then the use of natural hormones, the right diet, supplements and exercise can be very useful. For a free information sheet on phyto-estrogen Cream call Freephone 00800 8923 8923 or log on to www.pharmwest.com

- Most doctors recommend that you take twice the amount of calcium to magnesium, but some research has shown that in fact we need more magnesium than calcium. Dr Robert Trossell, a nutritional physician based in Europe and London, says, "We have found that a greater majority of women need more magnesium than calcium and I recommend at least equal amounts, or more magnesium than calcium. An optimum dose would be 1000mg magnesium and 600mg of calcium taken in a chelated (or citrate) form, as they are more easily absorbed. These minerals are known as nature's tranquillizers and are better utilized if taken at night."

- 10mg of vitamin K daily is very important for "gluing" the calcium into your bone matrix. Research has shown that vitamin K can reduce fracture risk by 65%. The beneficial effect of vitamin K is particularly noticeable in post-menopausal women who are not receiving oestrogen treatment. Most bone formulas contain some vitamin K.

- 1–2g per day of vitamin C with meals in an ascorbate form, promotes the formation of proteins required in bone and is also involved in the synthesis and repair of all collagen, including cartilage and matrix of bone.

- 15mg per day of zinc is necessary for bone building.

- Vitamin D, 400iu, is essential for calcium and phosphorus absorption.

- 3mg per day of boron is necessary for the conversion of vitamin D into its active forms. It also helps the body produce natural oestrogen. This mineral is vital for healthy bones. More women die from complications of a fracture of the femur in the USA than of breast cancer. Researchers also concluded that people living in countries with lower boron levels in the soil suffered much more arthritis.

- 100mg per day of vitamin B-6 , is a necessary co-factor for many enzyme reactions involved in bone building.

- All the companies listed on pages 13 and 14 make multivitamin/mineral and bone formulas that contain a balanced supply of most of these nutrients, which also includes HCl (stomach acid) to aid absorption. Don't be afraid to call and ask a nutritionist for help.

Helpful Hints

- Do not smoke. Women who smoke generally experience menopause up to a year and a half earlier than non-smokers, and thus face a longer period of oestrogen deficiency and accompanying bone loss. Smoking also hampers efficient processing of calcium. Smokers have a higher rate of spinal fractures than non-smokers.

- Chelation reduces the chances of developing osteoporosis (see *Chelation in Ageing p89*).

- Osteoporosis is a largely preventable disease and there are some common-sense things you can do to reduce the risk. The most important is weight-bearing exercise – swimming and cycling are great anti-ageing exercises, but they don't increase bone density as they are not weight bearing. Skipping, jogging, walking, aerobics and rebounding (mini-trampolines) are great exercises to beat osteoporosis. Tennis players have a 30% higher bone density in their serving arm compared to their non-serving arm. For anyone already suffering osteoporosis, join a local gym and begin exercising with a professional.

- Weight training also increases bone density. In an ideal world begin weight training in your 20s and 30s before your bones start to thin, but it is never too late.

- Ask in your gym about a Power Plate machine. You stand on the vibrating plate, which looks like a largish weighing scale. The vibration helps to strengthen bone tissue. It also reduces cellulite, increases secretion of human growth hormone and increases muscle strength. For details call Power Plate UK. Tel: 0208 450 8777, or visit: info@power-plate.co.uk

- Some clinics and doctors' surgeries in the UK have regular visits from mobile bone screening services. All you have to do is place your foot in a small ultrasonic device, which measures the bone density in the heel of the foot, and you have a full read out within 15 minutes. This simple and inexpensive test, while not as accurate as a full bone density scan from a hospital, is a great way to know where you stand! For details call 01923 857616, or visit: www.mobilescreening.org

■ Sunlight is needed to make active vitamin D in the body, so even if you are not a keen sunbather, then at least expose your skin to 15 minutes of sun regularly – but not between 11am–3pm. Vitamin D helps us to absorb calcium.

■ Dr Marilyn Glenville, one of the UK's leading experts on natural ways to cope with the menopause and osteoporosis, offers a postal consultation. For more information log on to: www.marilynglenville.com. For a consultation or an appointment in the UK call 01892 750511. Great bone recipes are in her book, *The Natural Alternatives to HRT Cookbook* by Dr Marilyn Glenville, Kyle Cathie.

■ Read *The Osteoporosis Solution* by Carl Germano, Kensington Publishing Corporation.

OTHER VITAL HORMONES

(Human Growth Hormone – See *Growth Hormone*, Oestrogen and Progesterone – See *Menopause* and *Women's Hormones*, Testosterone – See *Men's Hormones*. For Thyroid Hormones – See *Thyroid in Ageing*)

Please note that you should not self-medicate with hormones, always consult a qualified doctor or practitioner who can prescribe the correct balance for your individual needs.

CORTISOL AND AGEING

(See also *Low Blood Sugar p194* and *Stress in Ageing p293*)

Cortisol is a steroid hormone made by the adrenal glands and is produced in response to any stressful "fight or flight" situations. Aeons ago, this perfectly normal and natural response gave us the extra energy boost and mental sharpness to either run from our attacker or stand and fight. Either way, our bodies would utilize the cortisol and levels would then return to normal. Unfortunately, these days when we are stressed most of us don't tend to run away, we head for the coffee machine or the nearest packet of cakes and treats to cheer us up!

Cortisol is both good and bad. It is needed to help regulate blood pressure and cardiovascular function as well as regulation of the body's use of proteins, carbohydrates and fats. It is also released during times of infections, trauma, fatigue, temperature extremes, and crucially, when you worry too much.

In the short-term cortisol is a good guy, but if levels circulating in your body become, and remain, too high, i.e. chronically elevated, then cortisol damages tissues, organs and greatly affects memory and brain functioning. And stress hormones in the long-term contribute to bone loss.

Other common symptoms include palpitations, depression, sleep disorders, high blood pressure, anorexia, low blood sugar, insulin resistance, thyroid problems, menstrual disorders, osteoporosis and obesity (when combined with high insulin levels). You get the picture.

Too much stress and cortisol can kill you. Think of a Pacific salmon: after spawning it undergoes rapid cortisol-induced ageing, and death follows in a matter of days.

Obviously, we are all unique and what stresses one person can be a healthy challenge to another. You simply need to be aware that when you suffer negative stress, in the short-term your body can cope, but in the long-term, if you want to live to a ripe old age, you must deal with stress more effectively (see *Stress in Ageing*).

Foods to Avoid

- Don't underestimate how your diet can affect stress and therefore cortisol levels.
- Research has shown that drinking 2–3 cups of regular coffee per day can elevate cortisol levels.
- Avoid sugar, alcohol, fizzy drinks and all foods and drinks containing caffeine. They give you a quick energy hit, but in the long-term, will exacerbate the problem, as they cause even more cortisol to be released.
- See also *Friendly Foods* under *Low Blood Sugar p196* and *Stress in Ageing p294*.

Friendly Foods

- When you are stressed you burn up protein faster than normal, so make sure you eat quality protein: meat, fish, chicken, soya tofu or beans every day.
- Whey protein is a great source of easily digestible protein, add a dessertspoon daily to fruit smoothies.
- See also *Friendly Foods* under *Low Blood Sugar* and *Stress*.

Useful Remedies

- As a base, take a high-strength multivitamin/mineral supplement to support your system (see details of Kudos 24 on p348).
- PhosphatidylSerine, take 200mg per day. Take before bed to help the body stop over-producing cortisol.
- To support adrenal glands and compensate for the breakdown of protein by excess cortisol take a 100mg vitamin B-complex per day, plus an extra 500mg of pantothenic acid (B5).
- Your need for vitamin C increases with stress, so take 2 grams daily with meals.
- The mineral magnesium is greatly depleted by cortisol, so take an extra 400mg per day as well as the multivitamin/mineral.
- DHEA (see next heading) is also good for stress and in some ways protects against the negative effects of cortisol. DHEA works to build up body tissues, whereas cortisol breaks

them down.

- Good stress-busting supplements include homeopathic valerian, ignatia and avena sativa, try 6c or 30c. The German homeopathic company, HEEL, manufacture several anti-stress formulas, including Valerian-heel, Nervo-heel and Ignatia-homaccord. These remedies are available to order from Boots and Lloyds chemists and all homeopathic pharmacies.

- Try Bach Flower Remedies, which have important psychological benefits. Mimulus, for example, is great for fear, and if you feel overwhelmed, then Rescue Remedy can prove invaluable.

- See also *Useful Remedies* under *Stress in Ageing p295*.

Helpful Hints

- Oestrogen replacement, from orthodox HRT, can increase cortisol levels.

- One of the best methods for measuring cortisol levels is an adrenal stress index saliva test. This test measures cortisol levels from early morning to midnight. The results are plotted on a graph and compared with a normal daily output of cortisol. This test is available at The Individual Wellbeing Clinic, tel: 0207 730 7010, or visit www.individual-wellbeing.co.uk, or from your health practitioner.

- If you become over-excited, you also produce cortisol and in the long-term too much excitement (like a big shopping spree) can literally "excite" your cells to death – stay calm ladies.

- The best answer to stress, in all situations, is avoid it if you can. If you can't then you must find ways to minimize its damage. Meditation, regular exercise, yoga, t'ai chi or aromatherapy massage, etc. will all aid relaxation and reduce stress.

DHEA AND AGEING

DHEA is produced by the adrenal glands and is the most abundant steroid hormone in the body. It is made from cholesterol and can be converted into oestrogen or testosterone. By the age of 65, we make only 10–20% of what we made at 20. Many scientists, including Dr Samuel Yen at the University of California San Diego, and Dr William Regelson at Virginia Commonwealth University, agree that if you want to stay young, you need to maintain youthful levels of DHEA.

One 20-year study found that DHEA levels were far lower in men who died of heart disease than in healthier men. Low levels of DHEA have also been found in Alzheimer's patients. In fact, there is now little doubt that DHEA helps prevent the ravages of brain ageing. It protects against Alzheimer's and dementia and brings an improved overall sense of wellbeing which scientists have identified as being due to increased levels of endorphins (the chemicals we make naturally when we are happy and during exercise).

Tests have shown that DHEA can help prevent cancer, heart disease, bone and skin degeneration, it helps maintain brain function and gives powerful support to the immune system. It is anti-infections, anti-autoimmune disorders, anti-obesity, anti-diabetes and anti-stress. It's definitely anti-ageing!

DHEA has also been shown in numerous studies to improve mood and energy levels in both men and women and is therefore a valid treatment for depression and long-term negative stress. This effect was found to be particularly noticeable for post-menopausal women. One German study showed that DHEA considerably increased the libido and sexual satisfaction in the women taking part.

Also, at the menopause, women often undergo rapid age transformation and while most doctors suggest some kind of HRT, very few prescribe DHEA. It helps reverse many of the unfavourable effects of excess cortisol, creating subsequent improvement in energy, vitality, sleep, premenstrual symptoms and mental clarity.

Fortunately, DHEA is easy to supplement in tablet form and serum levels can be controlled with ease. But as always, before self-treating with hormones, have a blood test and find out what your levels are. If DHEA is lower than 300mgm/dL, you would need to take a supplementary dose. Men should consider 25–50mg daily and can go as high as 100mg until levels normalize and then a maintenance dose of 50mg should be fine. Adjust the dose until you get a definite beneficial response.

In women, anything more than modest doses, may trigger increased facial hair growth, spots and greasy skin. To avoid such undesirable side-effects, women should take no more than 25mgs daily. Generally, 10–15mg is adequate and still provides the benefits. When I was very stressed about 4 years ago, I had a blood test and found that my DHEA levels were almost nil and I began taking 10mg daily. Within 2 months I felt as though I had been re-born. After 4 months I started to get what I eventually learned were "DHEA" spots on my forehead and so I cut the dose. These days I only take 10mg twice a week which works fine for me.

A note of caution Because DHEA can be metabolized into testosterone and oestrogen, DHEA use should be avoided by anyone who currently has prostate cancer or breast cancer. Having said this, DHEA helps prevent cancer in those who do not have it. Also do not take this hormone if it you are pregnant, nursing, or have prior ovarian, adrenal or thyroid tumours. Women should avoid DHEA just prior to menopause because their levels typically increase around that time anyway

DHEA is not available over the counter in health stores in the UK as it is in the USA. You can purchase it for your own use from PharmWest by calling freephone 00800-8923-8923, or ask a friend travelling to America to bring some home for you. You can also order it by post from The Life Extension Foundation on www.lef.org.

Note that regular exercise increases DHEA levels naturally.

For further help and information on DHEA read *DHEA – The Ultimate Rejuvenating Hormone* by Hasnain Walji, Hohm Press, or *DHEA, A Practical Guide* by Ray Sahelian, Avery.

INSULIN
(See also *Carbohydrate Control, Diabetes – Late-onset* and *Insulin Resistance*).

Insulin is a hormone secreted by cells in the pancreas. Its major function is to lower blood sugar levels and promote the storage of sugars as fats. Its release is stimulated by the consumption of any type of carbohydrates from fruits and grains to starchy vegetables and cakes. It also slows the breakdown of any stored fats. Of all the hormones, insulin is the king player when it comes to ageing. By many mechanisms (which are explained in the sections on *Diabetes – Late Onset*, *Carbohydrate Control* and *Insulin Resistance*) high insulin levels cause ageing, disease, hormone imbalance and deterioration of virtually every body system.

According to American diabetes expert, Dr Ron Rosedale MD, almost everyone eating a typical western diet is overproducing insulin. The modern diet is based on far too many refined carbohydrates, which always causes an overproduction of insulin.

MELATONIN AND AGEING
(See also *Sleep p286*)

Melatonin, is secreted by the pineal gland located behind our eyes in the brain and many scientists now believe that this hormone may be the most powerful anti-ager of all. Melatonin is crucial for controlling our biological rhythms and is secreted mainly at night, see-sawing with serotonin, its counterpart, which is secreted during the day. Melatonin helps you to sleep whilst serotonin raises mood and makes you feel positive. Serotonin, called the "happy neurotransmitter", is converted to melatonin by the pineal gland.

Professor Richard Wurtmann of the Massachusetts Institute, proved to the scientific world that ageing is caused by healthy cells being attacked by free radicals when the pineal gland no longer secretes sufficient amounts of melatonin to protect them. Secretion of this natural anti-ageing agent starts at the age of 3 months and then drops before puberty. It continues to decline and falls dramatically around age 45. The other systems in the body seem to take this as a signal to slow down – and the ageing process begins in earnest.

In thousands of published studies, melatonin has been shown to protect against almost every disease associated with ageing including cardiovascular disease, as melatonin helps to lower LDL (the bad cholesterol) and lower blood pressure. It also helps reduce incidence of osteoporosis, and protects against Alzheimer's and Parkinson's disease, as well as against ageing itself. Further, melatonin boosts immunity, by increasing our "natural killer" cells (the ones which attack and destroy wandering microbes and cancer cells) and is one of the most effective antioxidants yet studied. One study found that as little as 2mg of melatonin led to a 240% increase in natural killer cell activity.

The strong relaxant effects of melatonin means that it can be helpful in schizophrenia, depression, anxiety, panic attacks and sleep disorders. The list goes on and on, melatonin also acts effectively against wrinkles as it enhances the elasticity of the skin, the suppleness of the joints, sexual activity and bone and muscular strength.

At least some of the anti-ageing benefits of melatonin may come from the fact that is also promotes the release of human growth hormone (see *Growth Hormone p156*), which is a master anti-ageing hormone. It seems no coincidence that both these hormones appear in our bloodstream only at night.

Some drugs also interfere with melatonin production, chiefly the NSAIDs, such as aspirin, ibuprofen and indomethacin.

Paradoxically, lack of sunshine during the daytime affects melatonin secretion at night. This is because during the daytime we are supposed to be making serotonin, a precursor of melatonin and sunlight is vital to make these hormones. Serotonin fights depression (Prozac and St John's Wort both work by inhibiting the breakdown of serotonin).

Foods to Avoid
■ Too much caffeine and alcohol inhibit the release of melatonin.

Friendly Foods
■ Tryptophan, which increases production of melatonin, is found in such foods as turkey, bananas, sunflowers seeds, and milk. You can now buy organic Slumber Milk from most branches of Waitrose, which helps increase melatonin levels.

■ If you are taking NSAIDs, you need to eat more essential fats, especially the omega-3s, eicosopentanoic acid (EPA) and dicosohexanoinc acid (DHA), which counter the inflammatory prostaglandins and are good for the brain. EPA and DHA are found in oily fish, egg yolks, animal organs and marine algae (for more information on essential fats see *Fats for Anti-ageing p139*).

Useful Remedies
■ Melatonin is not available over the counter in health stores in the UK as it is in the USA. You can purchase it for your own use from PharmWest on freephone 00800-8923-8923, or ask a friend travelling to America to bring some home for you.

■ The most common side effect of taking too much melatonin is feeling drowsy when you wake up. This can be prevented by taking less melatonin the next night. Begin by taking 1mg and see how you go, you can increase to 3mg and up to a maximum of 5mg. Keep a sleep diary and note which dose gives you the best night's sleep.

■ Tryptophan increases the production of melatonin and serotonin. Take 100mg at night before bed in the form of 5-HTP (for more details see *Sleep in Ageing p286*).

■ For good melatonin production you need B vitamins, especially B1, B6, B12, so take a B complex with breakfast.

■ You also need adequate magnesium, take 400mg daily at bedtime.

Helpful Hints

- Melatonin is naturally released during sleep. It is important therefore that you get around 7–8 hours of deep satisfying sleep. REM (rapid eye movement) sleep when we dream, is particularly important for melatonin production.

- It is vital to sleep in a properly darkened room. Even very low light levels can impair melatonin secretion. If your blinds and curtains are not adequate, consider a fabric sleeping visor and grow younger while you sleep.

- Electromagnetic radiation exposure during sleep can also cause the reduction of melatonin production. Therefore turn off the bedroom TV at the mains, use a battery operated clock and avoid sleeping with an electric blanket on unless it's really cold.

- Certain pain relievers such as aspirin and ibuprofen cause the partial suppression of melatonin.

- For further help read *The Melatonin Miracle* by Walter Pierpaoli, Pocket Books.

PREGNENOLONE AND AGEING

Pregnenolone is manufactured in the body from cholesterol and is a precursor to the production of DHEA, testosterone, oestrogens, cortisol and aldosterone, a kidney control hormone. Probably because of its involvement with many hormone pathways, pregnenolone tends to decline less dramatically than other hormones in later life. However, by the age of 75 our bodies produce 60% less pregnenolone than the levels produced in our mid-30s. For this reason pregnenolone levels are one of the important biomarkers of aging.

Also, strict cholesterol-controlled diets, vegan diets and the medical use of cholesterol lowering drugs, could impair your natural production of pregnenolone, with consequent negative ageing effects.

The best news about pregnenolone however is its mind-enhancing function. Studies have shown that this hormone increases memory, improves concentration, gives you quicker reaction times, helps protect the all-important myelin sheath around nerve fibres, increases resistance to stress and reduces depression.

Pregnenolone is therefore an ideal supplement for helping to reduce many conditions associated with ageing such as confusion, forgetfulness, loss of energy, apathy, decreased sense of worth and depression.

Another positive point is that pregnenolone converts directly to progesterone. Therefore if you suffer from oestrogen dominance (see *Menopause p212*), try supplementing pregnenolone before you try DHEA.

Useful Remedies

- There are no dietary sources of pregnenolone and supplemental pregnenolone is made from substances found in soya beans. A safe starting dose is 30mgm daily.

- Pregnenolone is not available over the counter in health stores in the UK as it is in the USA. You can purchase it for your own use from www.lef.org

■ For further help with balancing your hormones, contact your doctor, health professional or HB Health at 59 Beachamp Place London SW3 1NZ. Tel: 0207 838 0765, website: www.hbHealthOnline.com

OXYGEN IN AGEING

(See also *Breathing, Lungs in Ageing* and *Pollution Protection*)

For billions of years on Earth, the only life forms were blue-green algae, which excrete oxygen as a waste product and over the millennia they created the oxygen that enabled more complex life forms to evolve, including humans.

When you breathe in, oxygen is taken in through the lungs and transported via the tissues into the blood. When you breathe out, carbon dioxide from de-oxygenated blood is exhaled via the lungs. Oxygen has an alkalizing (healthy) affect on the body, whereas carbon dioxide is acid forming (unhealthy). Every time you breathe out, you exhale toxic waste from your cells. This waste is highly acidic, hence why ancient monuments are now being closed to the public – our breath acts just like acid rain. Low oxygen levels cause lactic acid build-up in our muscles, which triggers cramps during aerobic exercise.

The human body can survive for weeks without food, days without water, but only minutes without oxygen. Every cell in the body requires a continuous supply of oxygen to feed the chemical reactions that generate energy and detoxify both internally and externally derived waste products such as pesticides, heavy metals, and carbon dioxide build-up.

But in writing this section I have come across several schools of thought on oxygen. This gets rather technical, but at least you have a fuller explanation about oxygen in ageing. Some scientists state that too much oxygen can produce an excess of free radicals (oxidants) – that is if you have insufficient antioxidants to neutralize them (see *Antioxidants in Ageing*). They say that excessive oxygen being burnt in the body for energy, which occurs during strenuous exercise, produces more free radicals. And combined with the free radicals being produced by pollution, stress, fried food, and radiation etc, if you don't have sufficient antioxidants in your body, you may suffer more cellular oxidation. The result is faster ageing. This is the first school of thought.

For the more technically minded, Mark Lester, an authority on oxygen therapies, offers a second school of thought saying, "The body is perfectly designed to handle free radicals and the free radical scavenger enzymes in the body (glutathione peroxidase, superoxide dismutase, reductase and catalase) are easily able to handle any left-over free radicals from normal body processes. The prime generators of the harmful free radicals in the human body are pollution, toxicity from a poor diet and a lack of oxygen. The trouble comes when toxins are allowed to build up in the system because we do not eat, exercise and cleanse our bodies properly. These toxins prevent the enzymes from physically contacting the free radicals, allowing the radicals to escape their birthplace and do damage elsewhere, where the enzymes can't find them. So the cause of the problem is not with the free radicals themselves, but rather with the build-up of toxins that allows the free radicals to hide and escape neutralization by the scavenger enzymes." This is why Doctor William F. Koch, MD, Ph.D. and Professor of Chemistry at Wayne State University, stated, "The cause of (harmful) free radicals in the human body is a lack of oxygen." In other words oxygen is the "good" free radical, which cleans out the harmful "bad" free radicals.

Today, you can pop into department stores like Harvey Nichols, buy an oxygen mask and inhale oxygen for a few minutes to give you an energy boost. There are also numerous oxygen facials and creams that claim to boost the oxygen content of your skin. You can even buy an oxygen "pen" from major chemists that helps clear up skin spots.

You can also have ozone (an activated form of oxygen) therapy, that helps to kill viruses, bacteria, fungi (candida) and other pathogens (see *Helpful Hints* in this section).

These treatments will undoubtedly aid good health, as our atmosphere now contains less oxygen and considerably more pollution than it did in the past. Furthermore, as we age, our ability to store and transport oxygen in the blood is greatly diminished. This is because we tend to breathe more shallowly, sit for longer periods, don't take sufficient exercise, and so on.

Foods to Avoid and Friendly Foods
■ See *Foods to Avoid* and *Friendly Foods* under *Breathing p67.*

Useful Remedies
■ A powdered formula called Colosan, made up from oxygen bonded to magnesium, is an excellent way to get more oxygen into the body. And the more you take, the more you flood the body, especially the colon with oxygen, generating more energy and killing candida and anaerobic bacteria in the gut. Colosan will not harm the friendly intestinal bacteria because they are aerobic and thrive in a high-oxygen environment. Colosan has a gentle non-irritating, non-addictive laxative effect which for some people is an inconvenience but for others is a blessing. Depending on your tolerance to its bowels opening effects, the maximum that is usually practical/convenient to take is 1–3 teaspoons daily in water. Available from The Finchley Clinic, as below.

■ Hydroxygen Plus (also known as "Life Support") is an oxygen product that combines oxygen, hydrogen, minerals and enzymes that work together so that all the vitamins and other nutrients you ingest can be easily absorbed by your cells. It does not cause loose bowels. A monthly supply comes in a small bottle. It is not sensitive to heat and keeps indefinitely. It works regardless of whether it is taken near to or away from food, whereas Colosan is best taken on an empty stomach. For these reasons some people find it more convenient to take than Colosan. Adding 2 drops of Hydroxygen Plus to a gallon of water and setting the mixture aside for four hours sterilizes it. By supplying the body with oxygen, hydrogen, minerals and enzymes at the same time is especially good for candida and chronic fatigue syndrome. Available from The NutriCentre on 0207 436 5122, or contact the Finchley Clinic on 020 8349 4730.

Helpful Hints

- When the body is flooded with an activated, non-toxic form of oxygen – namely ozone – practitioners report that numerous age-related conditions, including some cancers, dramatically improve or disappear.

- Dr Otto Warburg won a Nobel Prize for discovering that normal cells when deprived of oxygen for a sufficient time turn into cancer cells. To get more oxygen into the body you can either have ozone therapy (such as in the use of an ozone steam cabinet) or some doctors are working with hydrogen peroxide injections, which provide an instant supply of oxygen oxidants to counter the effects of serious illness or toxicity.

- Many therapists who offer these treatments have been harassed by Government bodies, especially in America. Perhaps certain people are not keen for us to know that there are inexpensive non-drug based treatments that really can help. In Mexico, Dr Kurt Donsbach has used intravenous hydrogen peroxide for years and claims that the majority of his patients make a full recovery from illness. For details log on to www.hospitalsantamonica.com

- In the UK hydrogen peroxide injections (in conjunction with intravenous vitamins and minerals) are used by:

  • Dr Patrick Kingsley in Leicestershire – Tel: 01530 223 622

  • Dr Fritz Schellander in Tunbridge Wells – Tel: 01892 543 535

  • Dr Julian Kenyon in London – Tel: 020 7486 5588

  • Dr Wendy Denning at the Integrated Medical Centre in London – Tel: 0207 224 5111

  • Dr Rodney Adeniyi-Jones at the Regent Clinic Tel: 0207 486 6354

  • Dr Robert Trossell in London – Tel: 0207 486 1095

- Mark Lester, based in the Finchley area of North London, uses an ozone steam cabinet to treat patients. This method, which dates back to at least 1881, is relaxing and has a deeper healing effect than conventional saunas and steam rooms. He says that the non-toxic ozone treatment, which takes about one hour, opens the pores and the ozone is absorbed through the skin. Flooding the tissues with oxygen helps to inactivate viruses, bacteria, parasites, yeast fungal overgrowths and it helps to stimulate immune function. It also (like chelation) helps to clean the veins and arteries thus reducing the risk for heart disease and strokes. Mark says this treatment also helps to break down excess adrenalin in the body, which reduces stress and its ageing effects on the body, and chelates (removes) heavy metals such as mercury and aluminium. He sees especially good results with people with chronic fatigue syndrome (ME), arthritis, and viral diseases.

- Mark also uses other methods of ozone therapy described on his website. As this is a huge subject. I strongly suggest that you visit his site on www.thefinchleyclinic.co.uk, or call 020 8349 4730.

- For further information I suggest you read *Oxygen Healing Therapies* by Nathaniel Altman, Healing Arts Press, or *Flood Your Body with Oxygen – Therapies For Our Polluted World* by Ed McCabe, Energy Publications. Website: www.edmccabe.org

- For technically minded sports people who want to know more about oxygen and ageing regarding the school of thought that says strenuous exercise accelerates ageing, Ed McCabe, the author of *Flood Your Body With Oxygen* says, "To say that long distance runners age faster because they take in too much oxygen is wrong. Some long distance runners may age faster because after they run out of oxygen they start pulling energy out of their body's ATP reserves. Adenosine Tri-Phosphate (ATP) is the energy currency of the body. The body can make 2 types. "Aerobic ATP" and "Anaerobic ATP", depending upon how much oxygen it has to work with. Aerobic ATP = lots of power and little residue. Anaerobic ATP = poor performance lots of painful residue and harmful free radicals. If athletes have plenty of tissue and fluid oxygen reserves, then the athlete would only produce the high quality aerobic type ATP, enjoy the workout and stay younger longer. And Aerobic ATP leaves little lactic acid behind. Basically, what all this means is that oxygen is generally the good guy!

PANCREAS IN AGEING

(See also *Diabetes – Late-onset* and *Low Blood Sugar*)
Increasingly common in older people are problems with the pancreas. Your pancreas is a large gland situated behind your stomach towards your spine. It secretes digestive juices into the small intestine, as well as insulin and other hormones into the bloodstream, which are primarily involved in keeping your blood sugar (energy) levels even.

Common ailments affecting the pancreas are pancreatitis (inflammation of the pancreas), pancreatic cancer (the fourth leading cause of cancer deaths in the United States) and pancreatic scarring from alcohol-related damage.

Because the pancreas produces digestive juices and the hormones insulin and glucagons, which regulate blood sugar levels, problems with the pancreas often lead to digestive problems, glucose intolerance or late-onset diabetes.

Foods to Avoid

■ Don't drink excessive alcohol, keep intake to no more than 3 units a day, as alcohol can cause scarring of the pancreatic tissue.

■ Eat a diet low in fat and sugar to reduce the workload on the pancreas by reducing your need for pancreatic digestive juices and insulin. A high level of fat in the blood is a factor in pancreatitis, which can then lead to cardiovascular problems.

■ Reduce your consumption of meat, its concentrated protein and high fat content are difficult to digest and force the pancreas to work harder producing digestive juices. Some research has suggested that high meat consumption may be one of the risk factors contributing to pancreatic cancer.

■ Reduce your consumption of coffee, tea, cigarettes, refined (white) foods, sugar and other stimulants, they all disrupt blood sugar levels.

Friendly Foods

■ Eat more raw foods, 40% or more in summer, as they are much more easily digested and contain live enzymes that aid digestion, which are destroyed by cooking. Eat plenty of fresh fruits, vegetable crudités and salads.

■ Give your pancreas (and digestive system) a rest. soups and juices are an ideal way to get lots of easily digested and absorbable nutrients into your system.

■ Increase your consumption of zinc-rich foods, such as oysters, pumpkin seeds, nuts, wholegrains such as brown rice, millet, lentils, barley, seafood, and the occasional portion of organic calves' liver. Zinc plays a role in the manufacture of insulin.

■ Lecithin aids the digestion of fats, thus reducing the demands on your pancreas to produce digestive juices. Sprinkle a dessertspoonful of GM-free lecithin granules on your breakfast cereal every morning, or sprinkle over fruit salads, into yoghurts and so on.

■ Eat more bitter foods such as celeriac, artichoke, rocket and bitter salad leaves like radicchio.

■ Drink lemon juice in warm water before meals to stimulate the body's own production of digestive enzymes.

■ See also *Friendly Foods* under *Low Blood Sugar p194*.

Useful Remedies

■ Start with a good-quality multivitamin/mineral, which provides a baseline of nutrients you can then add to.

■ Chromium and vitamin B3 are essential for maintaining stable blood sugar levels, thus reducing the workload on the pancreas. BioCare's Sucroguard combines these and other nutrients, and helps reduce cravings and improve energy levels (take 1 with main meals). For details see BioCare on page 13.

■ Digestive enzyme tablets aid in reducing the strain on the pancreas by aiding protein digestion. Try BioCare's Polyzyme Forte, 1 with each main meal, or Solgar's Pancreatic Digestive Enzymes (see pages 13 and 14).

■ Gentian tincture will help to increase pancreatic enzymes naturally – take 15 drops in a small glass of water 15 minutes before food.

Helpful Hints

■ Pancreatic problems are serious and require medical supervision. Talk to your doctor if you have any questions or concerns about your pancreas.

■ Stop smoking and also avoid secondhand smoke. Recent studies point to a distinct link between poor pancreatic health and cigarette smoke.

■ Regular fasting can improve the health of all organs, including the pancreas (see *Detoxing*).

PARKINSON'S DISEASE

Parkinson's Disease affects some 120,000 people in Britain, including 1 in every 100 people over the age of 60. Affecting men more often than women, Parkinson's is a progressive disorder involving the deterioration of the nerve centers in the brain responsible for controlling movement. As the condition progresses, muscular movement is affected. Eventually coordination can become a nightmare and it's common for patients to experience tremors, rigidity and muscular spasms in different limbs to varying degrees. Other symptoms include unsteadiness, chronic constipation, impaired speech, a fixed facial expression and a shuffling gait.

The person knows what they want the muscle to do but the messages received by the muscle group are not properly coordinated to allow smooth movement.

The reason for this impaired muscle control is a lack of the brain chemical dopamine. No definitive cause has yet been identified, but nutrient deficiencies, heavy metal toxicity, especially from mercury and aluminium, over-consumption of the artificial sweetener aspartame, viruses and carbon-monoxide poisoning have all been mooted as possible triggers. Some prescription drugs can cause Parkinson's-like symptoms.

To replace the dopamine, most patients take a synthetic form of the amino acid L-dopa, which the body then makes into dopamine, helping restore proper brain function. Many of the drugs used to treat Parkinson's can cause lethargy and extreme mental confusion, or completely uncontrolled jerky movements if there is too much L-dopa in the body. As every case is unique, I strongly recommend that anyone with

Parkinson's consult a nutritional physician who is trained in PD Management, as this condition needs highly specialized care (see *Useful Information and Addresses p344*).

Foods to Avoid

- Reduce stimulants such as coffee, colas, tea and alcohol, as these foods can affect tremors.

- Cut down on animal fats, which impair the metabolism of essential fats (see *Fats for Anti-ageing p139*).

- Avoid sugar in any form, highly refined and processed foods and especially additives and preservatives such as monosodium glutamate and aspartame, because of their negative affect on the brain.

- With professional guidance you may also need to eliminate gluten containing grains such as wheat, rye, oats and barley, as the gluten can prevent absorption of nutrients and medication.

- Cut down on peanuts, bananas and potatoes, yeasty foods, liver and meat, which contain vitamin B6, which can interfere with the medication L-dopa. But if you are not taking L-dopa, vitamin B6 is important for Parkinson's.

- Don't fry food and avoid all hydrogenated and trans-fats, often found in margarines and pre-prepared foods. These fats are also found in most mass-produced cakes, biscuits, pies and so on. Always check labels.

Friendly Foods

- Ensure an adequate dietary intake. Because chewing can become difficult, loss of appetite is common and then nutrient deficiencies can speed the progression of the disease. Foods can be liquidized or meal replacements used.

- As much as possible eat only organic foods, which contain fewer pesticides and herbicides. A University of Miami post-mortem study in 1994 found pesticides more often than not in those who had died of Parkinson's Disease than in those who had died of other causes.

- Research has shown that restricting protein intake is helpful and that 90% of the daily intake should be eaten with the evening meal, when you're not having your L-dopa medication. This is extremely important advice not always given to patients on L-dopa. Protein competes for absorption with the L-dopa, so eating protein during the day, when most sufferers take their medication, can block the efficacy of the medication.

- Protein sources are meat, fish, eggs, beans, dairy foods, nuts and seeds, lentils, soya and wholegrains. The best sources for Parkinson's sufferers are small amounts of soya, eggs, oily and white fish, and poultry.

- Eat more corn-based foods and corn pasta.

- Include apples, pears, mangoes, kiwi fruit and vegetables such as cabbage, cauliflower, carrots and broccoli in your diet.

- Use unrefined, organic sunflower, sesame and olive oil for salad dressings and drizzle over cold foods. These oils are rich in essential fats, which are vital for healthy brain function as they enhance brain cell wall stability (see *Fats for Anti-ageing p139*).

■ Get into the habit of juicing, using organic carrots, beetroot and artichoke, which are high in vitamins and minerals and help to cleanse the liver (see *Liver in Ageing p189*).

■ If you have mercury fillings, eat lots of seaweed, apples and coriander, which detoxify metals from the body.

■ Dried or ready-to-eat fruits such as prunes, figs and apricots help to ease or prevent constipation, as does drinking at least eight glasses of water daily.

■ Begin drinking green tea, which is rich in antioxidants, or, if you don't like the tea, take high-strength green tea capsules.

Useful Remedies

■ As it is vital to take various nutrients in specific amounts for each individual case and the supplements you take also depend on the time of day and which medication you are taking. Again I strongly recommend that you see a qualified nutritionist or nutritional physician who can devise a programme specifically for you. Your own GP will need to refer you to a nutritional physician and they will be able to find the address of your nearest practitioner by contacting: British Society for Allergy Environmental and Nutritional Medicine (BSAENM), PO Box 7, Knighton, LD7 1WT. Tel: 01547 550 380

■ The following are some general guidelines:

■ Studies from the Birkmayer Institute for Parkinson's in Vienna has shown that NADH, a co-enzyme form of vitamin B3, can help increase energy levels, reduce depression and stimulate the body to produce more L-dopa. 5mg should be taken on an empty stomach at least 40 minutes before food. Professor Birkmayer's highly absorbable NADH is called Springfield Enada and is available worldwide. Anyone who is very stressed and suffers from palpitations should avoid this supplement. However, in some cases the intravenous form of this nutrient is more effective in Parkinson's – speak to your doctor about the intravenous form.

■ Taking antioxidants, such as vitamin C, up to 1gram daily with food and 400iu of full-spectrum, natural-source vitamin E, plus an antioxidant complex, may help to slow the progression.

■ 300 mg daily of co-EnzymeQ10 has been shown to slow the mental decline associated with Parkinson's disease.

■ L-methionine is an essential sulphur amino acid, which readily crosses the blood-brain barrier where it can be converted into the vital nutrient S-adenosyl methionine (SAMe). L-dopa supplementation reduces brain SAMe levels. For details contact the NutriCentre (see page 14).

■ Phosphatidyl serine is another vital brain nutrient that improves nerve cell health. The body can manufacture PS but only if you tend to eat lots of organ meats. 100mg can be supplemented two to three times a day.

■ For extra fibre to ease constipation and cleanse the bowel, try psyllium husks daily in warm water. They taste dreadful, but do help reduce constipation. Also available in capsules.

■ The herb, St John's Wort, can ease depression but should not be taken by people with Parkinson's as it can interfere with medication.

■ If you have mercury fillings take 500mg of vitamin C daily, which chelates with heavy metals and carries them out of the body, plus mercury antagonists: calcium – take 450mg a day – and zinc – take 15mg twice daily.

■ I strongly recommend that you read the section on *Essential Sugars p126*. I have interviewed some people with Parkinson's who have had excellent results after taking this newly-discovered essential food group.

Helpful Hints

■ Mercury fillings are linked to Parkinson's disease – have them checked by a holistic dentist and removed if necessary (with all the necessary protection during removal – otherwise you can become even more contaminated). See also *Toxic Metal Overload p317*.

■ As many of the world's oceans are heavily polluted, high levels of mercury are also being reported in some coastal fish.

■ Both aluminium and mercury have been linked to Parkinson's disease, therefore avoid all aluminium cookware or aluminium foil. Read labels carefully as cake mixes, antacids, buffered aspirin, self-raising flour, pickles, processed cheeses, most deodorants and toothpastes contain aluminium.

■ Monosodium glutamate (MSG), the food additive, and aspartame the artificial sweetener, have been linked to Parkinson's disease; therefore avoid all additives and preservatives whenever possible. Over 3,000 foods and drinks contain artificial sweeteners.

■ Reduce stress. At times of stress the body uses dopamine to make the stress hormones noradrenaline and adrenaline, using up your already short supply. Tools for reducing stress, apart from removing any obvious sources, include exercise, massage, relaxation techniques, meditation or enjoyable hobbies (see *Stress in Ageing p293*).

■ If tremors are worse at or after meal times, avoid protein (meat, fish, beans, nuts, seeds) at meals where you take your medication as protein competes with the L-dopa for absorption.

■ Constipation is a major symptom that must be dealt with to ensure the proper elimination of toxins. In addition to the dried fruits, flaxseeds and water recommended above, try abdominal massage in a clockwise circular motion to massage the bowel, walks after meals, or supplemented magnesium (take 150mg three times per day) to relax the bowel.

■ As organophosphates (OPs) from pesticides and herbicides, are now found in drinking water, use a good-quality water filter like Watersimple from The Fresh Water Filter Company. Contact The Fresh Water Filter Company, Gem House, 895 High Street, Chadwell Health, Essex RM6 4HL. Tel 0208 597 3223. www.freshwaterfilter.com or The Pure H2O Company on 01784 21188, or visit www.pureH20.co.uk

- A book well worth reading is *Parkinson's Disease, The Way Forward* by Dr Geoffrey Leader and Lucille Leader, Bath Press. To order call 0207 323 2382. This user-friendly book presents an integrated approach to the management of Parkinson's disease.

- Dr David Perlmutter, a neurologist in Naples, Florida, has pioneered the use of intravenous glutathione, which has had a dramatic effect on most of his Parkinson's patients. His book *BrainRecovery.com* makes fascinating reading. Published by the Perlmutter Health Centre. Available from the NutriCentre Book Shop (tel: 0207 323 2382), or log on to his website: www.BrainRecovery.com. In the UK doctors that administer chelation therapy usually work with glutathione – a list of these doctors is under *Chelation in Ageing p89*.

- For further help contact The Parkinson's Disease Society, 215 Vauxhall Bridge Road, London, SW1V 1EJ. Tel: 020 7931 8080. Helpline: 0808 800 0303. Website: www.parkinsons.org.uk Or the European Parkinson's Disease Society, 4 Golding Road, Sevenoaks Kent TN13 3NJ. Tel/Fax: 01732 457683. Website: www.epda.eu.com

PLASTIC SURGERY

(See also *Rejuvenation Therapies*)

I realize that plastic surgery is not what most people would term alternative, but I believe that if something can help you to feel more positive about yourself, and you are aware of the possible risks and still choose to do it – then why not. I sure have.

I first had plastic surgery to reduce my large nose when I was 21. Through my own actions and on a couple of occasions being operated on by poor surgeons – I ended up having eight further corrective operations on my nose.

But that initial surgery changed my life. I felt more positive about myself, I had more confidence and without a doubt it made me feel happier. As Joan Collins once said to me, "People can tell you that you look great, but it's how you feel inside, that determines whether you are happy or sad."

Once I finally found a good surgeon I could trust, at 39 I had my upper eyelids reduced as the skin overlapped my upper lids, a family trait, and at 48 I had a face-lift.

My surgeon Mr Basim Matti says, "These days women want more conservative surgery, the days of the face being over-stretched are hopefully behind us, and I have found that more subtle surgery gives the most natural looking results. Today with the use of botulism and collagen injections, plus various types of peels and creams (see *Rejuvenation Therapies*), we can hold back the years for longer, therefore the majority of patients don't have their first face-lift until their late 40s and beyond. A few patients may have a second or third face-lift, which usually last approximately 7 to 10 years each. The most popular operations are the upper and lower eyes, or a lower face-lift when we lift the cheeks, neck, jowl, jaw line areas. Obviously every face is unique and every patient has their own requests. Most brow lifts are done using an endoscope, keyhole surgery, so there is minimal scarring. Also thanks to

Botox injections, a forehead lift is often not always necessary, or is done much later in the 50s and onwards. Today, the new generation of face-lifts are targeted to the eye area, the lower eyelid and in particular the junction where the lower eyelid and face meet. As we age, you see a demarcation between the cheek and the eye, which makes older people look tired. In the past, we removed fat from the lower eyelid to try and reduce the bagginess or puffiness from under the eyes, but some surgeons went too far and if too much fat was removed, the eye looked too hollow and the patient could look tired or even older as a result.

These days we still remove a little of the excess fat under the eyes and if they have the demarcation line between the eyes and the cheek, then we spread the fat around this area, which makes this area look less hollow and shadowy.

We are progressing to injecting the patient's own fat, during the face-lift procedure, which adds a youthful plumpness to the patient's features."

Other surgery that is common for anti-ageing purposes is an Abdominoplasty, when the surgeon tightens the muscles in the abdomen and removes excess skin. Depending on how bad the tummy looks, you can either have a mini-lift or a full one. Either way this surgery is painful for at least a week and you'll need a minimum one night in hospital.

Liposuction is the commonest operation in plastic surgery, when excess fat is removed from under the skin, mostly from the outer thighs, the "love handles" on the abdomens or underneath the chin. If you still have good elasticity in your skin, it should respond by shrinking to give you a smoother line. Liposuction has to be done with maximum care, by a qualified and experienced surgeon. Mr Matti says "There needs to be a careful limit as to the volume of fat that can be removed, otherwise the patient can go into severe shock because of fluid loss and there is a risk of excess bleeding and other complications."

On this one ladies, I would say use it as a last resort, and only if you are fully aware of what could happen if things go wrong!

Breast implants remain as popular as ever and even after all the scares with silicone implants, mine have been fine for over 13 years, and dare I say it, with no problems whatsoever. But after 15 years they should be checked and perhaps replaced.

Soya bean implants were hailed as being safe, but the Government's Medical Device Agency have now banned their use and anyone with the soya oil implants (Trilucent) has been advised to have them removed.

There are also fat injections being offered to enlarge breasts, but Mr Matti does not recommend these, as fat tissue over time, can become calcified, which could be confused as being possible breast cancer tissue, during a mammography. Also injectable gels are being offered by some people directly into breast tissue, but again Mr Matti warns against such treatments. Techniques are being advanced almost monthly, talk to other women who have had the procedures and find a surgeon you can trust, and if it feels right to you, then you are free to choose.

Foods to Avoid Before Having Surgery

■ Avoid foods rich in vitamin E such as avocado, almonds, hazel nuts and wheatgerm for one week prior to surgery. Generally essential fats and oils thin the blood naturally, so cut down on large amounts of salad dressings or cod liver oil for just a week.

■ Reduce your intake of garlic which also thins the blood naturally.

Friendly Foods

■ Pineapple is rich in bromelain, a natural enzyme that reduces bruising.

■ Carrots, apricots dried or fresh, all green vegetables especially spinach, spring greens, parsley and watercress, tomatoes and tomato puree, sweet potatoes, cantaloupe melon and mangoes are all rich in natural source carotenes which aid skin healing.

■ Eat plenty of fruits rich in vitamin C: cherries, kiwi, strawberries, oranges, blueberries etc.

■ The mineral zinc is vital to aid skin healing, so include organic raw nuts, grains, oysters and liver in your diet.

Useful Remedies

■ One of the best ways to reduce the swelling from any surgery is to take homeopathic arnica, 30c. Take one under the tongue prior to going to the operating theatre and as soon as you wake – take 1 or 2 under the tongue away from food or water every two to three hours. Once dressings are removed apply arnica cream or gels onto any bruised areas.

■ Take at least 2 grams of vitamin C daily, plus a multivitamin/mineral to speed the healing process.

■ You can take a 500mg capsule of bromelain daily until bruises disappear.

■ Don't take any vitamin E, garlic or ginkgo capsules for at least 14 days prior to undergoing this type of surgery.

■ Also avoid aspirin and all anti-inflammatory painkillers such as Ibufren prior to surgery.

Helpful Hints

■ No matter where you are in the world, find a good surgeon. I have always found that personal recommendation from a friend who has had surgery (that you like the results of) is the best way forward.

■ When you go for an initial consultation, ask to see before and after pictures of their work.

■ I have found that the anaesthetic tends to cause me more problems than the surgery, therefore I always ask for intravenous sedation – when you are out cold, but not as deeply unconscious as if you have a general anaesthetic.

■ Discuss all concerns with your surgeon and anaesthetist. Make a list of queries, because if you are nervous, you tend to be forgetful.

■ In the UK, to find your nearest qualified Plastic Surgeon contact: The British Association of

Plastic Surgeons, The Royal College of Surgeons, 35–43 Lincoln's Inn Fields, London WC2A 3PN. Tel: 0207 831 5161, Fax: 0207 831 4041. www.baps.co.uk or The British Association of Aesthetic Plastic Surgeons at the same address as above, Tel: 0207 405 2234, Fax: 0207 430 1840, Website: www.baaps.org.uk. Mr Basim Matti's details are on this site. Or contact him at 30 Harley Street, London W1G 9PW. Tel: 0207 637 9595, Fax: 0207 636 1639. e-mail; basim.matti@bmplasticsurgery.com

■ A full face, neck, eyes and brow lift will cost you anything from £6,000 to £12,000 and beyond, depending where you go in the world and the surgeon's reputation and popularity.

■ Eyelids, top and bottom, cost from £3,000.

■ An abdominoplasty costs around £5,500–£8000, a mini £4,500.

■ Breast implants vary from £3,650–£4,500.

■ Following surgery, keep a couple of bottles of witch hazel in the fridge and apply cold pads soaked in the witch hazel to the injured areas as often as you can during the first 48 hours.

■ Ask to be fully informed of the risks and understand that every time you go under a knife, there are risks involved.

■ Get plenty of rest, as nothing aids healing faster than sufficient sleep. But don't lie around in bed for too long as you need to keep your circulation going.

■ Also avoid any blood thinning drugs, such as aspirin, prior to surgery, which can cause excessive bleeding.

■ Avoid smoking, which slows the healing process.

POLLUTION PROTECTION

(See also *Liver in Ageing, Radiation in Ageing, Toxic Metal Overload* and *Water in Ageing*)

Our bodies are now contaminated with some 500 man-made chemicals that were not in the bodies of our great-grandparents. Human ingenuity has produced around 10 million new chemicals – substances that have never before been part of our environment. Data from the US Environmental Protection Agency indicate that manufacturing firms released over seven billion pounds of toxic chemicals into the environment in 1999 alone. These toxins, many of which are carcinogenic, continue to be sprayed upon our food, they are in our water, they are in the air we breathe; and unless humanity, every single one of us, makes an effort to do what we can, where we can, to lessen the toxic load, then an even unhealthier future awaits us all.

Pollutants and toxins create free radicals that damage our cells, burden our immune system and detoxification mechanisms. Because exposure to environmental pollution is virtually inevitable, we need to be aware of environmental toxins and learn how to protect ourselves from them.

A major problem is hormone-disrupting chemicals. Our hormonal system controls many crucial aspects of the working of our bodies. It governs the way children grow into adults, our sexual characteristics, our day-to-day bodily functions and the way our bodies burn oxygen to make energy. Hormone disrupting chemicals are able to imitate or disrupt the action of these natural hormones. It is now known that more and more chemicals in everyday use are hormone disrupters. The chemicals involved include pesticides and industrial chemicals such as DDT, lindane, vinclozolin, phthalates and alkylphenols. The pesticides can be found in residues on food and the industrial chemicals are in many PVC plastics and in the linings of many food cans. The accumulation of so many toxins is having a devastating impact on our health. Lowered sperm counts, infertility, an increase in auto-immune conditions such as lupus, sexual organ mutations (in humans and animals), compromised immune function, multiple food intolerances and a massive increase in people who are allergic to household cleaners and so on. Governments in several countries have started to develop policies towards hormone-disrupting chemicals. Most of these policies involve research and screening of chemicals, rather than regulatory action on individual chemicals. The chemical industry is unwilling to accept that endocrine disruption is any more than a "hypothesis", but rates of testicular, breast and prostate cancers have all been rising in recent decades and sperm counts have been falling. A recent study, published in 2000, concluded that more than 40% of young Danish men have reduced sperm counts. Testicular cancer increased by 55% between 1979 and 1991 in England and Wales and scientists have found that 1 in 6 girls in Britain is starting to show signs of puberty at the age of 8, compared to 1 in 100 girls a century ago. I have absolutely no doubt that the rise in incidence of breast cancer is linked to exposure to hormone-disrupting chemicals. Prostate cancer increased by 40% between 1979 and 1991 in England and Wales. Although some of this increase may be due to improved diagnosis, hormone-disrupting chemicals are considered by many experts to be the most likely contributor.

If you are really healthy, then you can adapt to mild and periodic exposure to pollutants in our air, water, and food, and some chemicals are easier to avoid than others. We have considerable control over what we eat, drink and breathe, so healthy food choices, such as organic produce and purified water, and avoiding food additives, cigarettes, heavy traffic and home chemicals will certainly help reduce the toxic overload.

Foods to Avoid

- Because chemical bombardment can lead to a weakened immune system, an increase in allergies and a myriad of other diseases, avoiding foods high in chemicals is definitely important. Some people become hypersensitive to the chemicals in the environment as a result of chemical exposures and foods can be a major factor.

- Avoid artificial food colours found in a host of foods from desserts to ready-packed meals.

- Avoid cured meats, such as bacon, ham and salami. Artificial flavours and other food additives, especially monosodium glutamate and aspartame, should also be avoided.

■ Tea plants naturally accumulate fluoride from soil and drinking large quantities of tea will raise a person's fluoride intake.

Friendly Foods

■ See the *Friendly Foods* section in *Liver in Ageing p192*.

■ Eat organic foods as much as possible, which contain far less pesticides.

■ Eat more antioxidant-rich fresh fruit and vegetables such as organic berries, beetroot, carrots, sweet potato, tomatoes, peppers, and dark green leafy vegetables such as watercress, cabbage, broccoli, Brussels sprouts, spinach, chard and kale.

■ Add more fresh coriander to cooked meals, which helps to detoxify heavy metals from the body.

■ Cruciferous vegetables, such as cabbage, cauliflower, broccoli, and Brussels sprouts, are good sources of vitamin K and compounds called glucosinolates are known to be protective against cancer.

■ Foods rich in beta-carotene, such as cruciferous vegetables, as well as carrots, sweet potatoes, cantaloupe melons, apricots, swede etc, will add more antioxidant nutrients.

■ Miso, a fermented soybean paste used for soup broth, is known to help protect against pollution and radiation.

■ Seaweeds, high in natural metal-chelating algins, are likewise useful anti-pollution foods and they are also high in minerals. Available in good health stores and recipe ideas can usually be found on the packets.

■ Drink more clean water – six glasses daily to help flush toxins from the body.

Useful Remedies

■ Research from all over the world has shown that vitamins protect cells and biological systems from the harmful effects of chemicals and environmental pollution.

■ A good-quality "multiple" will provide many nutrients and help to counter the effects of "anti-nutrient" pollutants. A good antioxidant formula (see *Antioxidants in Ageing*) that also contains natural source carotenes will decrease the potential of free-radical toxicity. A multi-nutrient powder called Kudos 24 would be ideal (see page 348).

■ Vitamin C protects the body against the effects of water-soluble chemicals such as carbon monoxide, metals such as cadmium and metabolic by-products such as carcinogenic nitrosamines made from nitrites. Take 1 gram one to three times daily with food in an ascorbate form.

■ Natural source vitamin E, about 400–600iu's daily, and selenium, 200–300mcg daily, work together to protect the cells from pollutants including ozone, nitrogen dioxide, nitrites and metals, such as lead, mercury, silver, and cadmium.

■ Zinc helps to strengthen the immune system and the function of many detoxifying enzymes, thus helping to protect the cells from pollutant toxins. The recommended dose is 30mg per day.

■ Calcium and magnesium help to neutralize some colon toxins and decrease heavy metal absorption from the gastrointestinal tract. Recommended dose: calcium – 1,000mg per day and magnesium – 400mg per day.

■ Vitamin B3 (niacin) has an important role in the purification process, especially with many chemicals and pesticides. Recommended dose: 100mg per day

■ Alpha lipoic acid helps to protect the liver and aids in detoxification, particularly for the effects of radiation. Recommended dose: 60mg per day (see *Antioxidants in Ageing p38*).

■ N-acetyl cysteine helps to neutralize many heavy metal toxins and toxic by-products (aldehydes) of smoking, smog, alcohol, and fats. Recommended dose: 500mg per day.

■ Fibre, such as rice or oat bran and the more soluble cracked flax seeds (Linusit Gold) or psyllium husks, encourage natural detoxification in the colon, binding (chelating) toxins and reducing absorption of metals.

■ Organic source chlorophyll containing algae, such as chlorella and spirulina also provide a chelating effect.

Helpful Hints

■ Chelation therapy is a great way to eliminate most of the toxic heavy metals from your body (see *Chelation in Ageing p89*).

■ The only way to deal with smog, in the short-term, is to avoid it as much as possible. Don't jog beside busy roads, because aerobic exercise makes you breathe deeply and you draw pollutants deep into your lungs. In the long-term, consider living in a less polluted area and/or reducing your own pollution production. Many car trips are unnecessary and could be replaced by walking, using public transport, or car-pooling with friends and colleagues.

■ Don't smoke cigarettes and avoid the cigarette smoke of others. Smoking exposes your lungs to some of the same toxins found in smog.

■ Invest in a home air purifier. Air pollution inside the home, such as carbon monoxide (CO), nitrogen dioxide (NO2), benzene vapour, and volatile organic compounds (VOCs), can be a bigger problem than outdoor pollution. Plants also do a remarkable job of filtering indoor air, though make sure the soil doesn't become mouldy as mould spores can also irritate your respiratory system.

■ Drink a minimum of four to six glasses of purified water per day which helps keep everything moving and favours elimination of toxins. Remember, "dilution is the solution to pollution". To make sure our water, our most important nutrient, is pure it is worth investing in a good-quality, solid-carbon-block filter or reverse osmosis water purifier (for details of Pure H2O see *Water in Ageing*).

- Taking "medicinal" baths can also be used for detoxification of certain pollutants and radiation exposure. Try this salt-soda bath following airline flights or long hours at a computer: add 1 pound each of sea salt and baking soda to a warm bath and leisurely soak yourself. For an energizing detoxification bath add 2 cups apple cider vinegar to a warm bath; soak 15 to 30 minutes.

- Avoid over-use of chemicals such as cleaning products at home and reduce exposure at work whenever possible. Buy environmentally safer products such as Ecover, available from supermarkets and health stores.

- Avoid chemical-based hair dyes and sunscreens – ask at your health store for safer alternatives. Call The Green People on 01444 401444, or e-mail: organic@greenpeople.co.uk or visit www.greenpeople-organic-health.co.uk

- Be aware of the dozens of toxins and chemicals found in your cosmetics. Read *Drop Dead Gorgeous; Protecting Yourself From the Hidden Dangers of Cosmetics* by Kim Erickson and Dr Damuel Epstein, Contemporary Books.

- Don't microwave food and never place plastic or foil containers in the oven, as the hormone-disrupting chemicals can leach into your food.

- Use water-based paints where possible. Many household paints give off dangerous fumes as they dry. Water-based paints are better because they contain fewer "volatile organic compounds" (VOCs). Contact the Association for Environmentally Conscious Building on 01559 370908 for information on non-toxic paints, www.ecb.net

- There has been a marked increase in skin cancer, thought to be a result of the thinning of the ozone layer caused by air pollution. This means that the sun's ultraviolet rays are less filtered and more dangerous now than they were 25 years ago. Wear a sunscreen with 15–20 SPF whenever sun exposure will last longer than an hour (see *Sunshine in Ageing*).

- With any radioactive iodine tests or exposure to iodine fallout, take one kelp or iodine tablet daily for several weeks before and after the test to occupy the iodine-binding sites (unless, of course, this will interfere with the test) so that the least amount of the radioactive element will stay in the body. Regarding X-rays, see also *Radiation in Ageing*.

- Frequent high-altitude airline flights increase radiation exposure.

- Minimize your use of mobile phones to only what is strictly necessary (see also *Radiation in Ageing p265*).

- If you live near a nuclear power plant or an industry that uses radioactive wastes or toxic chemicals seriously consider moving, as more evidence is emerging confirming the higher incidences of cancers and other diseases in communities surrounding these installations.

- Become more environmentally aware – take out a subscription to the *Ecologist*, a highly regarded, authoritative magazine that keeps you up to date on all the latest environmental news and issues www.theecologist.org

- Read *How to Stay Young and Healthy in a Toxic World*, a brilliant book by Ann Louise Gittleman. Keats Publishing.

PROSTATE

(See also *Bladder Problems in Ageing*)

Approximately 50% of men over 55, and three-quarters of men over 70, suffer from enlarged prostate. That's more than 2 million men in the UK and 10,000 cases of prostate cancer are diagnosed in every year. The prostate is a walnut-sized gland that sits below the male bladder. Its job is to secrete seminal fluids and contract strongly during orgasm to cause ejaculation.

As men get older it is common for the prostate gland to gradually enlarge, up to two to four times its normal size, to about the size of a lemon. This is largely attributable to hormonal changes associated with ageing. After the age of 50 or so, a man's levels of testosterone decrease, while levels of other hormones, including oestrogen, increase.

Unfortunately, older men will have had a lifetime of exposure to plastics, petrochemicals and pesticides, which all have hormone-disrupting (oestrogenic) effects in the body and are linked to hormonal cancers. Although testosterone levels decrease with age, some of it is converted into a far more potent form – dihydrotestosterone (DHT) – and the normal process by which it is broken down is inhibited by the excess oestrogens. The potent DHT collects in the prostate and causes the overproduction of prostate cells, which ultimately results in prostate enlargement.

The tube that takes urine from the bladder to the outside (the urethra) passes through the prostate, so the enlarged gland places pressure on the urethra, impeding the flow of urine and triggering the need to urinate more often. Many men get up 3 or 4 times during the course of a night. Other symptoms include difficulty in beginning urination, poor stream, dribbling at the end of urination and sometimes pain. An enlarged prostate can also trigger urinary infections, bladder stones and kidney damage. The majority of prostate problems are due to this gradual enlargement, termed benign prostatic hypertrophy (BPH), but occasionally the prostate can be affected by cancer. The World Cancer Research Fund project has predicted that within 20 years one in four men could be affected by cancer of the prostate, and it is already the leading type of cancer in American men.

If you have blood in your urine, difficulty in passing urine, any swelling in your testicle area, please, please go and see your doctor. Although there is now a much greater awareness of this problem, many men are still dying from embarrassment – literally, when there is no need.

Foods to Avoid

■ Filter your main tap water supply before drinking. This is because hormone residues from the Pill and HRT, are found in most water supplies and they have an oestrogen effect in the body. One of the purest waters you can drink is reverse osmosis de-ionized water, which can be bought in health stores or plumbed in under your sink. For details of reverse osmosis water contact The Pure H2O Company on 01784 21188, or www.pureH20.co.uk. Or the Fresh Water Filter Company on 0870 442 3633, or www.freshwaterfilter.com.

- As pesticide and herbicide residues are now linked to prostate cancer, avoid non-organic foods as much as possible.

- Reduce your intake of animal fats found in meat, full-fat milks and cheeses, chocolate, hard margarines and fatty take-aways. Dairy foods and too much inorganic red meat (usually full of chemical residues) increase the risk for prostate cancer.

- Don't eat processed meat pies and pastries.

- Avoid fried and barbecued foods.

- Reduce your intake of caffeine, alcohol and sugar.

- See *Diet – The Stay Younger Longer Diet (see page 114)*.

Friendly Foods

- Eat organic foods as much as you can. Additionally, locally grown fruits and vegetables in season contain more nutrients than those flown thousands of miles.

- Sprinkle plenty of pumpkin, sunflower, sesame and linseeds over cereals, yoghurt, or into soups. They are rich in essential fats and zinc which are needed for a healthy prostate.

- Pumpkin seeds are rich in zinc, magnesium (a muscle relaxant) and essential fats, helping reduce the conversion of testosterone to the potent DHT – you should be eating 40–100g every day. Eat them raw or try lightly toasting them tossed in a little soya sauce to make a delicious prostate-friendly snack.

- Eat more oily fish, which are rich in essential fats, and use unrefined organic walnut, sesame, sunflower and olive oils for salad dressings, or drizzle over cooked foods (see *Fats for Anti-ageing p139*).

- Include plenty of fibre in your diet from fruits and vegetables, especially broccoli, kale, cauliflower and Brussels sprouts, which help to balance hormones naturally.

- Lentils, alfalfa, tomatoes, salad leaves, yellow peppers and organic carrots will help protect against cancers.

- Eat more brown rice, quinoa, millet, oats, cereals and oat and rice bran. The fibre helps remove excess hormones out of the body.

- Eat more pulses such as barley, kidney beans, soya beans plus lentils and corn, rice and lentil pastas.

- Have one serving of cooked, organic GM-free tempeh each week – Japanese men have a much lower incidence of prostate cancer until they adopt a Western diet. If you've never had tempeh before, you can try crumbling it, and adding it to stir-fries, soups or salads. But, if you have prostate cancer, then you really should try to avoid all types of soya based products.

- The carotene lycopene is the most abundant nutrient stored in the prostate and studies have shown that men who eat 10 or more cooked tomatoes (in a little olive oil) weekly are 45% less likely to develop prostate cancer. The lycopene in tomatoes is released when they are heated in a small amount of oil. A great way to do this is to cut tomatoes in half, brush them with a little olive oil and add chopped garlic and basil. Grill or bake for a few minutes and serve.

Useful Remedies

- The mineral zinc is more abundant in the prostate than any other organ in the body and its supplementation has been shown to reduce prostate overgrowth and symptoms of BPH. Zinc inhibits the conversion of testosterone to DHT, the primary hormonal trigger for prostate enlargement. Zinc deficiency is common in those with prostate problems. Take 20mg zinc two to three times per day. As zinc depletes copper levels, take a proportionate amount of copper, approximately 1mg of copper for every 15mg of zinc.

- The mineral selenium has been found to help prevent prostate enlargement and cancer. Taking 200mcg per day can significantly reduce your risk or either.

- The herb saw palmetto has been proven to reduce enlargement of the prostate gland and dramatically improve the symptoms of BPH. Take 150–350mg of standardized extract twice per day.

- Another good herb for enlarged prostate is pygeum, particularly for relieving symptoms such as frequent or difficult urination and associated sexual dysfunction. Take 50–100mg of standardized extract twice daily.

- One of the oldest remedies for enlarged prostates is nettle, taken either as a tincture or as tablets. Take 5ml of tincture, or 200–300mg of standardized extract two to three times per day in capsules. You can also try nettle tea with a little honey.

- Essential fats, especially omega-3, are found in fish oils. Taking 1gram of fish oil, or 1gram linseed oil, can also help prevent prostate enlargement.

- Many companies now make prostate formulas that include all these nutrients (see pages 13 and 14).

- Include a natural carotene-source supplement that is rich in lycopene – take 20–40mg daily.

- ProstaCol is a special formula that contains standardized extracts of saw palmetto, pygeum africanum and stinging nettle, all prized by the European medical community for treating BPH and improving impaired bladder functions. Safer than prescription drugs, studies show that ingredients in ProstaCol can help shrink and normalize the prostate. Recommended dosage: 1 capsule three times daily with meals. Call the Nutricentre or Sloane Health on page 14.

Helpful Hints

- An enlarged prostate is usually discovered via a rectal examination by a doctor. All men over 40 should have an annual rectal examination. Early detection greatly increases your chances of a complete cure.

- Ask your partner to see if they can feel any abnormalities, make this a fun thing, but try doing it once a month.

■ Regular exercise is vital as it boosts immune function and also reduces levels of stress hormones naturally. Do not bicycle too much, as this puts pressure on the prostate. Swimming or walking are great exercises.

■ To help improve circulation to the area and reduce inflammation, lie on your back, bend your knees, bring the soles of the feet together and bring the feet as close to your buttocks as possible. Relax your legs, letting the knees fall outwards towards the ground. Hold this position for five minutes. Only attempt this exercise if you are fit and have no joint problems in your hips and legs.

■ Massage essential oils of cypress, tea tree and juniper berry mixed with a little jojoba carrier oil, into your lower back and groin areas to help strengthen the prostate.

■ See an osteopath or chiropractor to check that the pelvis and spine are not misaligned, as in certain cases a major nerve connection from the lower part of the spine to the prostate becomes trapped and once this is released water can be passed normally (see *Useful Information and Addresses p338*).

■ If you have prostate cancer see *Useful Remedies* under *Cancer*.

■ There is a test for prostate health called a PSA, or Prostate Specific Antigen test. If your levels of PSA are elevated it can mean that your prostate is becoming enlarged or possibly an indication of prostate cancer. This is not a test for cancer per se, but indicates prostate cell activity. Other factors can raise the levels of PSA, for example ejaculation can raise it for two days, though in general, the higher the level the more likely it is to be a sign of cancer. Biopsies are needed to confirm this.

■ Enlarged prostate can be treated surgically with a procedure called a Trans-Urethral Resection of the Prostate (TURP). This very common procedure is more effective than drugs, although it can have side effects including impotence and incontinence, and one in 8 men who have the operation need another operation within 8 years. This highlights that surgery doesn't address the underlying cause, though if you've tried everything listed here and are desperate, discuss this and other options, including newer laser procedures, with your doctor.

■ For further help and advice, send a large SAE and two 1st class stamps to: The Prostate Help Association, Langworth, Lincoln, LN3 5DF. Website: www.pha.u-net.com. They also have self-help, informative books and CD-ROMS for sale. Shop website: www.prostatecharityshop.co.uk. Other literature can be obtained by sending an SAE with two 1st class stamps to the Prostate Research Campaign UK, PO Box 2371, Swindon SN1 3LS

■ If your prostate is enlarged, be cautious about using over-the-counter cold or allergy remedies. Many of these products contain ingredients that can inflame the condition and cause urinary retention.

■ Read *Prostate Cancer* by Philip Dunn, Ostrich Publishing.

RADIATION IN AGEING

(See also *Pollution Protection* and *Sunshine in Ageing*)

Every time you turn on a light switch or any electrical equipment, the rhythms of your brain change. Most people want the convenience of modern technology, but by over -exposing ourselves to excessive amounts of invisible, artificial frequencies we are inviting an avalanche of health problems.

Animals' sensory abilities are far more sensitive to these emissions, hence why whales, dolphins, insects and birds are also being affected. And the most likely cause of whales beaching themselves is the extremely low frequencies being used to communicate with submarines.

Electrical pollution is now thought to be a major contributing factor to many illnesses. People who live near power lines and sub-stations and whose homes and offices are packed with electrical equipment are more prone to illnesses such as ME (Chronic Fatigue), cancers, depression, migraines and insomnia.

Microwaves, TVs, videos, DVD players, computers and all electrical equipment affect our health. People are at last becoming more aware of the dangers of mobile phones and yet their use is still on the increase. A staggering 44 million out of 60 million people in the UK now (December 2002) have a mobile phone. When they are switched on, even when in your pocket, the base station pulses to your phone every minute or so to find out your location.

It's unfortunate that mobile phones need base stations, which are another source of harmful radiation. There are Chinese studies showing that children working and living near radio and microwave transmitters suffered from compromised immune function and slower learning abilities. Mobile phone masts are now being hidden in garage forecourt signs, church steeples, schools and hospitals. Simon Best, Editor of the *Electromagnetic Hazard and Therapy News Report* says, "If you are in close proximity to a base station, then over time, you are at risk, but without doubt using mobile phones exposes you to much greater doses of short-term radiation, because of the phones proximity to your head."

Being in an environment where others are using phones is equally bad for our health. Earpieces are variably protective, but those that simply connect the phone to the ear using an earpiece that you insert into the ear, can be worse than normal mobiles, if the radiation is being led directly into the brain by the wire. At least try and hold your phone a few inches away from your ear.

Roger Coghill, a bio-electromagnetics research scientist, based in Gwent in the UK, who is a leading authority on this subject, says, "It is imperative for people to understand that we are electrical beings in a physical shell. Every second, trillions of electrical impulses occur in the cells of the body, it is how they communicate with each other. But, mobile phones pulse artificial low and high frequencies directly into your brain which can kill brain cells, and at the same time they inhibit immune cell function, which means that immune cells are less likely to be able to destroy any cancer cells in the whole body – including the brain. The more you use a mobile phone the more quickly you age brain cells, which can result in memory loss, slowed reaction time, lack of focus and in extreme cases brain tumours and lymphatic cancers. Children's immune systems are significantly lowered and with the increasing numbers of children using mobile phones – we are sitting on a health time bomb."

Roger recommends that mobile phones should be used for no more than five minutes at a time and should not be used in cars or trains, as the signal (and therefore the health risks) are amplified.

Foods to Avoid

■ Believe it or not, all foods also emit frequencies and if you eat too many foods that emit a frequency that is incompatible with you own, then eventually symptons will arise.

■ Junk foods emit a dull energy field frequency, which will eventually trigger negative symptoms if you eat junk foods to excess.

Friendly Foods

■ Eat foods in as near a natural state as possible. For instance if you look at the energy field of a raw cabbage, it has a really bright energy field (which means you get more energy from that food), but once cooked the energy field is greatly reduced.

■ Organic and raw foods contain bio-photons (electromagnetic energy) which are reduced or destroyed in cooking and in over-processing. Living food is alive!

Useful Remedies

■ As electromagnetic fields trigger free radical production you need to take an all-in-one multi-nutrient formula that will help protect your cells and immune system against radiation and help slow ageing at every level. Try Kudos 24 Multi-Active Age Management Complex, see page 348.

Helpful Hints

■ Many people wonder whether safety shields are of any use. Roger has tested a few and says that the Mobile Phone Protection Chip has shown in his independent studies to help protect against harmful magnetic fields. These chips are available from Higher Nature. For further details call 01435 882 880.

■ Ask your phone dealer to fit a BioChip in your battery – a microchip that emits a weaker impulse when the phone is in use, which prevents the cells becoming so stressed. It has been developed after 4 years research for the US Military by Professor Ted Litovitz in America. The BioChip was developed to help reduce the negative effects of radiophones in soldiers' helmets.

- Roger says that very shortly new phones with headsets – which use radio infrared signals, that will be safer, will be introduced.

- Try an RF3 cellular headset, which delivers the sound to your ear through an air-filled wireless tube which reduces the radiation going into your head to almost zero. For details call Revital on 0800 252 875.

- Spending too much time under artificial fluorescent lighting, or in front of a computer screen can suppress the brain chemical melatonin. This can have negative effects as diverse as infertility, depression, insomnia and increasing the risk of cancer. Get out and walk in natural daylight and sunshine as much as you can.

- X-rays and scans ionize cells in the body, which create free radicals that are ageing (see *Antioxidants in Ageing p38*). If at all possible limit your exposure to no more than three X-rays or scans every year.

- Don't sleep with an electric blanket on (unless it's really cold, and obviously if you have a health problem that requires you to be extra warm, then for goodness sake keep it on). Turn off electric switches at the mains at night in the bedroom as much as you can.

- Use battery-operated clocks rather than electric ones by the side of your bed.

- Avoid microwaving food. Microwaves change the molecular structure of food and deplete nutrients. Microwaved food also creates free radicals and in the long-term has been proven to be hazardous to health. Use it for de-frosting but not for cooking and especially don't microwave children's food.

- Irradiating (X-raying) food could, in the long run, prove very dangerous. If any foods like strawberries and other soft fruits are still healthy looking after being in your fridge for a few days, then they have most likely been irradiated.

- Use magnetic mattresses as they make all the electrons in your body spin in the same direction. They calm the surrounding electric fields. Magnets improve circulation and bring oxygen to the cells. They also help to reduce pain and jet lag. Placing a magnet on your forehead for 20 minutes before landing helps reset the body's internal clock. When you travel long distances, your brain has to adjust itself to the new, local magnetic field and this is why a magnet helps to re-set this field – much like wiping a foreign video tape and playing it back in your own language. Some of the best magnetic beds are available from Sasaki, the leading manufacturers of magnetic beds, car seats, insoles etc. For details log on to www.sasakiuk.com

- Also when you fly, you are exposed to increased amounts of ultraviolet radiation, mostly UVB, which accelerates ageing. Under cabin pressure, which is very dehydrating, all body systems have to work harder to function. For instance the blood tends to thicken (hence deep vein problems) and the heart rate increases to compensate for the lower oxygen content in the atmosphere.

- If you have subterranean flowing water under your home or office, this often compounds health problems, as the water can create an inharmonious electromagnetic field known as geopathic stress. Hundreds of years ago, builders would watch carefully where sheep settled at night and would not build in places where sheep refused to sleep. If you think you maybe at risk, have your home dowsed by an expert. Send a SAE to The British Society of Dowsers, Sycamore Barn, Hastingleigh, Ashford, Kent TN25 5HW. Tel: 01233 750253. Office is open from 9am–1pm and 2pm-5pm. website: www.british dowsers.org. e-mail :bsd@dowsers.co.uk

■ Electricity can also be used to heal, for more information read *The Healing Energies of Light*, by Roger Coghill. Roger also makes Super Magnets that help reduce jet lag and pain. For details call 01495 752122, or log on to Roger's website at www.cogreslab.co.uk

■ For more information on how electrical equipment and radiation can damage your health log on to: www.em-hazard-therapy.com, or call Simon Best on the EM Hazard Helpline on 0906 4010237 (premium rate).

REJUVENATION THERAPIES

(See also *Cells in Ageing, Chelation in Ageing, Plastic Surgery* and *Skin*)

There are now dozens of therapies and treatments claiming to rejuvenate our cells and skin, thus helping us to stay looking and feeling younger for longer. If I wrote about them all, this book would be an enormous volume, rather than an easy-to-read book. Therefore I have included therapies that I have tried myself plus those that have some scientific research to back up their claims.

For most people, these treatments are an expensive anti-ageing luxury, for others they can make the difference between life and death.

I have met incredibly poised and elegant women in their 70s, who have never used Botox or had a face-lift, and yet they exude elegance and confidence. To be beautiful you don't need to eliminate every wrinkle from your face.

Magazines full of pictures of 18-year-old models and 20-something starlets don't help, and I'm thrilled that women like Catherine Deneuve are now being asked to front advertising campaigns.

In a perfect world, I'm sure that most men and women would love to retain the skin of a 30-something and believe me there are therapies that will help you do this.

Dr Jean Louis Sebagh, a consultant plastic surgeon based in London and Paris, encourages all younger women to begin practising more ageing maintenance in their late 30s, so that as wrinkles begin to show, "problem" areas can be treated, and the need for any face-lift can be avoided for far longer. He stresses, as I do, that to stay younger longer you also need to eat the right foods, take skin supplements (see *Skin p279*), maintain a regular weight, exercise, drink more water (he says that 80% of his patients are dehydrated), take more care in the sun and use moisturizers.

For ease of reference I have placed the following therapies in alphabetical order.

BOTOX INJECTIONS

These are now so common, that many high street chemists offer these injections. Most of the dermatologists and plastic surgeons I interviewed were concerned that some of the people giving Botox are often not sufficiently qualified or experienced. I have mine done by Mr Matti (see *Plastic Surgery*), Dr Sebagh or Professor Lowe (see *Skin Cell Therapy p273*). Unless these injections are given by a qualified, experienced doctor I would not have this treatment. Women as young as 25 are having this therapy, which greatly slows the onset of facial wrinkles, plus expression and frown-type lines. Dr Sebagh calls this Ageing Maintenance, saying that if more women would take preventative measures earlier (see *Skin p279*), they could hold back the years with greater ease and should not need to consider face-lifts until their late 50s.

Botulism is group of 17 deadly bacterial strains, which cause life threatening gastric illnesses. But botulism A, generally used for these treatments, is purified and greatly diluted before being injected into the face. In a few cases patients are resistant to the botulism A and so a B version is used, but the B toxin tends to last only half the time of type A. Once injected, after a few days the flow of nerve signals to the muscles slow and then stop, which leaves your face looking more relaxed. The secret to this treatment in my humble opinion is not to overdo it. Recently I met a woman of 34 who has had so much Botox, that she could not smile or frown. There was nil personality coming through and her face looked like an alabaster mask. Joan Collins calls it the "startled faun look". Costs vary depending on where you have it done, from £100 upwards. But some doctors are concerned about the accumulation of the toxin in the body; again, it's your choice.

CHELATION

Chelation is an intravenous drip therapy in which amino acids, plus high doses of vitamins and minerals are fed into the veins. There is now a large body of evidence to show that chelation, which is also being called Intravenous Antioxidant Therapy, is highly anti-ageing and rejuvenating (see also *Chelation in Ageing p89*).

CHEMICAL PEELS

These peels use various forms of fruit-based acids and must be done by a qualified plastic surgeon or dermatologist. Under sedation in a sterile environment the acid solution is "painted" on the face, which dissolves the top layer of skin. The results are similar to laser treatment (see p271). For details, contact the Cranley Clinic on 0207 499 3223 or see *Plastic Surgery p253*.

COLLAGEN INJECTIONS

Injectable collagen comes from bovine cowhide (mainly from America), which has been screened for problems such as BSE and CJD. The collagen plumps out deep lines and the look lasts from 6 to 8 months. It can also be used around the mouth. There can be some bruising, in which case use a little ice wrapped in gauze to dab onto the areas of the injections to reduce any swelling. Over time, the collagen disperses into the skin tissues and further treatments can be given.

A skin test is necessary in case of allergic reactions.

COSMETIC ACUPUNCTURE

In Japan and China cosmetic acupuncture has been used to help reverse and slow the visible signs of ageing for thousands of years. Most acupuncturists are not generally trained in this field – it's a specialization, but if you can find an acupuncturist who has trained in the Far East, they may know these anti-ageing techniques. One of my co-authors, Steve Langley, practises this type of acupuncture and was trained in China. When Steve told me that some of his patients' husbands thought they might be having affairs, as they looked so fresh, I asked him to have a go on me!

Needles are placed in specific points on the face to encourage blood and "chi" energy flow, which brings more oxygen and nutrients to the surrounding tissues. The effects are accumulative, but immediate results can be seen after even one treatment. After 45 minutes, the needles were removed and I was amazed to see that the dark circles under my eyes (from being at my computer writing this book for almost eight months!) had magically disappeared and I looked as though I had just enjoyed a really good sleep. If you need to look good for a special occasion, cosmetic acupuncture is well worth a try. Steve works at the Hale Clinic in London. Call 0870 167 6667 for more details (to find your nearest acupuncturist see *Useful Information and Addresses p338*).

Dr Sebagh is using electrical acupuncture – where the needles are attached to a machine, which pulses a current through the needle and into the skin to aid regeneration.

CREAMS, REJUVENATING SKIN
(See *Skin in Ageing p279*)

FAT INJECTIONS

Many plastic surgeons, including Dr Sebagh (0207 637 0548) and dermatologist Professor Nick Lowe (0207 499 3223) are now offering fat injections into the cheek and nasal fold areas, which fills out the face. As we age, the fat cells in our dermis begin to dissolve or "melt" away and unless you are overweight, you lose fat from your face after your 40s. Using a local anaesthetic, fat is removed from the outer thighs and stomach area and then carefully injected back into the cheeks for a fuller, more youthful look, which should last for a year or more. The face looks bruised for a few days, so take plenty of arnica. You may also need to use ice packs on the area for the first 24 hours. Dr Sebagh and Professor Lowe also offer fat injections into the backs of the hands, which are a dead give-away when it comes to guessing a woman's age. Unless done properly, injecting fat into the hands can cause unsightly lumps and considerable bruising.

INTENSE PULSED LIGHT THERAPY

Lasers emit a specific wavelength of light – but the new IPL machines deliver hundreds of wavelengths at one time. These 20-minute treatments encourage collagen production. They are also used to treat birthmarks and rosacea (a flushing of the skin). A cold gel is usually applied before the treatment and dark glasses should be worn. Women say it hurts about as much as a leg wax and there can be some slight reddening, but it should only last for a couple of hours. Contact Dr Sebagh (see *Skin Regeneration Injections p272*).

LASER THERAPY

Laser surgery has made great strides during the last 10 years. With lasers such as the Erbium Yag laser, a qualified surgeon removes the very top layer of skin. This needs to be done either under a local anaesthetic or intravenous sedation, in a sterile environment. Your skin looks pretty red after the surgery and most surgeons ask you to use sterile Vaseline for two weeks to keep the skin supple. As it heals, the skin becomes tighter and the lower layer of the skin – the dermis – begins producing more collagen and elastin, which gives you smoother, younger looking skin. With the newer lasers, healing times are much shorter and a great improvement can be seen after a week or so, with all redness disappearing in 1–4 months. Full-face laser surgery costs anything from £3,000 and upwards. But you can have isolated areas treated – such as the mouth. I have age spots and brown patches of skin removed every now and again by Dr Tom Bozek, who does laser surgery. For further details contact Dr Bozek at 18 Wimpole Street, London W1M 7AD. Tel: 020 7636 0357, fax 020 7436 1805, e-mail:tbozek@aol.com

Lasers can also be used to remove thread veins and facial scarring. Professor Lowe and his medical team also offer all types of laser surgery at the Cranley Clinic (for details see *Skin Cell Therapy p273*). For more gentle lasers for skin rejuvination etc. try looking at www.fraxel.com.

LIVE CELL THERAPY

In Europe, Live Cell Therapy has been used for over 50 years to help the body regenerate itself. This treatment involves removing cells from shark, sheep or bovine embryos – which are then treated to make sure that there is no possibility of transferring any disease. The cultured cells are then injected into the patient, which "wakes up" and rejuvenates cells that are fast approaching senescence (see *Cells in Ageing p85*). After four to six weeks patients say they feel renewed, invigorated and their memory improves. Joints no longer ache and skin looks fresher. It obviously worked for Sir Winston Churchill, who abused his body and yet still lived to a ripe old age, with a very sharp mind.

Clinique La Prairie was among the first to develop this treatment and their clinic is as popular today as it was 50 years ago. For details, log on to www.laprairie.com, or call (+41 21) 989 33 11, or contact Dr Claus Martin at the Four Seasons Clinic, in Germany on + (49) 8022 24041, fax 8022 24740.

SKIN FILLING INJECTIONS

See also *Collagen Injections*. Restylane, Perlane, Juvederm and Hylaform are all forms of hyaluronic acid (HA), which occurs naturally in our skin. But as we age, HA levels fall, and when you are injected with HA in a fluid form, it helps the skin to hold more moisture. This is why many dermatologists are now combining hyaluronic acid with other anti-ageing preparations, to fill and moisturize at the same time. Note that most of these fillers are derived from cockerel's beaks – so if you have a severe allergy to chickens, eggs or are vegetarian, ask for Juvederm or Perlane, which are not animal based.

There are now so many line "fillers" on the market, soft ones like collagen, liquid fillers like hyaluronic acid and also HA gels that can be used to fill out either lines or add volume to your cheeks. Dr Sebagh (details below) carries out this procedure, which gives you a fuller look for around 9 months.

Whatever you choose, ask about any side-effects, and ask whether if it goes wrong your implant can be removed (as some like Ultrasoft are permanent). I have seen a few beautiful women who have ruined their looks by having far too many fillers, especially in their lips, and in rare cases they look deformed. Ask to see pictures of work that the doctor and/or surgeon has already done – chat to other women in the waiting room. Professor Lowe's advice is to avoid lip fillers like Articol, Dermalive and Dermadeep, because they cannot be removed if they go wrong and you can be left with unsightly disfiguring lumps.

SKIN REGENERATION INJECTIONS

Dr Sebagh has combined hyaluronic acid with vitamins, minerals and homeopathic remedies that he and his fellow doctors inject into the dermis using a small "gun". This treatment is especially effective for the chest, neck and face areas that often suffer sun damage, as the skin is so thin on the chest bone area. When Dr Sebagh first told me about this therapy, I was extremely sceptical, as in my youth, I sunbathed far too much and the skin on my chest area was pigmented to the point where I could no longer wear a low evening dress. My chest was covered in large brown areas that alternated with white patches. It was a mess. Dr Seabagh "drags" the "gun" along the skin and you can feel the tiniest pricking sensation as the fluid goes into the skin. There is virtually no pain, more like a "tickling" sensation. After 4 treatments I noticed that the huge brown pigmentation marks on my chest had begun to fade. It took almost 6 months, but today after around 15 treatments, the skin on my chest is greatly repaired and regenerated. This treatment does not remove lines, it's not a filler treatment, but in time it regenerates the quality of the skin. Costs £200 per treatment and it takes 30 minutes.

In the UK this treatment is available via Dr Jean Louis Sebagh at the French Cosmetic Clinic, 25 Wimpole Street, London W1. Tel: 0207 637 0548. In Paris at 64 Rue De Longchamp, call (33-1) 47 04 65 75. In Los Angeles contact Dr Raj Kanodia, Camden Drive, Los Angeles. Tel: (310) 276 3106.

SKIN CELL THERAPY

This is an exciting treatment that is helping revolutionize facial skin ageing. Developed in conjunction with the American-based biotechnology firm Isologen, and Professor Nicholas Lowe, the Clinical Professor of Dermatology at UCLA in California – who also works in London as well as California. Basically, skin tissue is removed from either behind the ears, or below the bikini line. The proteins within the cells that keep the skin taut and youthful are extracted and held in a liquid, which can then be frozen until needed. So, if the cells are removed from a woman between 18 and 30, her cells can be frozen until she is older, then defrosted and cultured so that syringes of young skin cells and their collagan and elastin can then be injected back into her facial skin. Without the need for any other fillers, these young cells naturally increase collagen, elastin and hyaluronic acid production, thus making the skin look much younger, without the risk of allergic reactions.

The good news is that older women can also have this treatment. Professor Lowe simply finds a tiny area of skin that has not been over-exposed to the sun, and takes the cells from there. You can still get a good result. Studies in America suggest that a course of around 5 treatments gives the most benefits. Costs from £2,500.

For details of this therapy call the Cranley Clinic, 3 Harcourt House, 19a Cavendish Square, London W1M 9AD. Tel: 0207 499 3223. In America call (310) 828 8969. Cranley offers a full range of anti-ageing treatments, from Botox, collagen and fat injections into the face etc, to hair transplants, thread-vein treatments for the legs, laser surgery and chemical peels.

STEM CELL THERAPY See *Cells in Ageing p85.*

Helpful Hints

■ A good night's sleep is one of the least expensive ways to rejuvenate.

■ Treat yourself to regular facials and massage with essential oils – which help you to feel rejuvenated.

■ A walk in the park can do wonders for your skin.

■ See also *Helpful Hints* under *Ageing*, *Cells and Ageing*, *Oxygen in Ageing*, *Skin*.

RHEUMATOID ARTHRITIS

(See *Arthritis*)

SEX IN AGEING

(See also *Mid Life Crisis* and all *Hormone* sections)

It is no secret that consensual sex is one of the great human feel-good activities. Yet, as we age the passion can wane and sex can become infrequent, or just too much hard work. It doesn't have to be this way. Maintaining an enjoyable sex life well into old age is important because it's emerging that sex promotes living longer and staying younger.

Professor Pitzkhelauri, studied 15,000 long-lived individuals in the mountainous Caucasus region, which encompasses Georgia, Armenia, Azerbaijan, and south-western Russia, and found that, with very few exceptions, healthy married people over 80, were content with their relationship, and many continued active sex lives beyond the age of 100. Professor Pitzkhelauri concluded that marriage and a regular sex life were key ingredients in the recipe for attaining ages beyond 100. The majority of these individuals drank alcohol and many smoked, yet they survived far longer, on average, that supposedly healthy Westerners.

Pleasurable sex releases feel-good hormones, which help to boost immune function and reduce pain and stress levels. Some people think of sex as being tiring and it's true that after a satisfying orgasm, one does not usually feel like digging the garden or washing the car. But this is misleading. Although satisfying orgasm leads to a momentary energy deflation, over time it actually leads to increased zest and enjoyment of life. Both men and women report this important property of sex. The key word is satisfying.

So, if sex is so good for us, what gets in the way as we age? The most obvious factor is simply being with a partner for many years – the initial passion can turn into companionship, and there is nothing wrong with this. And we are all unique, while one man may constantly be thinking and talking about sex at any age, others have little or no interest. Women can be the same.

If you talk to anyone who has had an affair, the sex is like a drug – they say how they have forgotten how good the first thrill of passion (and lust) feels and simply cannot get enough. Some married people keep the fires burning all their lives, for others it wanes after several or so years. Also, many young couples who work long hours and may have young children admit that they only have sex seven or eight times a year. And what satisfies one person may be unthinkable to another.

Poor health, stress, lack of energy, hormone imbalances, a poor diet, impotence and vaginal dryness can all reduce one's sex life. Yet sex can be as satisfying at 60 with the right partner as it ever was. It is an invaluable part of bonding a relationship and can help keep you young.

A word of caution from nutritional physician Dr Keith Scott-Mumby who treats sexual problems in men and women, "Be sure you know what you really feel and where the real problem lies. I had one patient in her 50s who asked me if I would treat her husband to try to put some more (sex/passion) life into him. Apparently they had not had intercourse for three years. I prescribed hormone supplements and a series of IV antioxidant infusions (see *Chelation in Ageing p89*). It worked a treat. But she recoiled and later confessed to me that she found shopping far more exciting and interesting than sex!"

Personally, I think that too much emphasis is placed on sex these days and you see sexy models selling everything from paint to sticking plasters on TV. Almost 70% of women say they prefer shopping to sex, so if you are not getting any or enough, you can always head off down the high street!

Foods to Avoid

- Fast food is death to sexual desire.

- Cut down on sugar and stimulants like coffee, tea, cigarettes and alcohol – these foods make it harder for you to maintain consistent levels of energy and will tend to leave you tired or wired at the end of the day. Tiredness and excessive anxiety are both major sexual turn-offs (see *Carbohydrate Control p80*).

- Reduce your intake of animal fats in meat and dairy, fried foods and hydrogenated fats in processed foods. These "bad" fats can hinder the production of hormones from "good" fats and worsen your overall hormonal health.

Friendly Foods

- Choose organic foods as much as possible. Pesticide residues are common on non-organic foods and in combinations, even at very low levels, they're known hormone disrupters. Especially important are raw foods ,such as fruit and salad vegetables.

- Eat more oily fish. The good fats (EFAs) they contain are needed for hormone production and balancing hormone levels. These fats are known to reduce vaginal dryness if you have sufficient in your diet. Aim for 2–3 portions of salmon, fresh tuna, sardines, mackerel or herring each week and be aware that if you are low on EFAs, it can take a couple of months to restore proper levels. Regular consumption of EFAs can improve dry skin, inflamed joints and memory as well as your sex life.

- Eat a heaped tablespoon of ground seeds every day for essential fats, magnesium and zinc. Best are flax, pumpkin, hemp and sunflower seeds, which can be mixed together, ground in an electric coffee grinder fresh each day and sprinkled on breakfast cereals, soups or salads. To use EFAs efficiently in the body you need sufficient vitamin B6, zinc and magnesium – so seeds are an excellent addition to your diet.

- Oysters have a reputation as an aphrodisiac, mostly because of their very high zinc content – up to 15mg per oyster or 100% of the recommended daily allowance! – far higher than any other food source. Zinc is extremely important for sexual function, so other foods rich in this important mineral are lean meats, nuts, eggs and wholegrains.

- B vitamins are needed for energy, so make sure you eat plenty of brown rice, organic meat, eggs, low-fat dairy produce, mushrooms and broccoli.

- Foods rich in vitamin E that are needed for the manufacture of sex hormones are wheatgerm, eggs, soya beans, sprouting seeds such as alfalfa seeds, almonds, hazelnuts, dark green vegetables and avocados.

- Generally, eat more fruits and vegetables that are packed with natural source carotenes and vitamin C.

Useful Remedies

- Take a full-spectrum multivitamin/mineral/essential fats formula such as Kudos 24 (see page 348).

- Men, take extra zinc. Sperm is loaded with zinc and a man loses about 3mg of zinc with each ejaculation. The average daily intake of zinc is only 8mg (the EU recommended daily allowance is 15mg!), so you could easily be low in this important nutrient. Symptoms of zinc deficiency include more than three white flecks on your fingernails, depression and impotence, so more zinc may make an enormous difference to your sex life. Take a multi containing at least 15mg of zinc, and if it doesn't, add a 15mg zinc tablet to your daily supplement regime.

- DHEA is an energizing, anti-stress hormone that your body can convert into the sex hormones oestrogen or testosterone in men and women. It stimulates sexual response and the production of pheromones – the special chemicals our skin secretes in order to attract the opposite sex. Best taken under the supervision of a health care professional, DHEA is available over the counter (or Internet) in the United States on www.lef.org (see *Other Vital Hormones p239*).

- Dr Michael Perring, an expert on sexual problems, says, "Low dose testosterone supplementation, sometimes combined with DHEA, is useful for women whose levels are low. Testosterone can increase energy and libido, but these should be prescribed by a professional." (See also *Men's Hormones p218* and *Other Vital Hormones p237*).

- The herb gingko biloba increases circulation not only to your brain but also the peripheries, including the hands, feet, and even the penis. Studies have shown it to be helpful for impotence so gingko is gaining recognition as a natural alternative to Viagra. Try 1–3 capsules of 60mg of standardized extract daily.

- Korean (Panax) ginseng, can increase your energy, improve resistance to and recovery from stress and increase libido. Try 500–1000mg twice daily (capsule or powder) under the guidance of a health care professional, cutting back if you experience hot flushes or palpitations.

- Take essential fatty acid (EFAs) supplements daily. These healthy fats, known as omega-3 and omega-6, are vital for hormone balance and may help impotence by thinning the blood and can improve vaginal dryness (see *Fats for Anti-ageing p139*).

- Try ArgiMax for men and women. Trials have shown this combination formula improves sexual desire, performance and enjoyment – better erections and increased stamina for men, more arousal and satisfaction for women. Dr Mary Polan, at Stanford University Medical School in California, invited 94 women suffering low libido to test ArgiMax. Out of the group 46 were given ArgiMax and 48 were given a placebo. Within four weeks 71% of those taking the formula reported improvement in their level of sexual desire and 65%

were enjoying more frequent sex. Vaginal dryness was lessened and the quality of orgasm improved. The mind boggles. And thankfully, 87% of the men involved in the trials reported they were able to maintain an erection for longer. Nutritionist, Gareth Zeal, says, "The basis of the formula is L-arginine, an amino acid, that helps to lower cholesterol, as hardening of the arteries and poor circulation can trigger erectile problems for men and lack of heightened sensation for women. It also contains herbal aphrodisiacs such as Damiana, plus ginseng to boost energy, iron, calcium, zinc and selenium, and vitamins A, B, C, and E. Ginkgo biloba is added to both formulas for its proven ability to improve circulation. But anyone suffering from cold sores should avoid this formula as the virus that causes cold sores thrives on L-arginine, which is also found in chocolate, lentils, beans and nuts." Dosage: 3 capsules twice daily for four weeks. For your nearest stockists call Sundown Vitamins on 0870 7594003.

■ Another popular natural sex drive enhancer for men and women is Vigorex, which contains a substance found in oats (an extract of wild oats) that the manufacturers say helps increase sex drive by freeing up "dormant" testosterone in both men and women. It is available by mail order from www.vigorex.uk.com

■ The South American herb Muira Puama has a long history as an aphrodisiac. It is used by men and women in the Amazon to raise testosterone levels. Try one 500mg capsule twice daily. Available from the NutriCentre and Sloane Health Foods (see page 14).

Helpful Hints

■ If you have an under-active thyroid, sex hormones cannot work properly without the necessary thyroid hormones. This is especially common in women around the time of the menopause (see *Thyroid in Ageing p313*).

■ Reduce stress levels (see *Stress in Ageing p293*) – stress at any age is a major turn-off, and while many men find sex a good de-stressor, for many women stress and sex just don't mix. This is because stress can lower the already small amounts of testosterone in women that controls their sex-drive. Best of all is for everyone involved is to be relaxed, calm and tension-free.

■ Men, do you find housework sexy? Neither does your partner. Help her out and you might be surprised to find she has more energy for other activities.

■ Don't forget that there's a lot more to sex than sex. Set the stage and the performance is going to be more enjoyable. You may have heard of tantric sex that lasts for hours. The musician Sting, a well-known fan of tantric sex, recently gave a delightful explanation of just how that works – dinner at a restaurant for 1½ hours, a sexy movie followed by great sex.

■ If you have been married or together for many years and you have not had sex for ages – you may simply be embarrassed if your partner suddenly makes demands. Therefore one of the easiest ways to "get in the mood" is to both read sexy magazines or watch a sexy movie. And if this does not help, then seek professional help.

■ Never underestimate the importance of flowers, candle-lit dinners, bubble baths, soft lighting, romantic music, love notes and massage.

■ Smell is a powerful sexual stimulant so use it. Our skin secretes pheromones in order to attract the opposite sex and certain aromatherapy oils are known to enhance their effect – particularly ylang ylang, vanilla and musk. Sprinkle a few drops of these oils in the bath, on your bedding or lingerie, or make a naturally sensual perfume by diluting them in sweet almond oil, which you can also use for massage.

■ Performance anxiety is a key cause of impotence, so it's important to be comfortable with your partner and avoid placing too much importance on outcomes. Enjoy intimacy without thinking it has to lead to sex if the time isn't right for either of you.

■ Steve Langley, naturopath and acupuncturist says, "Professor Pitzkhelouri (see introduction, this section) doesn't mention how often the men ejaculate. A very important point, because a man can make love every day without ejaculating and can and should with practice be able to have whole body, more intense orgasms without ejaculating. This is good for qi (chi or essence) circulation and obviously as a man gets older he should retain his sperm but keep his qi circulating, which energizes him when he makes love. He doesn't lose zinc this way but can continue to make love whenever his partner desires. As to the woman, she should be encouraged to have orgasms, as this is also good for qi circulation. This is basic Taoist practice for longevity where the man will build his kidney yin qi through various herbs etc such as red and Siberian ginseng and velvet deer antler and not waste his qi, but preserve it and utilize it in lovemaking!

■ Acupuncture can help unblock stagnant sexual energy, Steve works from the Hale Clinic in London, call: 0870 167 667, or for details on how to find your nearest practitioner, see *Useful Information and Addresses p338.*

■ Steve recommends reading *The Multi-Orgasmic Man* by Mantak Chia, Thorsons.

■ Loss of libido can be dramatically affected by some prescription drugs such as blood pressure tablets, tranquillizers and anti-depressants.

■ Menopausal symptoms for women include fatigue, depression, weight gain, reduced sex drive and vaginal dryness, none of which are going to enhance your sex life (see *Menopause*).

■ Frequent sexual intercourse can help relieve vaginal dryness, but use a lubricant if necessary to avoid pain – a major turn-off.

■ Be wary of overly energetic sex, with the stresses this places on the body, if you're unfit or unhealthy. Your blood pressure and pulse rate rise considerably during stimulation and this might not be safe. Not to say sex is not possible – just take it easy and improve your health.

■ Don't be afraid to ask for professional help. If sex isn't a part of your relationship and you'd both like it to be, consider seeing a sex therapist – these professionals are very adept at getting to the root of the problem and helping you work through it.

■ Above all keep sex special – let it be something shared and enjoyed, and remember that it doesn't always have to mean intercourse.

- Dr Scott-Mumby does not recommend artificial excitants, such as sildenafil (Viagra) and apomorphine hydrochloride (men and women). They may work, but are not addressing the root causes of the problem and can have negative side effects, such as heart attacks. To contact Dr Keith Scott-Mumby www.alternative-doctor.com

- If you need professional help contact Dr Michael Perring who specializes in sexual problems at Optimal Health, 19 Milford House, 7 Queen Anne Street, London W1G 9HN. Tel 0207 436 7713 www.optimanalhealth.org.uk

- Contact a clinic that specializes in these types of problems such as The Whole Clinic, The Welbeck Hospital, 27 Welbeck Street, London WC1. Dr Stephen Hiew. Tel: 0798 555 7265, or visit: www.whole.org.uk

- Read In Bed With The Food Doctor by Ian Marber and Vicki Edgson, Collins and Brown – a great book for eating your way to better sex and sleep.

SKIN IN AGEING

(See also Muscles in Ageing, Plastic Surgery, Rejuvenation Therapies and Sunshine in Ageing).

Without doubt, finding a magic cream, injection, treatment or pill that can regenerate ageing skin is one of the ultimate "Holy Grails" for anti-ageing researchers. And scientists are getting closer all the time. Right now, you can have cell therapy, vitamin and mineral injections that regenerate skin (see under Regeneration Therapies), or take supplements such as carnosine, which not only extend cell life but also regenerate skin cells (see The Best Anti-ageing Supplements for Skin p282).

Your skin is made up of three layers: firstly the epidermis, the top layer, is made up of around 18 layers of dead protein (keratin) cells which are held together by fatty compounds like lipids – and sebum. The epidermis also contains melanocytes, the cells that produce melanin, which colours the skin. All races have similar numbers of melanocytes, but it's the amount of dark treacly looking melanin that is produced in the cells that determines the skin colour. Incredibly this top layer of skin is as thin as a human hair.

Beneath this lies the dermis, which is around 3mm thick, made up, when we are young, of approximately 85% collagen, 3% elastin, plus natural oils and water. This is where the blood vessels, nerve endings, hair follicles and the oil and sweat glands are situated.

Below this is the subcutis layer mainly made up of fat cells, plus blood vessels and nerve fibres. People who are overweight obviously carry far more fat, hence why they have plumper skin with fewer wrinkles.

The first thing I always notice about most young skin, is that it's clear, unblemished, plump and hydrated. And if you don't sunbathe to excess, which causes up to 85% of the visible signs of ageing, regularly eat more "skin foods", drink plenty of pure water and take the most effective supplements, it is possible for the skin to remain young for much longer.

Unfortunately when I had young, plump, hydrated skin, I presumed it was always going to stay that way. A *big* mistake. No wonder Oscar Wilde said that "youth, is wasted on the young". I sunbathed far too much and ate the wrong foods, which has taken its toll.

When we are young, skin cell turnover is very efficient, every 28 days plump, round new skin cells work their way up through the layers of the skin, and as they near the surface, the epidermis, they begin to flatten out much like a compact disc which gives us lovely fresh skin.

But over time, thanks to sunbathing, a poor diet, exposure to pollutants, stress, drugs and constant use in smiling, frowning and so on, this regeneration process begins to slow down. By your 30s, you produce less collagen and your skin begins to lose some of its elasticity.

In your 40s, you produce less sebum, for women with greasy skin, this is great, but for those with dry, fine skin – it heralds the onset of deeper wrinkles. Darker age spots begin to appear as the melanin begins to clump together. By your 50s, you may have lots of age spots, especially if you love the sun. Thread veins become established, the fat layer begins to "melt" away and your face becomes thinner. But, after the menopause your skin settles down and truly we can then enjoy many years of clear, glowing skin.

For this section, I have interviewed plastic surgeons, dermatologists, anti-ageing doctors and some leading beauticians. In the end I could have written a book on skin alone, and so I have written them all in alphabetical bullet point order under *Helpful Hints* for easier reading.

Foods to Avoid

- The single biggest culprit in ageing the skin is sugar. Sugar triggers cross-linking in the skin and ages the skin almost as much as smoking and excess sunbathing (see *Sugar in Ageing*).

- Of course you need treats but, if you want good skin, keep desserts to a minimum.

- Refined "white foods", breads, pastas, rice, cakes, biscuits and so on, will all accelerate ageing.

- Non-organic foods contain more pesticide residues and less vitamins and minerals.

- Avoid too much salt, which dehydrates the body and therefore the skin. Don't add salt to cooking and avoid processed, refined foods.

- Avoid fried, smoked and barbecued foods, which release more free radicals, and the more free radicals, the faster your skin (and body) will age (see *Antioxidants in Ageing p38*).

- Eating too many saturated fats especially hydrogenated/trans-fats place a large burden on the liver (as does HRT and the Pill) and if the liver is congested, then toxins can be dumped in the skin (see *Liver in Ageing p189*). Therefore cut down on fats from animal sources and don't use mass- produced fats and oils (see *Fats for Anti-ageing p139*).

■ Alcohol and caffeine dehydrate the body and the skin.

■ Avoid taking painkillers, which make your skin look dull.

Friendly Foods

■ As much as possible eat fresh, organic, locally grown fruits and vegetables which contain more vitamins and minerals.

■ Essential fatty acids are absolutely crucial for keeping your skin younger longer – they help you to tan better and burn less, lose weight and keep skin looking younger, more supple and hydrated. Therefore eat more oily fish, avocado and raw unsalted nuts and seeds plus olive oil (for full details see *Fats For Anti-ageing p139*).

■ All foods rich in vitamin A and natural carotenes will help to feed your skin from the inside out: organic carrots, spinach, all leafy greens, broccoli, pumpkin, sweet potatoes, apricots and tomatoes are all great skin foods.

■ Apples are high in pectin and vitamin C, which help to cleanse the liver and thus the skin.

■ Bananas are a rich source of potassium, vitamins A and C, iron, calcium, zinc and folic acid.

■ Figs are fabulous skin foods, especially green figs, but any fresh figs in season, rich in calcium, iron and magnesium, they also help to ease any constipation – which is often a factor in poor skin (see *Bowels p56* and *Elimination p120*).

■ For protein – eat more fresh fish and chicken and other meats. Try and make it organic. Eat more fermented soya-based proteins such as tempeh and miso, plus nuts, seeds and lentils.

■ Good-quality whey is also a great protein for the skin – use it in fruit smoothies daily to help increase new tissue growth. Good brands are Whey to Go by Solgar (in many flavours) or Twinlab Super Whey Powder. Call 0207 436 5122 for details.

■ Eat foods high in flavonoids: grapefruit, lemons, blueberries, bilberries, blackberries, cherries, strawberries and beetroot, all help strengthen fine capillaries in the skin.

■ Fresh lemon juice in warm water sipped before breakfast helps stimulate the liver to detox your system which helps to keep your skin clearer.

■ Dry, cracking skin can denote low vitamin B levels, so eat more low-sugar cereals and oats.

■ Papaya and pineapple contain digestive enzymes that will aid absorption of nutrients from your diet. You can also place a piece of papaya on a slow healing wound – it speeds up the healing process.

■ Silica is a great skin mineral, responsible for healthy collagen found in unrefined oats plus millet, onions, beetroot, wholegrains and potatoes.

■ Dry skin can be a symptom of a slightly underactive thyroid, therefore include sources of iodine in your diet such as seafoods and especially seaweed and kelp (see *Thyroid in Ageing*).

■ Hydration is crucial for skin – make the effort to carry a bottle of water around with you and drink six glasses a day. The purer the water, the fewer toxins it contains and the better hydrated your skin will be. For more details read about RODI water in *Water in Ageing p325*.

The Best Anti-ageing Supplements for Skin

- Carnosine – is one of the most exciting supplements for regenerating the skin that not only helps extend cell life (see *Cells in Ageing p85*) but also it has been shown to regenerate skin. For years, Soviet scientists secretly researched carnosine, a naturally occurring combination of two amino acids in our bodies that are also found in red meats and chicken. After the Cold War, scientists from other countries began to hear about carnosine. Australian, American and Japanese research concurred that this supplement can regenerate skin and the word is now getting out. Dr Marios Kyriazis, a gerontologist in the UK who has researched carnosine, states categorically that taking 100mg per day on an empty stomach, not only helps increase cell life, but definitely improves skin and in some patients their hair too. He says, "When we eat sugar, after digestion it passes into the bloodstream and attaches to proteins in the body – this process known as glycation – damages and breaks down proteins such as collagen, which triggers sagging and more wrinkled skin. Without doubt carnosine can slow this process not only in the skin, but also in the brain and the rest of the body." Dr Kyriazis has written about carnosine on the British Longevity Association's website on: www.antiageing.freeserve.co.uk Or read his book *Carnosine and Other Elixirs of Youth*, Watkins Publishing. You can buy carnosine from most good health stores or contact The NutriCentre or Sloane Health Shop (see page 14). Note that some practitioners suggest you need a minimum of 500mg of carnosine daily, but Dr Kyriazis says his research shows that 100mg daily is the most effective dose.

- Vitamin C is crucial for the formation and repair of collagen. Periods of stress and illness increase the need for vitamin C. A deficiency of vitamin C can lead to slow wound healing and broken capillaries. Take 1 gram a day – every day.

- Vitamin A, in the form of beta-carotene, helps protect the skin from the damaging effects of the sun. Vitamin A helps maintain soft, smooth disease-free skin. Rough, dry or prematurely-aged skin can be a symptom of vitamin A deficiency. Take 30mg of a natural-source carotene complex daily.

- Full-spectrum vitamin E helps counteract premature ageing of the skin. Take 200iu a day.

- Zinc, take 10mg per day. Zinc is important in skin growth and healing.

- Selenium, take 150mcg per day. Selenium works with vitamin E and helps to preserve the elasticity of tissue by delaying oxidation.

- All the companies on page 13 and 14 make high-strength antioxidant formulas that also contain grape seed extract, pycnagenol and other powerful antioxidants.

- Kudos 24 Multi-Active Age Management Complex is my dream anti-ageing skin formula and for full details see page 348.

- Active-H – you can also try taking Active-H, a really very potent antioxidant and many people have reported that by taking 250mg twice daily – their age spots have disappeared (see *Antioxidants p38*).

- Hawaiian Pacifica Spirulina contains high amounts of beta-carotene, as well as GLA for essential fatty acids, vitamins and minerals. (see Blackmores page 13 for details).

- For beautiful skin you definitely need to take essential fats (see also *Fats for Anti-ageing*).

- If skin is deficient in silica, it doesn't retain water as well and can become dehydrated, and your hair and nails can become more brittle. Take 75mg daily.

- Kelp is a good supplement for the skin, providing iodine and other nutrients. But don't take more than 500mcg of Iodine daily unless prescribed by a doctor as too much iodine can interfere with thyroid function.

- If you suffer scarring from acne, surgical scars or whatever, try Rio Rosa Mosqueta. This oil is extracted from the wild Andes rose and is rich in the essential fatty acid, GLA, which encourages new healthy skin to grow. Rosa Mosqueta is richer in natural GLA than evening primrose oil.

- If you suffer from acne rosacea, a flushing of the face, common in women after 35 – you are most probably lacking in digestive enzymes – see *Low Stomach Acid p199*.

Helpful Hints. Listed in alphabetical order

- **Acid-Alkaline Balance**. The natural pH of the skin is slightly acid which helps protect the skin against bacteria and pollution. Most soaps however are alkaline. Therefore ask for a pH-balanced cleansing bar or liquid formulas such as Johnson's Liquid Soap pH 5.5. And add half a cup of cider vinegar to your bath (see *Acid-Alkaline Balance p18*).

- **Anti-ageing creams** (see also *Rejuvenating Creams p285*). The most effective natural anti-ageing creams are those that are high in antioxidant vitamins, minerals and essential fats. In the UK and Europe you are allowed to label a cream as "natural" when only 4% may be natural. So, read the labels more carefully. If I gave a list here of anti-ageing creams that claim to reduce wrinkles and have you looking like a teenager within a month – I would fill this book! But a few of my favourite creams are:

  • Rose cream by the Organic Pharmacy which is packed with anti ageing nutrients. You can call on 0207 351 2232 or visit www.theorganicpharmacy.com

  • Espa products are extremely pure and packed with antioxidants, mineral, plant extracts and organic oils. Sold in all major department stores and Espa Salons.

  • HB Health in London make excellent vitamin C and anti ageing creams. These creams are packed with wonderful ingredients such as green tea and lipoic acid. To find out what is on offer and how to get these creams, you can call 0845 0725 825.

  • Jurlique creams, oils, and shampoos from Australia are great favourites. Made from organic plant-based ingredients, they really are fabulous and are the preferred label of Nicole Kidman. For stockists call 0208 841 6644 or log onto www.jurlique.com.au

• Rejuvenex cream contains RNA and DNA, vitamins A, C and E, aloe vera, ginseng, hyaluronic acid and sugar cane extract (glycolic acid). This cream is fabulous, order online from www.lef.org. They also make a cream with the anti-ageing hormones melatonin and DHEA, but if I use it more than twice a week, then the DHEA brings me out in spots.

• Body Shop skin cream, try Body Butter by The Body Shop. I use Brazil Nut and Shea Butter for dry skin. It's inexpensive and by buying it you help support the local cultures from where the ingredients were harvested. I also love the Extraordinary Skin Cream, and all the skin preparations from the Organic Pharmacy. You can telephone them for more information on 0207 351 2232 or find them at www.theorganicpharmacy.com

■ **Aromatherapy oils** – buy good-quality, preferably organic oils and for the face, dilute in a base of sweet almond, peach or apricot kernel, or avocado oil – 2 drops of pure oils to 5ml of base oil. For anti-ageing try Frankincense, Rose, Lavender, Neroli or Ylang Ylang.

■ **Avoid** using skin care products containing mineral oil, also called paraffin, or white paraffin. These ingredients are derived from petrochemicals and can rob your skin of fat-soluble vitamins – vitamins A and E. Instead make sure your skin care range contains natural, plant-derived oils.

■ **Chelation therapy** – an intravenous infusion of vitamins and minerals, helps to slow many of the visible signs of ageing, especially in the skin (see *Chelation in Ageing p89*).

■ **Chlorine** – it is worth noting that chlorine in swimming pools will also age the skin as it increases oxidative (free radical damage).

■ **Creams and oils** do penetrate the skin and the average woman absorbs 2 kilos of ingredients from creams and oils every year. Therefore, only use organic creams on your skin such as Dr Hauschka or Greenpeople organic creams; contact the NutriCentre on page 14.

■ **Cross-linking** – as we age, proteins in the body such as collagen, react with sugars, causing cross-linking of the sugars and proteins which is called glycation. When you roast a chicken, you can see cross-linking taking place as the chicken skin crisps and browns, and when you take too much sun, the same process happens in our skin!

■ The **Element**s. If you like sailing or skiing, then make sure that you wear a hat and apply high-protection, rich creams that will help slow the de-hydration caused by the wind, sun and/or salt.

■ **Exfoliate** – Susan Harmsworth, founder and owner of Espa, who make natural creams says, "The single most important thing you can do for ageing dry skin is to exfoliate. If your skin is greasy when you are young, then don't exfoliate so much. This is because when you strip away the excess oils, the skin works harder to produce even more oil and so by exfoliating you stimulate oil production. But, dry and older skin needs stimulating and the dryer it is, the more gentle exfoliating is necessary." After Sue told me this, and not having exfoliated for several months, I began either using exfoliating creams and gels once or twice a week and I then moved onto a loofah. The loofah was the quickest and easiest and although most beauticians would not recommend it for the face, I'm afraid I used it on my face, but more gently than on my body and I must admit that after three weeks of this thrice weekly regimen, my skin now looks and feels much fresher.

- **Humidit**y is great for the skin, as it increases the water content of skin. Use a steam room when you can and during the winter when humidity levels are low use a humidifier in the bedroom. Hot dry climates will add to dehydration.

- **Oxygen** is vital for healthy skin. Insufficient oxygen will leave your skin looking dull and tired. Numerous oxygen facials are now being offered, and once a month, these would be of benefit (see *Oxygen in Ageing p244*).

- **Reading**: For more help see *Rejuvenation Therapies p268* or read *Solve Your Skin Problems* by Natalie Savona and Patrick Holford, Piatkus, or *Skin Secrets* by Professor Nicholas Lowe and Polly Sellar. Collins and Brown.

- **Rejuvenating Creams That Help to Slow the Ageing Process.**

- The Environ Skin care range has been developed by a South African plastic surgeon, Des Fernandes FRCS, who wanted to help patients to reduce scarring and skin damage from burns, sun damage, skin cancers and scarring on the skin. He uses a mild form of vitamin A, and beta hydroxy acids (BHAs), extracted from pineapples, lemons and oranges, which have a mild exfoliating effect. They are gentler than Retin A prescribed creams (see below). They are also rich in vitamin C, which helps reduce pigmentation and rosacea (a facial flushing) plus beta-carotenes and vitamin E. For your nearest Environ stockists call – 0208 450 2020. www.environ.co.za

- Glycolic Acid Creams act in a similar way to AHA fruit extract creams, but glycolic acid is extracted from sugar cane. Anne McDevitt, one of Ireland's leading beauty therapists with over 20 years experience, says she can instantly spot skin that has been treated with prescription Retin A. She finds it too harsh and much prefers glycolic acid saying, "It doesn't have the sensitizing effects on the skin, and glycolic acid encourages the skin to function more normally, instead of leaving it red and sensitive. I have seen it time after time totally change the skin and the greater the damage the more dramatic the results. After several years of trying glycolic-based products, they gently remove dead skin, but also encourage the skin to hold more moisture. In the long-term they also help to prevent the melanin from 'clumping' together to form age spots." Anne uses the Danielo range from America. For details call 00353 1 6777962, or log on to her website: www.annemcdevitt.com.

- Retinoid is a term given to many creams derived from vitamin A, commonly known as Retin A or Tretinoin, and the milder versions are known as retinol or retinyl palmitate. These types of creams increase cell turnover bringing new skin cells to the surface more quickly – for as long as you keep using them! They can reduce wrinkles and thicken the skin which makes it look younger. Retin A itself (tretinoic acid) should only be used only under medical supervision as it can cause irritation and increase sensitivity to the sun. Use it at night as instructed, but if exposed to the sun, you will need higher factor protection.

- Another cream Tazarotene, (marketed as Avage in the USA) is another prescription vitamin A derivative which has been shown to be highly effective in reducing sun-induced skin ageing. For details contact The Cranley Clinic in London on 0207 499 3223.

e- mail cranleyuk@aol.com.

■ Syence Servitol Active Tissue Defence has been shown in medical trials at Guy's Hospital in London to thicken the skin– which reduces wrinkles, as where your skin thins first such as your hands, eyes, and so on, is where the wrinkles first appear. I now use this cream every day and am very impressed. The secret is to use it regularly. For stockists, call 0800 838 670; www. syence.com

■ **Smoking** starves your skin of oxygen. It also depletes the body of vitamins A, C and E – all needed for good skin health. Even being in a smoky room increases free radicals on the skin.

■ **Sleep on your back**, which over time greatly reduces the amounts of wrinkles that form on your face and chest area. A plastic surgeon told me this years ago, and I tried for months to sleep on my back and failed miserably. If you can master this, it really helps. Also, of course, get plenty of sleep which aids cell regeneration.

■ **Sun damage** (see *Sunshine in Ageing p305*).

■ **Water**. I have a girlfriend in her 50s who has the skin of a 35 year old. Her secret is bathing in cold (not freezing) water every single day. This really boosts circulation and brings fresh blood and oxygen to the surface without bursting delicate surface veins. I'm too much of a coward to even contemplate such bravery – but she has fabulous skin.Conversely, if you have the water too hot, then you bring too much blood to the surface and you can rupture surface veins. And the hotter the water, the more you will dehydrate your skin. Therefore enjoy a warm bath with added organic oils – but don't stay in it for more than 15 minutes. Have showers instead.

Drink more water. A new-born baby is made up of almost 80% water – in an older person this can drop to 55%. We need to drink more water but as we age, our "thirst mechanism" does not work as efficiently and we tend to drink less. So make the effort to drink six to eight full glasses of pure water a day which helps to re-hydrate your skin. For full details of the most hydrating way to take liquids, see also *Water in Ageing p325*.

Water also helps moisturize the skin, whereas a moisturizer helps the skin to retain moisture. Apply moisturizers to dampish skin for better penetration and hydration.

SLEEP AND INSOMNIA

Some people say that as we age, we need less sleep, but in fact the amount of sleep that suits our individual needs remains fairly constant throughout our adult life. For instance, I can manage for a few days on less sleep, but I still need and function best on eight hours a night. I only have to glance in the mirror to know if I have had insufficient sleep, the dark circles, the dull skin – you know what I mean.

In general, women cope better physically and mentally with broken sleep, but chronic loss of sleep can impair immune function by as much as 30% in a really bad night. Sleep loss can also reduce your ability to cope with pain, increase inflammation in the body, impair your coordination and make you very irritable. Lack of sleep ages you.

Before electricity, most people slept around 10 hours a night, but once we had light at the flick of a switch this gradually decreased to 8 and a lot of people today say they only get 5 to 6 hours a night.

We now live in a 24-hour society, but our bodies need sleep and it comes as no surprise to learn that in Britain alone 1 person in 11 suffers from insomnia regularly for longer than six months at a time, and one in every three adults feel they could use more sleep. Thirteen million prescriptions for sleeping pills are issued in the UK each year.

Sleeping pills can trigger abnormal sleeping patterns, nightmares, a dry mouth, memory loss, headaches, mood swings and in some cases depression. And if you go on taking them, they soon become addictive.

The main cause of insomnia is the laying awake worrying that you will not be able to get off to sleep and most people who say they hardly sleep at all, when tested at sleep laboratories, sleep a lot more than they think they do. And if you are very stressed, then the adrenalin pumping around the body prevents you from sleeping. Shift work, restless legs, and hot flushes during the menopause, are other sources of potential sleep problems.

The hormone melatonin (see *Other Vital Hormones p241*), secreted by the pineal gland, regulates our body's internal body clock – also known as the circadian rhythm, the cycles of day and night, summer and winter. Melatonin is produced within the brain once it gets dark, it's nature's way of helping us to feel more sleepy. As we age, especially after 60, we produce less melatonin, which could well be a contributing factor as to why older people say they are light sleepers. Melatonin, taken in supplement form, helps to decrease the time it takes to go to sleep and deepens the quality of sleep (see *Useful Remedies* in this section).

There are two kinds of sleep in a normal sleep cycle – rapid eye movement or dreaming sleep (REM) and quiet sleep (non-REM). For older people, the amount of time spent in the deepest stages of non-REM sleep decreases.

And while in deep sleep, your cells are being repaired and rejuvenated, your heart rate slows, blood pressure falls a little, your breathing becomes slower and your brain waves change to a relaxed alpha state. Human growth hormone, that helps slow ageing, is released during deep sleep. When you dream, neurotransmitters in the brain that are vital for learning, memory, organization skills, and for retaining newly learned knowledge are replenished.

Natural, regular, refreshing sleep is the cheapest and easiest way to slow the ageing process.

Foods to Avoid

- Caffeine taken too late in the day (in coffee, tea, colas, chocolate etc) can greatly affect your sleep. It's best to avoid caffeine after lunch, as caffeine stays in the system for a long time. It also takes longer for an older body to rid itself of caffeine. Having said this I have friends who can drink a double espresso after dinner and still sleep like a log, and yet if I take caffeine at night, I can easily be awake until 4am the next morning.

■ The food additive MSG often has the same effect as caffeine.

■ Avoid spicy foods at night as they are stimulating.

■ A large meal will make you temporarily drowsy, but prolongs digestion, which interferes with a good night's sleep.

■ Don't eat red meats and heavy, rich, fatty meals at night, as protein takes longer to digest and it also wakes up the brain.

■ Alcohol initially makes you feel sleepy, but it can greatly disrupt sleep, as it dehydrates the body. Even small amounts of alcohol can make it harder to stay asleep.

■ If you tend to wake during the early hours, this could signify that your liver is struggling, in which case you need to cut down on coffee, fats and alcohol (see *Liver in Ageing p189*).

Friendly Foods

■ As much as possible eat early and have light meals at night.

■ Carbohydrates such as wholewheat pasta, brown rice, barley, quinoa, couscous or a baked potato encourage the body to produce a brain chemical called serotonin, which in turn helps increase melatonin production, which aids natural sleep.

■ Include poppy seeds in your diet as they are a natural sleep aid.

■ If you wake in the night and cannot get back to sleep, have a small bowl of cereal (or porridge) with a chopped banana – which is rich in tryptophan, an amino acid that aids sleep. Use "Slumber Milk", high in tryptophan, available from Waitrose and many supermarkets. Otherwise eat a piece of wholemeal or rye toast and a cup of herbal tea, as carbohydrates make you sleepy. As a chronic insomniac, these remedies have worked for me on many occasions.

■ Other tryptophan-rich foods are fish, turkey, cottage cheese, beans, avocados, bananas and wheatgerm.

■ Eat more lettuce at night, it contains a natural sedative called lactucarium, which encourages deeper sleep. Lettuce can be added to stir-fries as well as being eaten cold in salads.

■ If you suffer from low blood sugar, eat a banana before going to bed and have a teaspoon of honey (rich in magnesium) in your camomile tea.

Useful Remedies

■ Melatonin is a natural hormone, which helps you to fall asleep more quickly and enjoy restful sleep. Begin by taking half to 1mg at night, and if this does not work after four to five nights, then increase the dose to 3mg, and up to a maximum of 5mg per night. Melatonin is a very important antioxidant that helps boost immune function and reduces

LDL cholesterol. Unfortunately, thanks to the Medicines Control Agency, you can no longer buy it in the UK (which is ridiculous), but it is freely available from overseas. You can order it for your own use by calling freephone 00800 8923 8923 or log on to www.lef.org. The Life Extension Foundation is in America and they run a very efficient postal service. Otherwise ask your GP for a prescription and you can fulfil this by posting it to The NutriCentre in London (see page14 for details).

- 5 hydroxytryptophan (5-HTP), is derived from the plant griffonia and has been found to encourage natural sleep, but again doses vary. Try 50mg to begin with every evening and if this does not help after four to five days then increase to 100mg and up to a maximum of 200mg per night. I find that a combination of 1mg of melatonin and 150mg of the 5HTP works well for me.

- Many people who wake in the wee small hours are lacking in magnesium, as calcium and magnesium are known as Nature's tranquillizers. Take a combined formula containing 400–600mg of each before bed. If you wake in the night take another.

- Niacinamide (vitamin B3) acts as a natural sleeping pill. If you try this remedy **please ask for no-flush niacin,** as this supplement can cause your skin to turn bright red because it increases circulation. Taking 500mg of the no-flush before bed is useful for people who fall asleep easily but cannot get back to sleep if they wake in the night. As all the B vitamins work together, take a B complex with breakfast to support your nerves.

- Nitebalm is a herbal complex containing lemon balm, passionflower, lavender, hops and valerian. In a trial of 225 patients who had difficulty falling and remaining asleep over 80% showed an improvement in sleeping after taking these herbs. Passionflower reduces nervous restlessness in adults and children and is widely used to help natural sleep. Valerian is a relaxant. In Europe, valerian is the most common non-prescription sedative. Hops can help a person sleep without causing a headache, but should not be used by people suffering from depression. Initially try 30–40 drops three times daily in a little water. It takes about three days to take effect. Then reduce the dose to 40 to 50 drops twice daily and then 40 drops before going to bed. Available from The NutriCentre and Sloane Health Shop (see page 14).

- These and other herbs such as California poppy, catnip and lemon balm are often blended together with camomile and peppermint in night-time formula herbal teas. Find one that you enjoy and if they are bitter, add a little honey to make them more palatable and sip before bedtime.

- Viburcol is a complex homeopathic preparation, which helps people who cannot get to sleep because the mind is too active or over-stressed. Take one ampoule before supper in water and another before going to bed but not with food. Valeriana is for those who tend to wake between 2 and 4am and cannot get back to sleep. Take 10 drops 3 times daily in-between meals. Neither of these products impairs judgement the next day. These preparations made by HEEL can be ordered via a homeopathic pharmacy, or through Boots and Lloyds Chemist.

- Naturopath Jan de Vries has formulated a Night Essence flower remedy, which you can use nightly. It is made by Bioforce, www.avogel.co.uk

Helpful Hints

- If you tend to wake between 3 and 5am you may be suffering from adrenal exhaustion and stress (see *Stress in Ageing p293*).

- The pineal gland can be affected by electromagnetic fields, so avoid using your mobile phone in the evenings (see *Radiation in Ageing p265*).

- Stop smoking. Nicotine is a stimulant and has been linked to sleep problems. In one study, smokers were more likely than non-smokers to report problems falling, and staying, asleep.

- Regular exercise aids sleep and if you have had a particularly stressful day, making lots of adrenalin, then go for an evening walk to help use up the adrenalin, otherwise you may lie awake for hours!

- Natural sunlight helps you to make serotonin and thus melatonin – which aids sleep.

- Go to bed at a regular time each night. If you want to look younger make it around 10pm as the two hours of sleep before midnight are truly anti-ageing. Our systems, particularly the adrenal glands, recharge and recover between 11pm and 1am.

- Don't watch violent or thought-provoking TV and movies just before bed, and don't take work to bed. Read a novel that completely takes your mind away from the day's events.

- If anything is on your mind, write it down and deal with it in the morning. Keep a pad by your bedside.

- The darker the bedroom, the more melatonin you will produce, which helps you to stay younger longer.

- For people who need to work odd hours or women with young babies, try catnaps, or power naps as they are now called, which can be really refreshing.

- If your feet are cold, it's virtually impossible to sleep, so wear socks in bed or have a hot water bottle to warm your feet. Thermoregulation – the body's heat distribution system – is strongly linked to sleep cycles. Even lying down increases sleepiness by redistributing heat in the body.

- Treat yourself to a massage using essential oils of lavender, marjoram, rosewood or sandalwood, add a few drops of any/or a combination of these oils to almond or jojoba oil and massage around your neck, back and shoulders to help relax you and aid natural sleep.

- Paul McKenna, the hypnotherapist, has made some great sleep tapes which you need to use regularly for best effects, especially if you are trying to get off sleeping pills. Call 01455 852233, or visit www.paulmckenna.com

- Read *The Melatonin Miracle* by Dr Walter Pierpaoli, Pocket Books, or *Freedom from Insomnia*, Alexander Stalmatski, Kyle Kathie.

STOMACH

(See also *Absorption, Digestion and Low Stomach Acid*)

Your stomach is situated below your chest area, just under the rib cage but above the tummy button, and it veers to the left hand side of the body; the liver and gall bladder are more towards the right.

Most people think of a protruding "gut" as being their stomach, in fact it is their bulging intestines which are packed with toxic faeces, plus layers of external fat covering their organs such as their liver, pancreas, stomach and so on (see *Bowels*).

Our stomach is naturally protected by a layer of mucin, a mucous-like substance, which lines the stomach walls. But as we age, this barrier can be eroded, leaving us more vulnerable to conditions such as gastric ulcers and helicobacter pylori infestation, the bacteria now known to contribute to conditions such as gastritis (inflammation of the stomach mucosa) and both gastric and duodenal ulcers. Helicobacter, of which there are several strains, is also linked to certain heart conditions. It is the only bacteria that can survive in our stomach acid (hydrochloric acid), levels of which tend to fall as we age, which triggers a whole host of problems from malabsorption and leaky gut, to skin complaints such as eczema.

Protein foods, such as meat and fish, are broken down in the stomach and if stomach acid is low, this makes more work for the pancreas and eventually food can pass through the gut undigested and therefore unabsorbed. Less absorption, means fewer nutrients, which in turn will speed the ageing process.

Low stomach acid can also be a contributing factor to pernicious anaemia, caused by a lack of vitamin B12.

Once food has been digested in the stomach, it then moves on into the small intestine, where further digestion and absorption occurs. What remains passes into the large bowel where salts and water are re-absorbed back into the bloodstream, and all residues are eventually eliminated.

Foods to Avoid

- Don't eat too much food at one sitting, as obviously it stretches the stomach, which reduces the efficiency of your digestive system. If you continually over-eat, and eat too fast over many years, this can cause a hiatus hernia.

- Heavy protein-based meals with red meat, game and organ meats take a long time to digest, so if you want to eat meat simply eat smaller portions.

- Fried foods and melted cheeses are extremely hard to digest.

- A little red wine can aid digestion, but too much alcohol can irritate the gut lining, especially hard spirits, as can nicotine, too much tea and coffee, caffeine, especially cola-type fizzy drinks.

- Fizzy water can trigger gas and indigestion.

- Too much water with food will dilute the stomach acid, again prohibiting proper digestion. Drink water in-between meals.
- For some people oranges (and the juice), mandarins and grapefruits, plus tomatoes may irritate the stomach. If you eat these foods and experience any burning-type indigestion pains, then avoid them.

Friendly Foods

- If you want your stomach to work for life, then it is better to eat smaller meals regularly rather than large meals at one sitting.
- Chlorophyll-rich foods such as alfalfa, cabbage, wheat grass, chlorella and all green vegetables, are all healing stomach foods.
- Raw cabbage juice contains L-glutamine, an amino acid that is very healing to the gut wall.
- Pumpkin, cantaloupe melon, apricots and carrots are rich in beta-carotene, which helps repair and regenerate stomach lining.
- All alkaline foods (see *Acid-Alkaline Balance p18*).
- Live, low-fat bio-yoghurts can help calm the stomach.

Useful Remedies

- Mastica gum can be taken in capsule form. Take 1gram before bed on an empty stomach.
- Find out if you have low stomach acid (see *Low Stomach Acid p199*) and if it is too low, then take a HCl, hydrochloric acid capsule, just prior to eating. (But not if you have active stomach ulcers).
- Alternatively take a digestive enzyme capsule with all main meals.
- Aloe vera juice is very healing. Stir half a cupful into a freshly made vegetable juice daily.
- Manuka honey is very healing, take 1 teaspoon three times daily at any time.
- Liquorice (deglycerinated), available from health shops, contains flavonoids, which are anti-inflammatory and aid healing of the mucosa. It should be taken 20–30 minutes before meals.
- L-glutamine 500mg also helps heal the stomach lining and can be taken last thing at night, or first thing in the morning on an empty stomach.
- Camomile, meadowsweet, calendula or marshmallow root tea will all calm the stomach.

Helpful Hints

- Aspirin, Ibufren (NSAIDS) and painkillers in general, including paracetamol, will irritate the stomach lining. If you must take these remedies, take them with food.
- When you are stressed or fearful, digestion is impaired, therefore never eat a large meal if you are under stress as this could further irritate the stomach lining.

STRESS IN AGEING

(See also *Depression in Ageing* and *Energy*)

More than 6.5 million working days are lost in the UK every year through stress. Stress is a major cause of accelerated ageing, and one of your best strategies for staying younger longer is to stay calm. Stress isn't all bad – it can help to keep you sharp and alert, but in the longer term how your body copes, depends on your reaction to the stress.

Aeons ago when our ancestors were faced with life and death situations, the hormones adrenalin and cortisol were released from the endocrine system, (pancreas, thyroid, pituitary and adrenal glands) to make the heart pump faster, and giving an instant energy boost to the body and brain. Muscles would tense, and cholesterol was released into the arteries to thicken the blood, so that if a person was injured their blood clotted more easily. Blood vessels would constrict, and endorphins, the body's own painkillers, would be released and oxygen consumption increases.

Known as "fight or flight" reaction, these responses saved many lives back then as our ancestors fought off marauding animals and invaders. Today our automatic responses to stress remain the same, but unfortunately these days they trigger heart attacks, strokes, cancers, stomach ulcers and even Alzheimer's. Why?

Because if we don't disperse stress hormones through regular exercise or relaxation, in the longer term they become highly toxic to every major organ, and set up inflammatory responses in the body. It's like putting rocket fuel in a scooter, you eventually burn out the engine. And these days instead of going for a walk, breathing deeply and calming down – we tend to head for the coffee/cola machine and drink another of the 154 million coffees or 250 million soft drinks that we consume every week in the UK. Or we eat another sugary "treat" to keep us going, which triggers even more adrenalin to be released, which exacerbates the situation. Make no mistake, stress can kill you – and that is definitely ageing.

The first signs of extreme stress usually show up in behavioural changes, such as feeling constantly irritable, a sense of humour failure, suppressed anger, trying to do more than one job at once, you begin to feel that you cannot cope, break down in tears, you are tired or wired.

Then come the physical symptoms, palpitations and headaches, lack of appetite/or cravings for sugary foods, insomnia, poor digestion, muscle cramps, frequent urination, constipation/and or diarrhoea, a dry mouth, constant thirst, feeling clammy or cold/ or too hot. Your brain doesn't work properly and you forget simple words or names. That's because stress creates more ageing free radicals (see *Antioxidants*) and research at Stanford University has shown that raised cortisol levels damage the connections between brain cells, affecting brain functions. Luckily, if you stop the stress, the connections grow back. Long-term stress makes the body more acid and vital minerals are then leached from the bones to re-alkalize the body (see *Acid-Alkaline Balance p18*).

If any or all of these symptoms sound familiar, you need to stop and rest, because the next stage could be total burn-out, a heart attack or stroke. Whether your stress comes from a bad relationship, your work, children, an illness, lack of money, whatever it is, if possible make a space and time between what is stressing you and your reaction to it. Talk to someone and tell them how you are feeling, ask your doctor to send you for counselling. If more people could do this, thousands of lives could be saved.

Research has shown that if you think negatively, tend to be angry a lot of the time and are under stress, especially after 50 – then you are more likely to suffer heart and arterial disease.

This is because so many of us hold in emotions that we should get off our chest. Remember, the more indirect you are – the more stressed you become. Emotions held in for long periods will eventually cause a fuse to blow.

There are also those infuriating (but wise) souls who are always positive, they love some stress and positively thrive on it. However, we are all unique and you need to learn what your limits are and listen to your body. And there are many things you can do to reduce the negative effects of stress on your body and enjoy a healthier, more productive and longer life.

Foods to Avoid

- Never underestimate just how much your diet can affect your stress levels and your ability to cope with it. Avoid any foods and drinks containing alcohol, caffeine, sugar and artificial sweeteners, especially aspartame, as these are all stimulants that cause the adrenal glands to overwork and interfere with normal brain chemistry, making you more nervous and worsening your sleep quality.

- Reduce refined (white) and processed foods, they're high in additives/preservatives and sugar, and usually low in nutrients. The more refined and processed food you eat, the more stress you place on your liver, digestive system and ultimately your adrenal glands.

- Cut down on heavy meals especially red meat, which is hard to digest, and when you are stressed digestion is one of the first things to be affected. Don't eat in a rush.

Friendly Foods

- Stress breaks down protein in the body very quickly, this is why most people who are very stressed lose weight. Make sure that you eat around 100–175g (4–6 oz) of quality protein daily – preferably at breakfast and lunch, which helps to balance blood sugar levels.

- Whey is an easily absorbed form of protein. Solgar make an excellent formula (see page 14).

- Eat oily fish and unrefined sunflower, pumpkin and hemp seeds – all rich in essential fats that reduce inflammation triggered by stress hormones (see *Fats for Anti-ageing p139*).

- Liquorice tea helps to support adrenal function and echinacea tea will help support your immune system which is greatly affected by stress. Valerian and camomile teas with a little honey help to calm you down.

- Make sure your eat breakfast, a low-sugar muesli, eggs or wholemeal toast would be fine. Oats especially porridge made with rice milk, as oats are a rich source of B vitamins that help you to stay calm.

- Wholewheat pasta, noodles and breads, couscous, quinoa, amaranth or oat crackers, brown rice and barley are all calming foods.

- Avocados, turkey, cottage cheese, bananas, potatoes, ginger, yoghurt, leafy green vegetables, lettuce and low fat milks will also help to calm you down.

- Generally, increase your intake of easy-to-digest foods such as homemade vegetable soups, mashed sweet potatoes, poached fish, stewed fruits and so on, which helps take some of the burden off your digestive system.

- Eat smaller meals regularly – as low blood sugar is common in people who are stressed (see *Low Blood Sugar p194*).

- See also *Diet – The Stay Younger Longer Diet (see page 114)*.

Useful Remedies

- If the stress has been induced by shock or trauma, use homeopathic Arnica 30c – and take it every two hours in-between meals for a few days. Give the shocked person some sweet tea, as at times of shock the brain uses more glucose.

- Jan De Vries has formulated Emergency Essence for Shock, use as directed. Available from all health stores, or visit www.bioforce.co.uk

- Meanwhile, pronounced stress uses up nutrients more quickly, placing heavy demands on your nutritional resources. To support your body and immune system, begin taking a high-strength multi-nutrient powder that contains vitamins, minerals, antioxidants and essential fats, such as Kudos 24. Take 2 scoops daily in juice or put into yoghurts etc. For more details see page 348.

- For general long-term stress, try the herb rhodiola root. In Siberia, where the root is made into a tea, many local people live healthy lives to well over 100. This could be because rhodiola root has been proven to decrease the release of stress hormones, improve mood, help to lower blood pressure and aid memory. Take for one month, then stop for a month and then start again. It's now available in the UK in one-a-day high-strength (900mg) capsules. For details call Kudos on 0800 389 5476 – or ask at your local health store.

If you are not taking a high-strength multivitamin/mineral then these are the nutrients you need for stress:

- Begin taking a high-strength B-complex to support your nerves. Even if you are taking a multi, for two weeks, in cases of severe stress, also take 500mg of vitamin B5 pantothenic acid one to two times a day which really helps adrenal function.

- Urinary excretion of vitamin C increases with stress, so take 1–2 grams of vitamin C plus 400iu of natural-source, full-spectrum vitamin E to thin your blood naturally, as stress also thickens the blood.

- Bio Care's AD206 contains vitamins C, B5, Siberian ginseng and other nutrients involved in the support of the adrenals in one convenient capsule. Taken three times per day (see Biocare, page 13).

- You need additional calming minerals, so take 750mg of calcium and 500mg of magnesium, which are known as nature's tranquillizers, and are usually very depleted in a stressed person. Take this supplement at night.

- 5-Hydroxy Tryptophan (5HTP) taking 50–200mg daily helps to increase levels of the hormone serotonin in the brain to raise mood.

- Take a high-strength fish oil (1gram) which thins the blood naturally and helps to keep blood pressure down.

- For calming anxiety, try a herbal formula containing the herbs valerian and passionflower. Take 1–3ml of tincture daily, 500–1500mg in tablets, or 3–4 cups of tea per day.

- L-theanine is an amino acid found in the tea plant and in the mushroom xerocomus badius. It is a natural relaxant that increases alpha-waves, which help you to feel more relaxed without inducing drowsiness. Studies show that L-theanine is effective in single dosages in the range of 50–200mg. For details call The NutriCentre or Sloane Health Shop (see page 14).

Helpful Hints

- If you tend to wake regularly between 3–5 am, this is a sign that your adrenal glands and/or your liver are struggling See *Liver p189*.

- Take stock of your life. An important first step is to identify sources of stress. Keep a diary and write down what is winding you up. After a month, you will see it's most probably the same things over and over again. Take steps (if possible or practical) to remove what stresses you from your life.

- Laughter releases stress – learn to lighten up and don't take life too seriously.

- Stop worrying so much. Dale Carnegie once said that 85% of the things we worry about, never actually happen, so trust that things will turn out for the best.

- Keep a pet. Studies with cat and dog owners have shown the considerable stress-reducing abilities of a furry companion. When cats purr, they produce calming alpha waves, so stroke your cat and de-stress!

■ Concentrate on what you can change in your life and let go of the things you have no control over.

■ Doctors agree that if we could all practise a pleasurable hobby, that requires a fair amount of concentration, by taking our minds off what is stressing us, it reduces the release of stress hormones and helps calm us down. At the very least watch a movie that makes you laugh.

■ Make sure you get at least 8 hours sleep every night. Sleep deprivation is a major stress in itself and lowers your tolerance to other stresses.

■ Avoid obvious pressures, such as taking on too many commitments and deadlines. Learn to see when a problem is somebody else's responsibility, and refuse to take it on.

■ Learn to say *no* and mean it – stop feeling guilty.

■ If you are in a very stressed situation, if possible walk away. Go for a walk, take some deep breaths, calm down and then go back. If you do this, you will feel more able to cope.

■ Get plenty of exercise, as relaxed muscles mean relaxed nerves, which reduces stress. A brisk walk or vigorous exercise session is good instant first aid for feelings of stress. If this is impossible, you will still benefit from regular exercise.

■ Take a deeper breath every 20 minutes, this helps to re-alkalize the body and slow the release of stress hormones (see *Breathing p67*).

■ Learn how to relax. Try a simple progressive muscle relaxation exercise to free the body of physical tensions and distract the mind. Lay down flat on the floor with your palms up, breathe into your tummy, then beginning with your feet and calves, tense the muscles as hard as you can and then relax. Work your way up your body until you reach your head and face. Then just stay there for 5 minutes imagining that you are simply empty space and just let go.

■ Learn to meditate, it's one of the best antidotes for stress. Studies have shown considerable positive effects, including reduced anxiety, increased peace and contentment, better stress tolerance, quicker recovery from stress, lower blood pressure and heart rate and more stable brain wave patterns (see *Meditation p207*).

■ Have a regular massage using essential oils of lavender, valerian, frankincense, neroli, jasmine or ylang ylang, which will all help to calm you down as the oils are absorbed into the body. Leave them on overnight to increase their effectiveness.

■ Hypnotherapy on a weekly basis will really help to calm you down (see *Useful Information and Addresses p338*).

■ If you have an emotional problem that you cannot solve or can't handle the stresses in your life, seek outside help and advice. Simply talking with a trusted friend can be very beneficial, although it is often better to find a professional counsellor who can help you handle your problems and learn effective stress-reduction techniques, in a completely objective manner.

- For an excellent guide on how to lower the stress in your life read *Don't Sweat the Small Stuff…and it's all small stuff* by Richard Carlson PhD, Hyperion Books.
- Read *500 of The Most Important Stress Busting Tips You'll Ever Need*, Suzannah Oliver, Cico Books.

STROKES

(See also *Cholesterol, Heart in Ageing* and *High Blood Pressure*)

Strokes are the third most common cause of death in the West and account for the disability and dementia of approximately 150,000 people every year in the UK. Children and young people can also suffer a stroke, but 9 out of every 10 cases occur in the over 55s – and the risk for stroke increases with age.

The good news is that most strokes can be avoided. A stroke occurs when there is a loss of blood supply to the brain that damages or destroys an area of brain tissue. Depending on the part of the brain affected, there may be sudden loss of speech or movement, heaviness in the limbs, numbness, blurred vision, confusion, dizziness, loss of consciousness or coma. Stroke often causes weakness and paralysis on one side of the body, involving the arm and/or leg and face. Symptoms can last for several hours or the rest of one's life depending on the severity of the stroke. "Mini" strokes may even go unnoticed and can contribute to subtle reductions in mental function. Many people who suffer a stroke go on to make a partial or even complete recovery.

So what causes them? As we age, arteries gradually narrow due to a build-up of sticky cholesterol-like substances. Arterial blockages cause 9 out of 10 strokes (called ischemic strokes). The blockages may be the result of thickening of the arteries (atherosclerosis). Sometimes blood clots travel from another part of the body such as the heart or neck, to the brain, causing a cerebral embolism. The other 10% of strokes (called haemorrhagic strokes) are caused by bleeding into the brain from a ruptured blood vessel, which is most commonly caused by high blood pressure.

The risk of having a stroke is higher among people with an unhealthy lifestyle. Smoking, eating too much salt and too much saturated fat, high oestrogen levels, stress, high LDL cholesterol levels and being overweight can all contribute. People who tend to be angry or aggressive a lot of the time are also at a higher risk. This is because stress and anger raise LDL (the bad) cholesterol levels, that thicken the blood.

The first step towards heart disease and stroke is damage to the delicate inner lining of your arteries, which leads to the development of plaque, thickening and the eventual risk of a total blockage. But what causes the damage in the first place? We know that a lack of vitamin C weakens the matrix of the artery wall, making it more prone to damage. Free radicals, for example from smoking or eating fried foods, may lead to increasing arterial damage, especially if the person is deficient in antioxidants such as vitamin C and E (see *Antioxidants in Ageing p38*). But there is another, more insidious factor produced by the body that many doctors now believe to be more dangerous than having high cholesterol – it's called homocysteine.

High levels of homocysteine, a toxic by-product of the metabolism of proteins, are known to damage arteries and the link to heart disease and strokes is now beyond question. Researchers from across Europe have found that a high level of homocysteine in the blood is as great a risk factor for cardiovascular disease as smoking or having a high blood cholesterol level. However, if you have sufficient vitamin B6, B12 and folic acid, your body will convert homocysteine into less toxic substances and studies have confirmed that the less vitamin B6 and folic acid in your blood, the higher your levels of homocysteine. Hence why taking a B-complex daily could save your life.

Foods to Avoid

■ Avoid refined grains. According to a 12-year study, higher intakes of wholegrain foods are associated with a lower risk of ischemic stroke. Replace refined grains (white bread, pasta, rice, couscous, cakes and biscuits) with wholegrains such as brown rice, wholegrain breads and pastas, quinoa, and oats. Whole grains contain more vitamin B, which has often been removed in the processing of "white" products.

■ Reduce your intake of saturated fats from red meats, full-fat dairy produce, cheeses and chocolates – goats' cheese is extremely high in saturated fats.

■ Avoid fried foods or hard margarines. Those most at risk of having high homocysteine levels are high protein (meat) eaters with a poor dietary intake of vitamin B6, B12 and folic acid.

■ Reduce your intake of dairy products – they're associated with an increase in cardiovascular disease, especially strokes. While high in calcium, dairy foods are relatively low in magnesium. Calcium requires adequate magnesium to be deposited in the bones, otherwise it is usually deposited in soft tissues including joints and arteries. Secondly, dairy foods are high in protein so raise homocysteine levels, but lack adequate levels of B vitamins needed to process it into less toxic substances.

■ Avoid all fizzy drinks because of the sugar content that causes damage to the circulatory system and leads to an increase risk of strokes.

■ Caffeine can drive up blood pressure. Cut down on coffee, tea, cola and other caffeine-based drinks and foods such as chocolate cake! Good alternatives include green tea, peppermint tea, fruit teas, or diluted fruit juices.

■ Eliminate sodium-based salts from your diet because of the effects on blood pressure. Replace them with magnesium or potassium-based salt such as Solo salt. Ask at your local health food store.

■ Avoid all highly preserved meats, salted nuts and smoked foods.

Friendly Foods

■ Eat plenty of fresh fruits and vegetables and their freshly made juices for the vitamin C and other protective antioxidants they contain. Especially good are wholegrains such as brown rice, quinoa, barley and lentils, plus broccoli, sprouts, carrots, watercress, fresh and dried apricots, spinach, cabbage, spring greens, mangoes, cantaloupe melon and tomato puree.

■ Potassium-rich foods help prevent strokes and a recent study showed that a low potassium intake can increase the risk of stroke by 50% in the over-65s. Therefore, eat more potassium-rich foods. Bananas, low-fat yoghurt, baked potato with skin, prune juice, tomato juice, Swiss chard, spinach and all leafy greens, squash, asparagus, dried apricots, oranges, kidney beans, and lentils are all rich in potassium. (Note: if you have kidney disease or take a diuretic medication to lower blood pressure, check with your doctor before taking any extra potassium.)

■ Eat more beta-carotene rich foods such as carrots, sweet potatoes, watercress, mangoes, cabbage, broccoli, cantaloupe melon, pumpkin and tomatoes.

■ Vitamin B6 and folic acid help prevent the build-up of homocysteine and can be found in citrus fruits, bananas, tomatoes, green leafy vegetables, beans, nuts, seeds and wholegrain products. Many breakfast cereals are fortified with additional folic acid. Enjoy organic porridge oats for breakfast made with half skimmed milk and half water, and add a chopped apple to sweeten plus a few raisins and some wheatgerm.

■ Make sure you eat a serving of greens, especially dark green leafy vegetables, every day. Spinach, cabbage, spring greens, kale, chard, broccoli, peas and watercress are all good. Greens contain vitamin C, B6, beta-carotene and folic acid, all of which can reduce your risk of stroke.

■ Lettuce, spinach and green vegetables are also rich in vitamin K, which helps to keep calcium in your bones and out of your arteries. You naturally produce vitamin K (K2) in your gut, so if you have taken antibiotics, make sure you eat a live, low-fat yoghurt daily, which in turn will aid vitamin K production.

■ Eat more foods rich in essential fats such as oily fish and use unrefined olive, walnut and sunflower oil for salad dressings. Eat more raw, unsalted nuts and seeds – especially flax, pumpkin and sunflower seeds (see *Fats for Anti-ageing p139*).

■ Eating fish at least twice a week significantly reduces risk of strokes caused by blood clots.

■ Garlic and onions help to thin the blood naturally.

■ Magnesium-rich foods include honey, kelp, raw wheatgerm, dates, winkles, almonds, Brazil nuts and curry powder.

■ Sprinkle raw wheatgerm over cereals and soups, as it is high in vitamin E.

■ Cayenne pepper is a powerful heart and circulation tonic and has been known to reverse plaque formation on the arterial walls.

Useful Remedies

■ Magnesium relaxes constricted arteries and reduces the risk of a blockage. 400mg per day. Many doctors have found that anyone who has suffered a stroke caused by a clot in the brain should be given intravenous magnesium as soon as possible after the stroke.

Magnesium has a powerful dilatory action on the arteries and helps restore blood flow to the damaged tissue.

■ Take a B-complex to help lower the level of the toxic amino acid homocysteine. Participants who consumed at least 300 micrograms of folate each day had a 20% lower risk of stroke. Folic acid 400–1,000 micrograms and vitamin B-complex 50mg per day.

■ Take fish oils, 1–3grams daily, to thin the blood naturally. Don't take fish oil supplements, if you are on blood-thinning medication, without first consulting your doctor.

■ Take 1 gram of vitamin C, plus 400iu of natural source vitamin E, which protect against clotting. Don't take vitamin E supplements, if you are on blood-thinning medication, without first consulting your doctor.

■ Co-EnzymeQ10, take 30–60mg per day, to help strengthen the heart muscle. People high in CoQ10 are less prone to strokes.

■ Bioflavonoids, 1000mg taken daily, help to strengthen capillaries.

■ Ginkgo biloba helps to increase circulation to the brain. Ginkgo is known to inhibit platelets in blood from sticking together. Kudos make a one-a-day high-strength capsule (see page 14). Again, if you are on blood-thinning drugs, tell your doctor about taking any supplements as over time, and under guidance, your medication may be reduced.

■ Take a good-quality antioxidant formula that contains at least 200mcg of selenium.

■ Vinpocetine is an extract of the periwinkle plant that is used in more than 35 countries in the treatment of stroke and dementia triggered by poor blood flow to the brain. It helps to increase oxygen levels in the brain by increasing blood flow and in one study was shown to improve the transport of glucose (brain fuel) into the damaged brain tissue caused by the stroke. Try 10mg twice daily with food. Because this remedy can reduce the ability of blood to clot, never take vinpocetine if you are on blood-thinning drugs. For more information speak to the nutritionist at The NutriCentre on 0207 436 5122.

Helpful Hints

■ Research shows that people living in soft water areas are more prone to high blood pressure, which can lead to strokes, as soft water is low in minerals including magnesium. Therefore, if you live in an area of soft water, supplement with around 400mg of magnesium daily, and drink more bottled water (see *Water in Ageing p325*).

■ Stop smoking – it doubles your stroke risk. Smoking damages blood vessel walls, speeds up the clogging of arteries, raises blood pressure and makes the heart work harder. The damage can be undone, research shows that the risk of stroke for people who have quit smoking for 2 to 5 years is significantly lower than people who still smoke.

■ Certain types of combined oral contraceptives can make the blood stickier which increases the risk for clotting. Orthodox HRT is also linked to an increased risk (see *Menopause p212*).

■ Control your blood pressure (see *High Blood Pressure p170*).

- Take regular exercise, which makes the heart stronger and improves circulation. It also helps control weight. Being overweight increases the chance of high blood pressure and stroke.

- Homeopathic Arnica 6x – taken three times daily between meals for 3 weeks helps to reduce the effects of shock on the body.

- Read *After Stroke* by David Hinds, HarperCollins. A very useful book for anyone who is nursing a relative or friend who has suffered a stroke.

- For more help, contact the Stroke Information Service, The Stroke Association, 240 City Road, London, EC1V 2PR, Tel: 0845 3033 100, or visit: www.stroke.org.uk

SUGAR IN AGEING

(See also *Carbohydrate Control, Diabetes, Essential Sugars* and *Insulin Resistance*)

Most of us know that eating too much sugar can make us fat and yet we still manage to swallow around 14kg (30lb) each annually.

Being overweight increases your risk of various diseases that can shorten your life (see *Weight Problems in Ageing p330*). But sugar can age you in other ways too: by directly harming vital molecules, it makes your skin wrinkle faster!

This is because glucose, the simplest form of sugar, binds to proteins in a process called glycosylation, which can "cross-link" proteins that are not supposed to be connected, making them less flexible. Cross-linked, inflexible collagen proteins in your skin appear as wrinkles, but this wrinkling isn't confined to just the skin. The effects of glycosylation can be seen everywhere in the body where collagen is found – including arteries, tendons and the lungs. Glycosylation in arterial walls makes them less flexible too, which results in higher blood pressure.

Once glycosylation has occurred between proteins and sugars, more damage follows, including oxidation (see *Antioxidants in Ageing p38*), forming "advanced glycosylation end-products", appropriately known as "AGEs". AGE formation is the chemical equivalent of the browning of food in the oven, and as AGEs build up, tissues lose tone and organs degenerate. For example, AGEs are now recognized as an important factor in heart disease, cataracts, Alzheimer's disease, and of course loss of skin elasticity. AGEs cause a 50-fold increase in free radical production which all starts when you have too much sugar in your body.

The obvious remedy is simply to reduce our sugar intake, although this is only the beginning. Keeping your blood sugar levels even is also very important (see *Carbohydrate Control p80*). You should know also that some foods release their sugars quickly, which can cause too-high levels to be circulating around your body. Others release them more slowly, at a rate your body can use them, so levels don't get too high. Nutritionists have studied the effects of different foods on levels of sugar in the blood and devised a "glycaemic index" that compares them against the simplest form of sugar – glucose (set at 100 for comparisons).

Unsurprisingly, Mars bars (68), table sugar (sucrose: 59) and many commercial honeys (87) all score highly. Fructose, the sugar in fruit, has much less of an effect (just 20). Of the fruits, melons (72), bananas (62) and dried fruit (64) release their sugars most quickly, while apples (39), pears (39) and cherries (25) are the slowest.

Wholegrains have a small effect on blood sugar, unless they are refined into foods such as baguettes (95), rice cakes (82), white bread (70), white rice (72) or white pasta (50), which all have increased effects compared to their whole counterparts. The best bread is wholegrain rye bread, such as pumpernickel (41), oatcakes also have a small effect (55) compared to bread.

Cornflakes (80) come out badly for breakfast cereals, muesli is better (66), and porridge oats are the best (49).

Pulses: peas (51), beans (31) and lentils (29), don't have substantial effects on blood sugar.

Milk products, which contain the sugar lactose, are also good (36).

Vegetables, when cooked or highly processed, can have a surprisingly large effect on blood sugar. Baked potato (85) or French fries (75) have a stronger effect than a Mars bar. Carrots (49) and parsnips (97!) are the sweetest vegetables, however, if eaten raw or lightly cooked, have a much less dramatic effect.

The important thing to remember about the glycaemic index is that all foods will affect your blood sugar levels. They're supposed to provide us with energy, but some provide more sugar more quickly than others, so choose those foods, where you can, that have a lesser effect. A general rule is to eat foods in their whole form, or those that contain more fibre, which slows the sugar release down. Another strategy is to mix high GI foods with low GI foods. The low GI foods will slow them down, for example, rice cakes (82) with houmous (36), or toast (70) with baked beans (48). You don't have to avoid anything with a high score, but you should make it a habit of choosing lower GI foods more often. And then you and your skin will age more slowly.

Foods to Avoid

- Keep in mind that sugar is highly addictive and it's going to take you around six weeks to kick the habit. Once you have "lost the craving" for sugar, of course you can enjoy odd treats, but be careful not to become addicted again!

- Alcohol and stimulants like tea, coffee, chocolate, cola drinks and cigarettes also upset blood sugar levels. These substances work by releasing sugar stores and raising blood sugar levels, to give our muscles and brains a boost of energy.

- Avoid sugar and foods containing sugar such as fizzy drinks, chocolate, sweets, cakes, biscuits and ice-cream.

- Dilute fruit juices and only eat dried fruits infrequently in small quantities, preferably soaked for a short while, to reduce the sugar content.

- Reduce your consumption of high glycaemic index foods such as processed breakfast cereals, white bread, white rice, bananas and dried fruit, choosing low glycemic index alternatives where possible.

- Honey, rice syrup, maple syrup, maltose, dextrose and so on, are all high GI sugars. If you need sugar just use small amounts of these foods, or use a little fructose, which has a lower GI and is many times sweeter than ordinary sugar. Stevia makes a great sugar alternative, but is no longer available in the UK, but freely available from health stores in America.

- Be aware that many low-fat foods are high in sugar, which if not used up during exercise, will convert to fat in the body and you will wear excess sugars on your stomach and hips!

Friendly Foods

- Choose more low glycaemic index foods such as beans, peas and lentils, oats, brown rice, wholegrain rye bread, apples and pears. These foods are high in complex carbohydrates and contain special factors that help release their sugar content gradually. They are also high in fibre, which helps normalize blood sugar levels, as well as assisting digestive processes.

- Eat whole, fresh fruit for snacks instead of sugar-laden morning and afternoon tea favourites. Apples and pears are best.

- Oat and rye biscuits can be spread with a little butter and low-sugar jam.

Useful Remedies

- See *Carbohydrate Control* p80 for remedies to help balance blood sugar levels

- Pycnogenol (pine bark extract), is a free radical scavenger that strengthens collagen and helps protect it from glycosylation. Hence why it protects against excessive cross-linking. Grape seed and pine bark extracts possess an antioxidant activity 20 times greater than vitamin C and 50 times that of vitamin E against certain free radicals. Take daily and ask in your health store for creams based on these antioxidants.

- The protein supplement carnosine is by far the safest and most effective natural anti-glycating agent. Carnosine inhibits protein glycosylation and AGE formation. It does this by becoming glycated itself, sparing other proteins from the same fate. Carnosine not only inhibits the formation of AGEs, it can also protect normal proteins from the toxic effects of AGEs that have already formed, stopping protein damage from spreading to healthy proteins. It has been extremely well researched, and as well as helping your cells to live longer, carnosine has a proven ability to regenerate skin. Some scientists say that you need 500mg daily, but Dr Marios Kyriazis, a gerontologist in the UK says he has seen the best results when people take around 100mg daily. Check out his website on www.antiageing.freeserve.co.uk. For optimum benefits it needs to be taken daily for life! For details contact the NutriCentre or Sloane Health Shop (see page 14), or visit: www.lef.org

- The mineral chromium is vital for reducing sugar cravings and is greatly depleted by eating to much sugar. Take 200mcg daily.

- It's natural to like sweet foods, but this can become extreme if we have concentrated sweetness all the time, especially during childhood. If sweets are used as a reward or to cheer someone up, the desire for sweetness can take on an emotional component. To break the habit, nutritionist, Patrick Holford, advises avoiding all concentrated sweetness in the form of sugar, sweets, sweet desserts, dried fruits and concentrated fruit juice. Instead dilute fruit juice and get used to eating fruit instead of having a dessert. Add fresh chopped fruit to cereals and have fruit instead of sweet snacks. If you gradually dilute the sweetness in your food you'll get used to it. After a while, a tea with three sugars will be undrinkable. It's just a matter of what you're used to. But if you are desperate, use a little fructose.

- Artificial sweeteners may seem like a good solution, but do nothing to reduce your sweet tooth and bring their own list of problems to the table (see *Brain in Ageing p59*).

Helpful Hints

- Reduce your stress levels, which cause wild fluctuations in your blood sugar levels, causing fatigue and making you more likely to crave fast-energy foods laden with sugar (see *Stress in Ageing p293*).

- Stop smoking. Smokers have a far higher incidence of wrinkling skin, because smoking accelerates glycosylation in two ways. Firstly, because nicotine is a stimulant, it triggers the release of body stores of sugars into the blood, resulting in the excess sugar binding to proteins, and secondly, the free radicals produced by smoking then further damage these cross-linked proteins creating AGEs. Look at any elderly smoker and you'll see exactly what I'm talking about.

- Read *Get The Sugar Out* by Ann-Louise Gittleman, Three Rivers Press.

SUNSHINE IN AGEING

(See also *Rejuvenation Therapies* and *Skin in Ageing*)

We all know that the sun is ageing – in fact 80% of age-related skin damage comes from too much sun exposure. But it makes you feel so good. If you don't expose your skin to sufficient sunlight, then you can become depleted in vitamin D, which is vital for healthy bones and teeth. Too little sunshine can trigger SAD Syndrome as the body produces less serotonin – the feel-good hormone. Full spectrum light in natural daylight is vital for good health and your state of mind. Sunlight helps to lower cholesterol and increases hair and nail growth, but too much will lower your immune function. People who live in colder climates and have little sun, tend to suffer a higher incidence of internal cancers.

I have always adored the sun and up until my 30s I sunbathed far too much. When

I was a stewardess, I remember being stranded at New Delhi airport in India. It was over 100 degrees. What did I do? I took a blanket, removed my uniform and lay on the runway. No suntan creams and no dark glasses, such was my keenness to be tanned, and my skin has suffered as a result. I don't do that anymore!

Because the sun has had such bad press over the years and skin cancer rates are rising, we are all supposed to have become more sensible in the sun. But most people haven't changed a bit. Whether I'm in England or on a sunny beach in another country, people of all ages continue to literally cook their skin, as I once did. I see children on the beach in the midday tropical sun, without hats, with no tee-shirt and I think their parents must be mad. But they are there, soaking up the rays with beetroot-coloured skin.

On the other extreme you have people like Nicole Kidman who never sunbathes. She lives consciously – she chooses to keep her skin as young as she can for as long as she can and I hope she takes plenty of vitamin D!

When the skin turns red in the sun, this is the red blood cells response to the heat that is being generated on the skin. Your blood is basically trying to cool your skin.

What we need to do, as always, is to find a healthier compromise. For instance if you expose your skin to just 15 minutes of sun a day – then you can produce several days supply of vitamin D.

Sunshine gives off a cocktail of frequencies, but principally ultraviolet radiation. The UVA are the ageing rays, UVB are the burning, plus UVC, which is the most dangerous. Both UVB and UVC are mostly absorbed by the ozone layer (what's left of it). UVA can penetrate deeper into the skin than UVB or C and UVA causes damage down into the fat layer of your skin – 2.5mm into the dermis.

Black and Asian skins contain more melanin, the thick treacle-like substance that resides in your epidermis. The darker the skin, the more melanin it contains and the more easily it can reflect UV rays. Also darker skin is able to resist the penetration of the sun's rays down to the dermis up to five times more effectively than white skin.

People with greasy skin make more sebum, which helps to block the UV rays, hence why people with dark and oilier skins are able to tan better and suffer less wrinkling.

Basically the fairer you are the easier you will burn, the faster your skin will age and the greater the risk for skin cancers. To try to protect itself, your skin begins to thicken and of course it turns brown. And the slower you tan, the more you reduce the ageing effects on your skin.

Our cells can divide about 80 times in each cell's lifetime and too much radiation make cells divide more quickly. Once you reach that critical limit, the cell becomes useless and your skin ages even faster.

Foods to Avoid

■ Avoid foods and drinks that will trigger dehydration, alcohol, caffeine and too many fizzy drinks.

■ See *Foods to Avoid* under *Skin in Ageing* p280.

Friendly Foods

- Obviously, if you are out in the hot sun, you will sweat more and you can quickly dehydrate which can lead to low blood pressure. Drink plenty of water and if it's really hot, then add some extra sea salt to your food.

- The most important foods you need to eat more of to help protect your skin from the inside out are essential fats and carotenes.

- Eat lots more sunflower, pumpkin, sesame, hemp and linseeds and use their unrefined oils in salad dressings and drizzle over cooked foods (for more details see *Fats for Anti-ageing*).

- When you are in the sun, eat plenty of local grilled oily fish and enjoy avocado and salads with added olives.

- For carotenes eat more organic or fresh locally grown carrots, tomatoes and tomato puree, asparagus, mustard and cress, raw parsley, red peppers, steamed spinach, apricots, pumpkin, spring greens, sweet potato, watercress, mangoes, canteloupe melon and persimmons.

- See *Friendly Foods* under *Skin p281*.

Useful Remedies

- See *Useful Remedies* under *Skin p282*.

- Take a high-strength multivitamin/mineral and antioxidant powdered supplement that is also high in carotenes and essential fats (for details see *p348*).

- Take 30mg of natural source carotene complex for a month before and a month after your holiday in the sun.

- People who take 2 grams of vitamin C daily along with 400iu of vitamin E appear to have added protection. Obviously use a sunscreen!

- Melanin is made up from the amino acid L-tyrosine, and taking 1000mg daily can help the body tan naturally. Take in divided doses before food.

- Pine bark extract, known as pycnogenol, has been proven to reduce inflammation on the skin triggered by UV radiation.

Helpful Hints

- For details of vitamin and mineral injections that have rejuvenated my sun-damaged skin see *Rejuvenation Therapies p268*.

- Skin cancers are on the increase, especially in countries and latitudes that enjoy hot sunshine all year round. And as the ozone holes become larger and more widespread, skin cancers are increasing proportionately, especially after the age of 50. The most dangerous type is malignant melanoma, which is a tumour of the melanocyte (the melanin producing cells). They are usually pigmented either black or brown and can evolve from an existing mole or simply appear. It begins to itch, grows larger, and the skin can break down around the "mole". The secret to surviving melanoma, is to see a doctor, dermatologist or oncologist as fast as you can. If caught before the cancer spreads internally, it can be treated successfully. The good news is that if you have reached your 60s and have no skin cancer, the incidence of melanoma reduces.

- You may see small skin ulcers, tiny flaking patches, or small areas of skin that start to bleed, keep scaling and won't heal. This could be a squamous or basal cell carcinoma. These are not so dangerous, but again they need prompt checking. For useful remedies see *Cancer p72.*

- If you are using rejuvenating creams based upon Retin A, glycolic acids, AHA's etc, then wear a higher sunscreen factor and be really careful not to let your skin go red. I use these creams during the autumn and winter months and I stop using them one month before I go away on holiday.

- Don't allow your skin to go really red. This can trigger skin cancers and cause broken and unsightly capillaries on the face.

- If you suffer skin conditions such as eczema or psoriasis, moderate sunbathing and the seawater will help your skin.

- No matter how much people tell you that sun beds are safe, they are not, and continued use greatly increases the risk for skin and other cancers.

- If you carry the Herpes simplex virus, too much sun can trigger an attack of cold sores, in which case begin taking 500mg of the amino acid lysine and 1gram of vitamin C daily for two weeks before travel. Also keep away from chocolate, it contains arginine, another amino acid that makes cold sores more likely.

- Many scientists now believe that chemical-based sunscreens (containing ingredients such as sodium lauryl/laureth sulphate, octylmethoxycinnamate (OMC), benzophenones, synthetic fragrances and colourants, may do more harm than good. Certain preservatives in sunscreens such as parabens, mimic the affect of oestrogens, which can disrupt hormones and are linked to hormonal cancers. If you develop a rash after sun exposure, check out the ingredient list in the cream. PABA is also a problem for many people.

- I always use Green People's organic sunscreens which are fabulous. The UV protection comes from titanium dioxide and extract of cinnamon. Edelweiss, from the Alps, helps protect against skin cancers and is high in antioxidants. They also contain green tea extract, avocado oil, echinacea, myrrh and calendula that help soothe the skin. They really are fabulous and come as a No 8, 15 or 22 protection factors. They are sold in all good health shops and department stores, or order via www.greenpeople.co.uk. They also make wonderful shampoos, conditioners, face and body creams.

- Another favourite is Dr Hauschka sun products. Again they use titanium dioxide, combined with rice germ oil (rich in vitamin E), chestnut bark extracts, quince seeds and jojoba oil. They are sold at major department stores worldwide, or call 01386 791 022 or visit www.drhauschka.co.uk.

- Liz Earle makes great chemical-free creams; for details call 01983 813914 .

- After you have been in the sun, to help reduce the damage, try Jurlique's Calendula C cream (Nicole Kidman's favourite cream): the calendula reduces the inflammation and the carrot oil helps nourish your skin. For details call 0208 841 6644, or log on to www.jurlique.com.au.

- To help avoid cataracts and ageing eyes, wear good wrap-around sunglasses that block 99–100% of the UVA rays.

- Wear a hat, which greatly reduces the UV radiation to the eyes.

- Avoid the sun between 11am–3pm in an English summer – and make that 11am–4pm in hotter climates.

- Please try and be sensible; wear a light wrap or tee-shirt in the heat of the day and always re-apply the creams after swimming.

- Certain antibiotics, arthritis drugs, diuretic drugs and antihistamines (like Benadryl) can trigger extreme reactions. If you are taking any such drugs and you are going away to the sun, check with your doctor.

TASTE AND SMELL – LOSS IN AGEING

Babies have many taste buds in their mouths, including in their cheeks, but once we become adults the sensitivity of all our taste buds is diminished and in old age, greatly diminished. Your tongue is covered with tiny projections called papillae, inside which are the sensory nerves that enable you to taste. Saliva is needed for taste and without it our diet would be virtually tasteless.

The average nose can detect approximately 4,000 different odours, while an especially sensitive one can recognize around 10,000. Inside the nose we have two small receptor sites, which are yellow-brown patches of mucous-covered membrane found in the roof of the nasal cavities. They are covered in millions of hair-like antenna. As we age, these antenna become less effective. When you have a cold, your ability to taste and smell can be reduced by up to 80%. And loss of taste and smell occurs frequently if we have a cold or blocked sinuses.Also if the nose becomes too dry and "stuffed up" then the sense of smell can be impaired. It is generally easier to smell and taste in warm moist atmospheres rather than cold, dry ones. Hay fever, allergic rhinitis, nasal polyps and smoking can all interfere with taste and smell. Lack of zinc is greatly associated with this condition. Certain heart drugs can also cause a loss of taste and smell.

Foods to Avoid

- Generally as you age, you really need to avoid mucus-forming foods such as full-fat milk and dairy produce from cows and goats. Soya milk is also a problem for many people, as are chocolates, full-fat cheeses from any source, pastries and cakes, especially high-fat croissants.

- Sugary foods will also make the situation worse.
- See *Diet – The Stay Younger Longer Diet* on page 114.
- Avoid fried foods and heavy, rich, creamy meals.

Friendly Foods

- Make sure you eat plenty of fresh fruits and vegetables, salads and lightly steamed vegetables.
- Eat more brown rice, barley, lentils, low-sugar cereals, oats and wholemeal bread and pastas.
- Zinc-rich foods include lean steak, lamb and beef, wheatgerm, calves' liver, raw oysters, fresh peanuts, hazelnuts, ground ginger and dry mustard.
- Sunflower, pumpkin, sesame and linseeds all contain fair amounts of zinc.
- Try organic rice milk as a non-dairy substitute.

Useful Remedies

- Zinc – take 15–30mg of chelated zinc, or zinc picolinate, which can be useful in helping to restore the sense of smell.
- Lack of potassium sulphate can also cause loss of taste and smell. Take 75mg daily with food (see Blackmores page 13).
- If an infection has triggered the loss of taste and smell, take 10,000iu of vitamin A, which helps support the respiratory tract. If you are pregnant, take no more than 5000iu.
- Include a high-strength multivitamin/mineral, plus 1gram of vitamin C.
- Again if linked to an infection take Echinacea 500mg twice daily to boost your immune system (see *Immune Function in Ageing p175*).

Helpful Hints

- Acupuncture has proven quite successful for helping to restore the sense of smell (see *Useful Addresses* on page 338).
- Tap water is often contaminated by chemicals, which can exacerbate this problem. Invest in a good-quality water filter such as Watersimple from The Fresh Water Filter Company, they can be contacted at Gem House, 895 High Street, Chadwell Health, Essex RM6 4HL. Tel 0870 442 3633, www.freshwaterfilter.com. Or contact The Pure H2O Company on Tel: 01784 21188, or visit www.pureH2O.co.uk
- See a qualified nutritionist who will help to rebalance and detoxify your system.
- Homeopathic Nat Mur, Silica or Pulsatilla are also very useful for loss of taste and Belladonna or Hyos are useful for loss of smell (see *Useful Information* for further details).

TEETH IN AGEING

See also *Toxic Metal Overload*

By the time you are 35 you should have 28 teeth, plus 4 wisdom teeth which can arrive at any age after 18. Your teeth are made up of enamel, a dentine core and a root canal, which contains the nerve that serves the tooth.

As we age, gums tend to recede, teeth are worn away and jaw problems can arise from grinding of the teeth, which we tend to do at night, especially when stressed.

Headaches, migraines, neck and facial pain, back problems, jaw pain and tinnitus (ringing in the ears) are a few of the symptoms that can result from neuro-muscular imbalance, which is what triggers the grinding in the first place.

Over time, your cheeks move inwards giving the face an aged, hollow look and wrinkles develop around the mouth area. Sounds great doesn't it?

After years of dental problems and much surgery, my face and jaw caused me tremendous pain, until I could hardly smile. Then a chiropractor told me about dentists who specialize in facial pain and I went along to Mr Richard Dean, at Harcourt House, 19 Cavendish Square, London W1. Richard made a brace that fits properly and in the eight months that I have worn it, my facial pain has been greatly relieved. The treatment is not cheap, but to be free of pain, it's been worth it.

These treatments can also help Trigeminal Neuralgia, which causes excruciating facial pain. If you cannot get to London, then Richard is happy to recommend other colleagues around the UK – for details call 020 7580 2644.

Also, gum disease is now linked to heart disease. Sometimes bacteria from the mouth are absorbed into the bloodstream and can end up in the heart valves, triggering various heart conditions. Good oral hygiene will help you avoid such problems. Root canal work also needs to done thoroughly. David Hefferon, a holistic dentist, says, "The root needs to be thoroughly cleaned to make sure that no infection remains in the canals before the final root filling takes place, otherwise the jaw bone can become infected, and the patient carries a chronic area of local infection, producing toxins that will find their way into the bloodstream causing symptoms such as low-grade chronic fatigue, energy loss and recurring illnesses such as colds, but these bacteria can also travel to the heart, placing patients at risk of heart disease." And with advances in stem cell therapy, false teeth and implants could soon become a thing of the past. Professor Paul Sharpe, Head of Craniofacial Development at King's College, London, has now set up a company called Odontis, (www.odontis.co.uk) which is offering bio-engineered teeth. They will be able to take a few cells from your mouth, engineer them, and then they are replaced back into the site where the tooth is missing and a new tooth will grow.

Foods to Avoid

- When you ingest sugary foods and drinks, colas, concentrated fruit juices, white wine, vinegar, rhubarb, oranges, lemons, grapefruit and so on, the acids in these foods weakens tooth enamel and allows bacteria to enter the tooth, which is the cause of tooth decay.

- Boiled sweets and sticky toffee-type desserts are the worst foods for your teeth.

- If you brush your teeth immediately after eating these types of foods you can brush away the weakened enamel and cause erosion. Simply wash your mouth with water to help neutralize the acids and clean your teeth later.

Friendly Foods

- All fresh fruits, especially apples and vegetables are good for your teeth. Just be aware that when you eat "acid" tasting foods such as pineapple, rinse your mouth with water afterwards and avoid cleaning your teeth for a couple of hours.

- If you drink lots of concentrated fruit juices, dilute at a ratio of one part juice to four parts of water.

- Drink water in-between meals, which helps to normalize the pH balance of your saliva.

- Thai foods containing lemon grass, coriander and garlic make great bone foods and coriander also helps to detoxify heavy metals from the body.

Useful Remedies

- CoEnzymeQ-10 is an antioxidant that helps keep gums healthy. Take 60mg daily.

- Vitamin C, 1 gram a day, also helps to keep gums healthy.

- Vitamin B12 and vitamin K may be lacking if your gums tend to bleed. Therefore take a B- complex and 10mg of vitamin K daily.

- Replace fluoride mouthwashes with lukewarm salty mouthwashes. A teaspoon of sea salt is best as it is rich in minerals – table salt contains aluminium, which is linked to Alzheimer's disease.

- A supplement called Active-H helps to stop the build-up of dead bacteria, which stick to our teeth and becomes plaque. This is a very important breakthrough (for more information see *Antioxidants in Ageing p41*).

Helpful Hints

- Regular brushing, plus flossing daily will help keep your teeth and gums healthier; see an oral hygienist at least twice a year.

- Garden sage makes a great mouth wash for inflamed and bleeding gums (gingivitis), an inflamed tongue, mouth ulcers or a sore throat. Grow some of this wonderful anti-inflammatory and anti-bacterial herb in your garden and simply pour a cupful of water over 1–2 teaspoonfuls of the chopped leaves, allow to stand for 15 minutes and sip. To make up a mouthwash add the same amount of leaves to half a litre (one pint) of boiling water.

Cool and place in a screw-top jar and use two or three times daily. As a gargle, make the stronger tea solution and gargle while the water is still warm. As sage stimulates the muscles of the uterus – it should not be used during pregnancy.

■ As we age, we also lose bone mass and the gums follow the bones, hence why looking after your bones will help your teeth (see *Osteoporosis p233*).

■ Try Gengigel, a gel and mouthwash that contains hyaluronic acid (HA). As we age levels of HA fall in the body and it is an important component of skin and gum tissue. This gel helps to hydrate the gums and promotes new gum formation. It also reduces gum inflammation associated with gingivitis. For details call Revital on 0800 252 875 or 01895 629950 or visit www.revital.com.

■ Fluoride is a by-product of the fertilizer industry and is known to be carcinogenic. It has ruined many children's and adult's teeth thanks to fluorosis – a mottling and browning of the teeth. It also accumulates in our bones which can make them more brittle. Fluoride is absorbed through the gums and eventually ends up in the pineal gland, which controls production of the hormone melatonin, which aids proper sleep. And proper sleep helps slow the ageing process! Fluoride also causes free radical reactions in the body that accelerate ageing. If you have fluoride in your local tap water, do not use fluoride-based toothpastes.

■ There are plenty of healthier toothpastes now on the market, such as OralFresh Toothgel by Comvita, which is free from fluoride, preservatives, artificial flavours and sodium lauryl sulphate. It is made up from peppermint oil, propolis, tea tree oil, eucalyptus and chlorophyll. It is available from most health stores or call 01730 813642.

■ I also use Aloe Dent which is based on aloe, CoQ10 and tea tree. Kingfisher also make a fennel toothpaste.

■ If you suffer jaw and facial pain, see a chiropractor (see *Useful Information and Addresses*).

THREAD VEINS
(See *Veins in Ageing*)

THYROID IN AGEING
(See also *Other Vital Hormones*)

Your thyroid is often the most ignored gland in your body. Situated in your neck, just below the Adam's apple, it produces hormones that affect every major organ, the metabolism and repair of every single cell, and has a major influence on hormonal function. Every drop of our 8–10 pints or so of blood circulates through our thyroid every hour, bringing with it the substances the thyroid needs to do its work. The most important thyroid hormone is thyroxine (also known as T4), which outside the thyroid is converted to T3 (tri-iodothyronine), which is the active form of the hormone. Basically, the more T3 you produce, the faster your metabolism works. If you don't produce sufficient thyroid (T3) hormones, many systems in your body slow down – heartbeat, circulation, blood pressure, energy levels, metabolism and temperature. A slower metabolism will mean that you don't burn calories as efficiently as you could, so you gain weight more easily.

Up to 20% of the population is probably suffering from some degree of hypothyroidism (under-active thyroid) and the older you get, the more prone you are to the condition. But it needn't be that way. Look after your thyroid and it will look after you well into old age. Symptoms that should make you investigate whether your thyroid may be under-active include low energy, mental "fogginess", depression, cold hands and feet, even in summer, weight gain even with a poor appetite, high cholesterol even if you eat sensibly, a slow pulse, low blood sugar (see *Low Blood Sugar*), headaches, infertility, dry and sometimes puffy skin, brittle nails, poor vision and memory, constipation, sore throat, nasal congestion, thinning hair, low libido and heavy periods. An under-active thyroid is seven times more common in women than in men. Unfortunately, because some of the symptoms associated with an under-active thyroid are so often attributed to the menopause, thousands of women go undiagnosed or are offered orthodox HRT as a one-stop cure-all. But there is so much you can do to help yourself.

If you have your thyroid tested by a doctor its very likely they'll report that everything is fine. Unfortunately the tests are rather crude and your thyroid would have to be very under-active indeed before it would show up as altered blood levels. The quoted "normal" range is so wide it is relatively meaningless, you could be 50% down on "average" and still said to be within normal limits.

To test your own thyroid, there's a simple temperature test developed by Broda Barnes that's now widely used by nutritionists. Here's how it works. Shake out a thermometer and keep it by your bed. When you wake up in the morning, and before getting up, put the thermometer under your arm and lie there for 10 minutes. Your temperature should be 36.5 to 36.7 degrees Celsius. Do this for at least 2 days. (Women should do this test on day two and three of their period as body temperature fluctuates during the cycle.) If either of your temperature readings are below 36.5, take it again over a longer period, say a week, to see if it is low on a fairly regular basis. If it is lower than 36.5 you're probably hypothyroid, and your thyroid gland is under functioning. For more help, log onto www.brodabarnes.org. In many cases, a low temperature will not necessarily indicate a condition that would be medically diagnosed as an under-active thyroid (and treated with synthetic thyroid hormones), but nevertheless, you could benefit from the following guidelines.

If you take steps to improve your thyroid efficiency, take your early-morning temperature again for a couple of mornings every month or so. As it starts to increase, you should find that some of your symptoms also start to improve.

An overactive-thyroid (excess T3 production) is known as hyperthyroidism and is relatively rare. In this condition, the thyroid produces too many hormones, which can trigger symptoms such as goitre – when the thyroid becomes more prominent and the eyes bulge. Other common symptoms are anxiety, insomnia, an inability to relax, shakiness, excessive sweating, feeling warm even on cold days, rapid heartbeat, palpitations, breathlessness and weight loss even with a hearty appetite. If you are diagnosed with an overactive thyroid, you need the help of a competent physician or nutritional practitioner.

Foods to Avoid if you have an Under-active Thyroid

- Certain foods are known to inhibit thyroid function including soya (soya milk, tofu, etc), apples, cruciferous vegetables such as cabbage, broccoli, mustard, kale, spinach, peaches, pears and turnips. Also avoid walnuts and peanuts. These foods are generally good for you but just avoid them until the thyroid has stabilized.

- Avoid all foods and drinks containing caffeine which stimulate the release of adrenalin that can affect the thyroid.

Friendly Foods for an Under-active Thyroid

- Iodine (a mineral) and tyrosine (an amino acid i.e. a component part of protein) are the two nutrients the body uses to make thyroid hormones.

- Iodine can be found in seafood and seaweed (for example kelp, nori, arame), mushrooms, Swiss chard, butter beans, pumpkin seeds and sesame seeds (tahini), egg yolk, lecithin, minced beef, artichokes, onions and garlic.

- Use organic sea salt.

- Tyrosine is in all protein-rich foods, especially fish, butter beans, pumpkin seeds, bananas and avocados. If you have adequate protein in your diet you should be getting enough tyrosine.

- Essential fatty acids, the healthy fats, are essential for proper thyroid function, so include oily fish, seeds and cold pressed oils in your regular diet. See *Fats for Anti-Ageing p139.*

- Eat more radishes, watercress, wheatgerm, Brewer's Yeast, mushrooms, tropical fruits, watermelon, seeds and sprouted foods such as alfalfa. Make your own watermelon juice and add aloe vera juice, a great thyroid blend.

- Use coconut oil for cooking and for flapjacks, it helps stimulate the thyroid.

Useful Remedies for an Under-active Thyroid

- A high-strength multivitamin/mineral complex taken every day provides a baseline of nutrients for the body to work with.

- Kelp tablets contain iodine; follow the directions on the label, aiming for around 150mcg of iodine a day. But don't take more than 500mcg of iodine a day, unless under your doctor's instruction, as too much iodine can upset your thyroid balance.

- The body makes thyroxine from the amino acid L-tyrosine, so take 500mg twice daily on an empty stomach (plus 50mg B6 and 100mg C to help absorption).

■ Siberian ginseng: take 1–3grams (or 2–6ml of tincture) daily, for a month, then leave off and start again a month later. This can help reduce the effects of stress on your adrenals (see below), your thyroid and your health in general. Avoid Korean ginseng if you suffer from high blood pressure.

■ Taking 1gram of vitamin C, as well as 100mg of CoQ10, can help raise energy levels within the body.

■ Thyro Complex is a formulation by naturopath Martin Budd, an established authority on thyroid health. He has spent 15 years researching the nutritional support required for healthy thyroid function, and his formula contains all the nutrients needed to help support the thyroid. Take 1–3 tablets daily 30 minutes before food. Available from The NutriCentre and Sloane Health (see page 14).

Helpful Hints

■ Stop smoking – smoking is known to make an under-active thyroid worse. Cigarettes aren't an easy addiction to give up but worth the effort.

■ Avoid stress. Stress stimulates the adrenal glands to produce the hormone cortisol, which is known to hinder the conversion of the thyroid hormone T4 to the more potent T3. Learn to relax, ensure you have "down time" regularly, try yoga, t'ai chi, massage or meditation, and exercise regularly (see *Stress in Ageing p293*).

■ Support your digestion. One possible reason the thyroid slows down as we age is linked to our digestion. It is well established that our enzymatic function and digestive capacity decline with age, not to mention our chewing as our dental health declines. Tyrosine, needed to make thyroid hormones is a component of protein. Protein is relatively difficult to digest, so less digestion means less tyrosine and therefore less thyroid hormones. The answer is to chew well, relax over meals, and ensure you have an optimum level of nutrients in your diet to support digestion. If you have low stomach acid (needed to digest protein), you'll find that beetroots give you pink urine, in which case take a digestive enzyme.

■ Consider food intolerances. Dr James Braly has reported in his latest book *Dangerous Grains*, Putnams, a surprising correlation between wheat intolerances or allergies and thyroid problems. You can test for food intolerances with a kinesiologist or a simple at-home blood test from York Laboratories, call 01904 410410. It is also available through a nutritional practitioner (see *Useful Information and Addresses p338* for further details).

■ Exercise regularly. Exercise stimulates thyroid function, so take 30 minutes of aerobic exercise at least three times per week. If you are just starting an exercise programme, start gently and build up. Over-exertion is a sure way to give up on an exercise regime before you've had a chance to get used to it.

■ Avoid fluoride (in toothpaste) and chlorine (in tap water) as they are both chemically similar to iodine and block the iodine receptors in the thyroid.

- If an under-active thyroid is diagnosed early enough and the patient is otherwise vigorous, homeopathic thyroid treatment can be very useful. One such product is called Thyroidea Compositum, made by the German company HEEL, it is one of the most powerful and useful non-drug substances in the holistic physician's repertoire. For further information call Bio Pathica on 01233 636678.

- Try reading *Hypothyroidism, the Unsuspected Illness* by Broda O'Barnes and Lawrence Galton, Harper and Row Tel: 0207 323 2382, or *Why Am I So Tired – Is Your Thyroid Making You Ill*, by Martin Budd, Harper Collins.

- For further help, log on to www.brodabarnes.org

TOXIC METAL OVERLOAD

In recent years it has become increasingly obvious that "metal pollution" in our environment is a major health hazard. At least six cancer-causing metals have been identified and undoubtedly there will be more. Metals poison our metabolic systems and can block important enzyme pathways, by which our cells live and breathe.

Most toxic metals do not really belong in our environment, and the metal forms that are now so common, such as lead, iron, mercury, cobalt, arsenic, thallium, aluminium and others, have been put there by science, food manufacturers and industry.

There are metals that we need for good health, but only in certain forms and in minute quantities, such as copper and iron.

Dr Stephen Davies, a leading UK research doctor and Medical Director of BioLab in London, told the 1992 annual conference of the American College for the Advancement of Medicine that his researchers in Britain had revealed, from 30,000 hair, sweat and urine samples, that the vast majority of the population in the industrialized world has tissues laden with lead, cadmium, aluminium and arsenic.

Iron overload, a condition called haemochromatosis, although relatively uncommon, gives a good indication of the dangers of excess metals. Complications of this disease include liver enlargement, skin diseases, diabetes, heart failure and neurological dysfunction, such as dementia and Alzheimer's disease.

Toxic metals accumulate in the brain tissues, kidneys, liver and in the gut. Mercury and other toxic metals prevent you from absorbing nutrients into the nerve cells, which prevents energy production. If energy production is impaired your cells dehydrate and skin ages more quickly.

Also, the environmental protection agency in America have issued a warning that many fish such as tuna, swordfish and some mackerel contain high levels of mercury. But without doubt mercury-based amalgam dental fillings are doing the most damage to our health.

Dr Jack Levenson with David Hefferon are specialist dentists based in London who remove amalgam fillings and Dr Levenson says, "Around 2 million people in the UK alone are sensitive to amalgam. Mercury is proven to pass through the blood-brain barrier, it deposits and accumulates in the brain, which can trigger memory loss and symptoms that mimic senile dementia. Other illnesses we have seen that are a direct result of mercury toxicity are chronic fatigue, ME, multiple sclerosis, fibromyalgea, heart disease, motor neurone disease, migraines, infertility, joint and muscle pain, visual disturbances and so on."

When I had my mercury fillings tested by Jack five years ago, two of my fillings were emitting 10 times over the supposed safety limit of mercury emissions and I had them all removed on the spot. And the chronic fatigue that had plagued me on and off for over 20 years gradually disappeared.

Most dentists are afraid to speak out as the British and American Dental Associations still use amalgam fillings. In the UK around 20 million amalgam fillings are carried out by the NHS every year.

Foods to Avoid
■ If you have mercury fillings then avoid larger fish like cod, haddock, tuna and swordfish, which often contain higher mercury levels.

■ Commercial chocolate, ready-made desserts, baking powders, processed cheese, most chewing gums and pickles, plus ready-made meals in aluminium containers should be avoided. If you buy a ready meal in an aluminium container, transfer the contents to a glass or stainless steel oven-proof type dish to reduce the amounts of metals that would otherwise leach into your food during heating.

Friendly Foods
■ Organic apple pectin and kelp have mild chelating (metal-removing) properties.

■ The herb coriander (also known as cilantro) helps to remove toxic metals. For best effects, use the fresh herb, don't cook it.

■ Eat more wholegrains such as brown rice, barley, quinoa and amaranth.

■ Help keep your bowel healthier by taking acidophilus/bifidus powder daily, which again helps to detoxify heavy metals.

■ All organic foods, especially green foods such as parsley, cabbage, kale, kelp, grapefruit and all fruits rich in antioxidants, will help to detoxify the body.

■ Small amounts of alcohol, especially red wine, helps to release mercury vapour from the lungs.

■ Eat more garlic and onions, which also help to remove metals from the body.

Useful Remedies
■ Ask at your health shop for an organic source of chorella, a green algae, that binds neuro toxins from your cells and excretes them from the body. Generally take 500mg twice daily

or check with your health professional.

- MSM (an organic form of sulphur) 500mg, plus a multivitamin/mineral can be taken daily, which help to displace any mercury.

- The amino acids cysteine and methionine are also important. Take 500mg a day of each.

- All metals compete so putting back the healthy ones will squeeze out the poisonous ones. Magnesium, chromium, selenium and zinc are important in this respect. Selenium is outstanding against mercury, and selenium from cold-water fish is thought to be the reason cancer was unknown to Eskimos in their traditional way of life. Take selenium 100–200mcg daily.

- The supplement ProAlgen contains over 20 minerals and trace elements including iodine and selenium. These minerals bind heavy metals and radioactive substances to its own molecules. It cannot be broken down by bile or saliva to be absorbed, so it is secreted from the body together with heavy metals and radioactive substances. Developed in Norway in 1986 as an aid in removing radiation from victims of the Chernobyl nuclear accident in Russia. Recommended for anyone on a detoxification program due to heavy metal poisoning. Take 1 capsule three times daily before meals with 4–6oz of liquid (Nutricentre)

- Vitamin C is a recognised chelator. Be sure to take plenty if you are on an oral chelation programme – at least 2grams a day with food.

- The full list of metals which have entered our environment is very large. But the list includes at least some of the following:

Antimony, Cobalt, Manganese, Thallium, Aluminium, Copper, Mercury, Tin, Arsenic, Gallium, Nickel, Uranium, Cadmium, Gold, Platinum, Vanadium, Cerium, Iron, Silver, Zinc, Chromium, Lead, Tellurium

- Note that some of these metals are essential to health in small (trace) quantities, such as chromium, cobalt, iron, manganese, vanadium and zinc. But all can become toxic if taken to excess.

Helpful Hints

- Read *Toxic Metal Syndrome* by Richard H. Casdorph and Morton Walker, Avery Publishing.

- As with any pollution source, the first step to take is to cut down or eradicate exposure. Cadmium poisoning (bad for the kidneys) comes almost exclusively from cigarette smoking. You only have to stop smoking to begin the healing process.

- If you have mercury fillings, I suggest you have them removed by a dentist who specializes in mercury removal.

- For a free mercury information sheet and a list of dentists who specialize in the removal of mercury fillings, send a large SAE with 3 first-class stamps to The British Society for Mercury Free Dentistry, 221 Old Brompton Road, London SW5 OEA. Or call their information line on 020 7373 3655, or visit www.mercuryfree.co.uk *Menace in the Mouth* by Dr Jack Levenson is available to order by calling the Society.

■ Consult a nutritionist (see *Useful Information and Addresses* on page 338) or contact a specialist like David Hefferon who can test you for metal toxicity. David is on 020 7935 5281.

■ Chelation therapy is an effective way to remove most of the toxic metals from the body. It is a safe treatment and used worldwide as the treatment of choice for most metal poisoning. Chelation must only be administered by a qualified doctor. For further information (see *Chelation in Ageing p89*).

■ The following table from Dr Keith Scott-Mumby lists key sources for common metal pollution:

Lead
Old plumbing, old paints, pottery glazes, motor emissions, batteries, solder, roofing, insecticides.

Mercury
Amalgam fillings are the most dangerous, fish, some Chinese herbs, dyes, electroplating, cosmetics and antiseptics. Many vaccines contain a form of mercury that is used as a preservative. These have now been banned in America. Many fungicides sprayed on fruit and vegetables are mercury-based.

Cadmium
Tobacco products, smelting (releases 3.1 million tons of cadmium dust into the atmosphere annually), black polythene and rubber, ceramics, fungicides, cadmium vapour lamps, processed foods, foods from soils contaminated by cadmium fertilizers, copper refineries.

Aluminium
Aluminium cookware, "tin" foil, tea (Assam, Darjeeling and Ceylon), cows' milk, alum water precipitant (added by many water companies to your tap water), food additives (anti-caking agents, pickling salts), talcum powder, processed cheeses, chewing gum, baking soda, cat-litter, cement and industrial emissions.

Arsenic
Semiconductor manufacture, petrol refining, wood preservative, animal feed additives, herbicides, and contaminates ground water supply.

VEINS IN AGEING

(See also *Circulation, Elimination, Heart in Ageing, High Blood Pressure*)

The most likely venous problem you may suffer in later life is varicose veins, which are caused by poor circulation and weakened valves in the veins, allowing blood to accumulate and stretching the vein walls.

When I became pregnant at 18, after working long hours standing in a supermarket I developed varicose veins. Because I had no idea how to stop them they got worse. In my 20s I worked for nine years as an air stewardess and often had to be on my feet for 18 hours at a stretch. Today I tend to sit at a desk for 10 hours at a time, which also restricts circulation. Vascular surgeons are now seeing children as young as 11, who are "couch potatoes" and sit at computers or watch TV all day.

My mother and father both had vein problems. Yes, you can inherit a tendency for veins, but if I had known then what I know now, I could have definitely prevented their onset. In my 40s, I had some veins stripped, but the problem has returned. But today, thanks to more efficient diagnostic techniques and improved surgical procedures, you can in many cases eliminate varicose veins, but how much better to prevent them in the first place!

The most commonly affected areas are the legs, where eventually the veins can be clearly seen on the skin. Over time they bulge, become bluish and lumpy looking, can be painful, and if not treated can also ulcerate. Anything that slows the return of the blood from the legs to the heart will aggravate varicose veins.

This condition is closely linked to constipation and if you strain when you go to the toilet, then blood is forced into your lower body, which makes the problem worse. Vein problems are also linked to standing or sitting for long hours, being overweight, pregnancy and crossing your legs too much. Another common condition, thread or spider veins, involves chronically dilated and overly permeable capillaries near the surface of the skin. While they're harmless and rarely cause any problems, they can be distressing for cosmetic reasons. You can prevent them developing or worsening with much of the same advice below (see *Helpful Hints*).

Foods to Avoid

- Cut down on heavy meals, red meat and cheeses which are low in fibre and take a long time to pass through the bowel, potentially contributing to constipation. Furthermore, saturated, fried and hydrogenated fats thicken the blood and make it travel more slowly through your veins and arteries, increasing the risk of vascular problems.

- Foods made with flour from any source tend to block the bowels, so reduce your intake of flour-based foods especially croissants, meat pies, pizzas, cakes, biscuits and so on. Choose wholegrains instead where possible, for example German wholegrain breads, brown rice, rolled oats and barley grains.

- Coffee, tea, colas and especially alcohol will dehydrate the bowel and exacerbate leg problems.

- Reduce your salt intake, which can trigger water retention.

Friendly Foods

- Bilberries, blueberries, blackberries, sweet potatoes, pumpkin, squash, cherries, apricots, squash, spinach, spring greens and cabbage. Citrus fruits, broccoli, red grapes, papaya, tomatoes, tea and red wine are all rich sources of flavonoids and vitamin C — powerful antioxidants that help to strengthen capillaries and reduce the risk of haemorrhoids, thrombosis and bruises.

- Rose hips (try rose hip tea), buckwheat and apple peel contain the bioflavonoid rutin, which also helps to strengthen your veins. Buckwheat makes great pancakes and can be added to breads and biscuits.

- Avocados, sprouted seeds such as alfalfa, plus eggs, raw wheatgerm and unprocessed nuts are rich in Vitamin E, which reduce stickiness in the blood.

- Garlic, onions, ginger, and cayenne pepper all aid circulation.

- Eat plenty of fish, especially oily fish. The essential fatty acids (EFAs) they contain reduce pain and keep blood vessels soft and pliable. Aim for 2–3 portions per week. Eat more sunflower, pumpkin, sesame and linseeds, which are all high in essential fats and fibre (see *Fats for Anti-ageing p139*).

- Drink more water – six to eight glasses a day of bottled or filtered water. Water maintains blood pressure and reduces constipation.

- Make sure that your diet contains plenty of fibre to prevent constipation. Fruits, vegetables, wholegrains such as brown rice and quinoa, beans and lentils are your best sources. If you feel you need more than you're getting in your diet, skip the bran – a harsh, insoluble fibre – and use instead soluble fibre-rich (cracked) flax seeds such as Linusit Gold or psyllium husks, both available in your local health food store.

- If constipation is a real problem for you, in addition to the fibre, water and exercise recommended above and below, eat 4 prunes or a fig prior to each meal.

Useful Remedies

- For centuries plant extracts such as butcher's broom and horse chestnut seeds (commonly known as conkers) have been used to reduce inflammation and swelling associated with leg problems and science has now validated these age-old remedies. Dr John Wilkinson, Head of the Phyto Chemistry Discovery Group at Middlesex University in the UK, says, "We have found that saponins, a group of active agents found in the roots and seeds of these plants constrict and strengthen veins, have anti-inflammatory properties, and reduce swelling, thus making venous return to the heart more efficient. The compounds in these plants can be taken internally in capsule form daily (but not during the first three months of pregnancy, or by people on blood thinning drugs). Plant extracts can also be used topically in a cream or gel. We have found that butcher's broom is highly effective even when taken in isolation, but its effects appear to be amplified if combined with horse chestnut, vitamin C, and the flavonoid rutin." I used John's valuable quote here because at the time of going to print, various EU bureaucrats have stated that supplements containing herbs and vitamins are now illegal. Others remain under threat. And yet scientists have proof that these products work. Most health shops sell butcher's broom, which also reduces heaviness, tingling and cramping associated with varicose veins. Take 100–300mg standardized extract two to three times daily, or try V-Nal combination capsules made by Bional, available at most chemists and health shops worldwide.

- Horse chestnut seed extract can also be taken either as a combination or on its own. Clinical trials have confirmed its ability to aid vein contraction, reduce vein fragility and permeability and significantly reduce lower limb swelling. You need 50–75mg of aescin twice daily – the active ingredient in horse chestnut. If you prefer a tincture, take 1–4ml twice a day.

- Another herb, gotu kola, has also shown impressive clinical results in treating both varicose veins and varicose ulcers by improving circulation in the lower limbs and stimulating connective tissue repair. Try 500mg twice daily.

- Bioflavonoids help reduce swelling and strengthen the vein walls. Take 1000mg of the bioflavonoid rutin daily. .

- Silica is an excellent mineral for toughening up veins. Take 200mg of silica compound daily. It is available from Blackmores (see page 13).

- An antioxidant complex containing vitamins A, C, E, selenium and CoEnzyme-Q10 helps prevent free radical damage to the blood vessels as well as aiding in connective tissue repair. Take 1–2grams of vitamin C daily with meals and 400iu of natural source vitamin E, which also enhances circulation through its anti-clotting effects.

- If veins are sore and swollen, buy some witch hazel in tincture form and apply directly to the veins. Witch hazel in capsules and tincture can also be taken internally to reduce the swelling.

- Apply a little vitamin E cream mixed with 2 drops of juniper oil where the skin is sore.

- If you have facial thread veins, try Jason Vitamin K Cream for the face, which contains bioflavonoids, ginkgo biloba, and calendula, available from most good health and department stores worldwide. For your nearest stockists call Kinetics on 0845 0725 825.

Helpful Hints

- As we age, we tend to become less active and as younger people are also suffering vein problems, it's vital for your overall health and for anti-ageing that you stay active. Even brisk walking for 45 mins to an hour a day will help. Otherwise rebounding, skipping, tennis, jogging and dancing are all wonderful exercises for supporting veins. And if your legs ache, no matter what your job, swimming is the best all–round exercise for keeping legs healthy.

- For those on their feet all day, physiotherapist Geraldine Watkins recommends lying on the floor, bending the knees and placing the lower legs on a chair or bed for 15 minutes daily to give the leg valves a rest and encourage excess fluid to be absorbed back into the system. If the legs are swollen, then a cold compress should be applied.

- Also if you stand a lot all day, wear insoles to support your arches (available from John Bell in London on 0207 935 5555, or any good chemists or back shop), avoid heels over 5cm (2in) and at the first sign of vein problems wear support tights or socks.

- If you are at a desk for much of the day, take regular breaks, look for some stairs and climb them! Make sure you move for at least 30 minutes a day. But while seated use a D-shaped foot rest (available from The Back Shop on 0207 937 9120), as bending and circling the feet keeps circulation moving. When at your desk, make sure your knees are lower than your hips, which reduces compression in the arteries and veins in the groin area. Also avoid wearing tight fitting trousers, which adds to compression in the groin and back of knee areas when seated for long periods.

- Avoid crossing your legs, doing heavy lifting, or putting any unnecessary pressure on your legs.

- Reflexology, acupuncture and a firm massage can all help to increase circulation (see *Useful Information and Addresses* on page 338).

- If the veins are sore and throbbing make a warm water compress with added cypress and geranium essential oils. Use cold compresses to reduce swelling.

- Avoiding constipation and/or straining to pass stools to avoid varicose veins. Straining to go to the toilet forces blood into your lower body, which makes the problem worse. Haemorrhoids are actually varicose veins of the anus – follow the dietary guidelines above to avoid constipation and see also *Elimination p120* and *Bowels p56*.

- There is a minimally invasive laser treatment by a company called Diomed, in which lasers are used to thermally close off the faulty vein (the greater saphenous vein), often the underlying cause of many varicose veins. The treatment takes about one hour, under local anaesthetic and you can walk out. Not everyone is suitable for this type of vein treatment, but your doctor can advise. This treatment has been hugely successful in America and is now becoming available in the National Health and private sector. For further details log on to www.diomedinc.com.

- Facial thread veins can be treated using a fine needle. Often called Red Vein, the needle is quickly inserted into each end of the vein and a current passes through the needle, which cauterizes the tiny capillary, then the needle is quickly injected down the length of the vein, which makes the vein disappear. Available at most beauty salons. You then need to keep the treated areas dry for several days.

- You can also have thread veins lasered, which I found more effective. The laser literally "smashes" the thread vein and although you may have some bruising for a few days, it works very well. For details, contact Lasercare who have several clinics around the UK. Tel: 0800 028 7222, or visit: www.lasercare-clinics.co.uk

- To avoid facial thread veins in the first place, don't use very hot or very cold water on your face, as any extremes can cause delicate veins to rupture.

- Avoid strong winds and if you are out on a boat or skiing, wear thick protective creams.

- Avoid too much sunbathing.

- Finally, get a proper diagnosis says Mr John Scurr, a consultant vascular surgeon based at The Middlesex Hospital in London. "Many people believe there is little point in having veins, haemorrhoids and so on treated, thinking they will return. But these days newer diagnostic and treatment techniques are giving good long-term, and in many cases, permanent relief." For any further queries on all aspects of vein problems, Dr Scurr's website is excellent: www.jscurr.com.

WATER IN AGEING

(See also *Toxic Metal Overload*)

A baby's body is made up of approximately 75% water, and breast milk contains 87% water, so it is no wonder they have such smooth, hydrated skin and sparkling eyes. Unfortunately, as we age, our cells' ability to absorb water is impaired and levels in the body drop to around 55% by the time you are 65–70.

Why? Because over time we ingest considerable amounts of toxins, not only from our diet, but also from water, which contains more than 350 chemicals such as chlorine, fluoride, pesticides and herbicides, nitrates, plus antibiotic and hormone residues from the Pill and HRT, and heavy metal residues, such as aluminium and lead. These toxins accumulate in our bodies and eventually clog our cells, which reduces their ability to absorb water and eliminate the toxins. Paradoxically, even if you are one of the 5% of the population that drinks the recommended six to eight glasses daily – without optimum absorption, you could still be dehydrated.

Therefore, the purer the water you drink, the easier it can permeate your cells and the more hydrated and youthful you become (see Reverse Osmosis under *Helpful Hints p328*.

We lose around 3 litres of water a day: 1.5 litres of water are excreted in urine; 750ml through the skin (and more during exercise), 400ml from simply breathing, and 150ml from faeces.

We get just under a litre from food and we generate about half a litre by burning fats and carbohydrates, so we need to drink about one and a half litres, around six large glasses, every day simply to cover our losses. Very few people make the effort to drink more water, hence why 7,000 people die every year in the UK alone from kidney failure and kidney stones, and urinary tract infections are on the increase.

Dr Sebagh, a plastic surgeon in London, tells me that 80% of his patients are dehydrated and their skin could greatly improve if they would just drink more water.

Also, as we age the mechanism that triggers the feeling of thirst becomes less effective and if you wait until you are very thirsty, then you are already dehydrated.

Even the smallest degree of water loss can impair physical and mental function. And the body siphons what it needs from the colon, and faeces become hard and dry, triggering constipation. Other symptoms include headaches, lethargy and mental confusion.

The mucosal lining of your stomach and digestive system also needs water to protect it from stomach acids and if you don't drink sufficient amounts, then gastric ulcers may develop. Also, the liver is less able to perform one of its primary functions—metabolizing stored fat into usable energy, which means, if you don't drink enough, more fat remains stored in the body. Your joints and cartilage are dependant upon sufficient water for optimum functioning and to relieve joint pain.

But if you have a constant thirst this is a common symptom of diabetes; it can also denote a lack of essential fats (see *Fats for Anti-ageing p139*).

Many people have switched to bottled water believing that it is cleaner and safer than tap water. "However," says Dr John McKenna, a nutritional physician based in London and Ireland, "It depends on your definition of safe. The majority of waters are safe from a microbiological standpoint, in that chemicals like chlorine kill harmful organisms before we drink it, but once inside the body chlorine destroys the healthy bacteria in our guts which are vital for immune function. Most jug-type filters remove some of the chemicals, but many remain. Certain bottled waters are no better than tap water and you can often taste the chemicals."

He says that if you read the labels on some bottled waters, you will see they still contain nitrates which are harmful for our health and Dr McKenna says the best bottled water he has come across is SPA from Belgium (for further information visit their website: www.spa.co.uk).

Chlorine is bad for your skin, hair and for your internal organs. And in many cases chlorine levels in tap water are higher than those allowed in swimming pools!

Then, there is the question of minerals in water.

Soft water is high in sodium but low in the minerals, which are vital for good health. Whereas hard waters contain high concentrations of calcium carbonate, potassium carbonate and magnesium carbonate. The fact that some studies show a higher incidence of heart disease in hard water areas may be because high concentrations of calcium carbonate will over time harden the arteries (like furring up your kettle). Calcium carbonate (or lime) is an important ingredient in making cement or concrete.

Most people believe that if you drink mineral-rich waters, these are healthier waters. Minerals are indeed essential to health and you can absorb some of the minerals from water – but they are in an inorganic form which is not easily utilized in the body.

However, plants, vegetables and fruits, with the help of sunlight, transform inorganic minerals into organic minerals which humans can absorb and utilize far more easily. Some scientists now believe that excess inorganic minerals found in hard water can end up in your joints, which contributes to problems such as frozen shoulder. And too much calcium in your arteries adds to the plaque deposits that trigger heart and arterial diseases. Excess inorganic minerals also contribute to gall bladder and kidney stones.

Meanwhile, an excellent way to gauge if you are drinking sufficient water is by the colour of your urine. If it is a strong-coloured very dark yellow then you are not drinking enough liquids. Remember that vitamin B2 turns your urine a yellowy/orange colour, but this is normal. When you are drinking sufficient liquids your urine should be a light, white wine colour.

As you can tell, water is a big issue and if you want hydrated young skin – you need to drink more water, the purer the better.

Foods to Avoid

- Avoid or reduce alcohol and eating too many flour-based foods which can contribute to dehydration.

- Cola-type fizzy drinks, including diet drinks, affect blood sugar levels and can make you even thirstier.

- Don't drink more than 2 litres daily (under normal circumstances) as this will overburden the kidneys!

- The carbon in artificially fizzy drinks and waters grabs hold of (chelates) and removes minerals from the body, which can cause poor bone density.

- Distilled water is acidic and acidity within the body depletes minerals and accelerates the ageing process. When you boil a kettle and the steam vapour covers your window and then turns into water again, this is distilled water. It is fine for a short period especially during detoxification, but is not a long-term health strategy.

- Avoid fluoridated water. The fluoride that is added to our drinking water is a toxic, industrial waste product from the phosphate fertilizer industry. Fluoride accumulates in the body and is linked to bone and liver cancer, genetic damage and skeletal and dental fluorosis, a brown mottling that destroys teeth and eventually bone. If I lived in a fluoridated area, I would have an RO or RODI filter fitted – see *Helpful Hints*. For more help, contact the National Pure Water Association on www.npwa.freeserve.co.uk.

- Be aware that protein breakdown requires water and if you eat too much protein, you can become dehydrated.

- Don't drink too much water or fluids with main meals as it dilutes stomach acid, the very substance you need to digest your food. Drink water in-between meals.

Friendly Foods

- We absorb water more efficiently from freshly squeezed organic juices. This is live water as it is part of the "vital force" of the plant and is rich in natural enzymes and electrolytes which help transport water across the cellular membranes. You can test this yourself by drinking an eight ounce glass of freshly juiced organic fruit or vegetables, which will quench your thirst for longer than simply water. My favourite is watermelon juice, which is 90% water and great for your immune system and skin.

- If you eat 4 pieces of fruit and 4 servings of vegetables every day, this will provide almost a litre of water.

- Whether it's from a tap, in a hot drink, bottled, naturally carbonated, from a filter, reverse osmosis (see below) or whatever – please, if you want to stay younger longer – drink more water! Water re-alkalizes your system and helps to hydrate every cell in your body. The ideal amount is six to eight glasses a day.

- Increase the amount you drink if you exercise, or if the weather is hot and dry, or if you have a fever.

- Tea and coffee are OK in moderation. Caffeine does cause a loss of water, but you still get some hydration. Keep in mind that regular tea, coffee and colas are acid forming (see *Acid–Alkaline Balance p18*).

■ Organic foods contain more organic minerals that are more easily absorbed and utilized by the body.

■ Herbal teas are fine.

■ Tomatoes and lettuce are 95% water; melons, oranges broccoli and carrots are 90% water; apples, pears, berries and many other fruits are 85%, as is yoghurt. Ricotta cheese, bananas and sweetcorn contain 75% water; cooked long-grain rice, potatoes and white fish are 70% water; meat is 50% water.

■ Eat live, low-fat yoghurt to replenish healthy bacteria in the gut if you drink tap water.

Useful Remedies

■ See *Oxygen in Ageing* for a remedy that helps to sterilize water when you are travelling.

■ If you suffer with a consistently dry mouth, you are most probably lacking in potassium phosphate. Take 75mg daily it is available from Blackmores (see page 13).

■ Dry, cracking skin denotes a lack of water, B vitamins and essential fats.

■ To make sure there is sufficient moisture in the air, especially during the winter months when the heating is on, use a humidifier in the bedroom which helps to keep your skin younger longer.

■ The combination of so many chemicals in tap water destroys many vitamins in the body, so make sure you take a full-spectrum vitamin/mineral/essential fats formula daily, such as Kudos 24 (see details on page 348).

■ As chlorine destroys healthy bacteria in the gut, take an acidophilis/bifidus capsule daily with meals.

Helpful Hints

■ If you decide to use a water jug, charcoal or carbonfilter, then remember to change it regularly and be aware that many contaminants such as heavy metals, viruses and hormone residues (from the Pill and HRT) will still get through. Wash jugs regularly.

■ You can have various types of water filters such as ceramic filters plumbed under your sink that will help remove many impurities and toxins. But even these will let fluoride and some metal pollutants through. Or install a reverse osmosis (RO) water system, which passes through microscopic filters, to remove all minerals and toxins including pesticides and herbicides. However, you can still get minute seepage of some nitrates (from fertilizers) and fluoride, and depending on the RO system you choose, you will get between 80 and 95% purity, which is far better than tap and certain bottled waters. The RO units I recommend are supplied by The Fresh Water Filter Company, tel: 0870 442 3633, visit www.freshwaterfilter.com, or email: mail@freshwaterfilter.com.

- One of the purest waters is "reverse osmosis de-ionized (RODI) water". If you want 99.999% pure water, like the rain water that fell through unpolluted skies aeons ago, then you need RODI water. It is similar to reverse osmosis water, in that it is passed through microscopic filters, but then it is also passed through a resin which attracts and removes any remaining impurities. RODI water will even filter anthrax spores. This water called Pure H2O is available in bottles from most supermarkets and health stores. Or you can treat yourself to a plumbed in unit under your sink. The water tastes great. However as this water is totally pure and no longer contains minerals, this would mean that you would need to take a multi mineral daily (excluding iron if you are over 50). For details of your nearest stockists of RODI water, contact The Pure H2O Company on 01784 221188, or on www.purewater.co.uk. RODI units are available in more than 40 countries worldwide.

- From all the experts and scientists I have spoken to whilst researching this book, several of them recommend either Spa or Fiji water (rich in absorbable silica which is great for your skin) which are both widely available in stores and supermarkets.

- Soft water is acidic; it's therefore better for the skin externally and lathers easily.

- Remember that all tap waters contain chlorine and the steam we inhale while showering can contain up to 50 times the levels of chemicals that are in tap water, which are absorbed via our lungs directly into our bloodstream. And the inhalation of chlorine is now a suspected cause of asthma and bronchitis. Chlorine in shower and bath water also robs the skin and hair of moisture. Therefore if you love hot, steamy showers consider installing a whole house filter near your stopcock. Both the above companies can advise you on whole house systems. As I write, I am horrified to discover this about chlorine as I have just fitted a large steam shower – as the steam helps detoxify the body (or so I believed) and helps me to breathe better during the winter when I'm prone to occasional chest problems. So now, I shall have to have the marble tiles smashed out, to make way for a filter, so that the steam will be free of toxins!

- Drinking sufficient water every day is the best treatment for fluid retention. If you drink less than your body needs, it perceives the shortage as a threat to survival and will begin to retain every drop. Water reserves are stored in the spaces outside the cells and you may get swollen feet, hands and legs. The best way to overcome water retention is to give your body what it needs—plenty of water—only then will stored water be released.

- In Indian hospitals, it is common practice to magnetize the water, which "energizes it", and enables easier absorption into the cells. For details of good magnets, you can always ask at your local health store.

- Dr Batmanghelidj MD, has discovered that many modern diseases are due to dehydration of the body. In his book *My Natural Miracle Cure Program* and his most famous book *Your Body's Many Cries for Water*, Tagman Press, he has shown that with an increased intake of pure water he has been able to cure a large number of serious diseases. These books make enlightening reading.

WEIGHT PROBLEMS IN AGEING

(See also *Blood Type in Ageing, Carbohydrate Control, Calorie Restriction in Ageing, Diabetes – Late-onset* and *Thyroid in Ageing*)

Few factors are so critical to ageing as being overweight. Insurance actuaries are under no illusion: every extra pound of flesh measurably reduces your life expectancy. You may see obese people in their 50s and 60s, but you rarely see obese individuals in their 70s and onwards, as they have usually died of a heart attack or stroke.

More than 300 million people worldwide are obese and the problem is accelerating at an alarming rate. One in five adults is clinically obese, which causes more than 30,000 premature deaths a year in the UK alone.

Research shows that women who gain more than 20 kg (44 pounds) after the age of 18 (above the weight they should be for their height and age) are two and a half times more likely to eventually suffer a stroke. People who are significantly overweight are five times more likely to develop diabetes. More than 85% of people with Type 2 diabetes are overweight when first diagnosed. Obese men are 33% more likely to die of cancer and this rises to 55% in women.

The basics of finding your perfect weight and then maintaining it are: controlling your blood sugar levels, eating a varied diet that contains plenty of fibre and taking sufficient exercise. If you feel that you have truly tried every diet and you are still finding it hard to lose weight, then you may have an under-active thyroid, a chronic food intolerance that is causing water retention, or an overloaded liver that's allowing toxins to accumulate, which your body is then storing away in fat cells. Steroids are well known to trigger weight gain.

The human body contains 30 to 40 million fat cells and any extra calories we eat are stored as fat. As we age, the majority of us become less physically active, our metabolism slows down, and toxins begin to accumulate. The net result is "middle-age spread", we slowly gain weight, which makes us more prone to health problems that can shorten our life and reduce our quality of life along the way.

This book is about living consciously – you can choose. Choose what you put in your mouth and you can choose your weight. And if you choose to lose weight, then do it for yourself - and if you are happy being "overweight" then so be it.

Meanwhile I believe it is important to stop thinking "diet" and start thinking "eating more healthily for the rest of our lives". There are cabbage diets, zone diets, protein only diets, eat a twinkie only at night diet – and so on. And almost half of women between 25–35 are on a diet – but in the long-term they don't work. For example, if you go on a diet trying to survive on only 1,000 calories a day, your brain will begin craving more glucose which is the only form of fuel it utilizes and the more sugar you eat, the more this disrupts blood sugar levels and the more you will go on craving sugary foods. When you suddenly restrict your calories to less than you need, your body thinks there's a famine on and your metabolic rate slows down to protect your energy reserves to help you survive the shortage. When you come off your diet, which you surely will because you can't live successfully on a crash diet, and start eating as you were before, your slowed metabolism means you put anything you lost straight back on, and it's now harder than ever to lose it. This yo-yo dieting experience is all too common. Yet many studies show that 90% of dieters regain every ounce lost and 30% of these people become heavier than before their diet.

Rather than going "on a diet", I recommend simply changing the one you are already eating.

If you are 20% or more over your ideal weight, you are technically obese. This extra weight puts undue stress on the back, legs, joints, circulation and internal organs. Obesity increases the body's susceptibility to infection, the risk of heart disease, high blood pressure, arthritis, diabetes, stroke and other serious health problems that can result in premature death.

So how do you know if, for your height, build, age and sex, you're "normal", overweight or obese? There have been numerous charts produced, but the most recognized method, that's easy to do, is the Body Mass Index (BMI). Simply, the ratio of your weight in kilograms to your height in meters squared; it's a good rough guide and is widely used. The "normal" range is 20–25; over 25 is considered overweight, over 30 is moderately obese, and over 40 is very obese. As an example, a 1.8m- (6-foot-) man weighing 80 kilograms (177 pounds) has a BMI of 24 (80 divided by (1.83x1.83) and is a normal weight, but a 1.5m- (5–foot man-) weighing 177 pounds (80 kilograms) has a BMI of 34 and is regarded as obese – his normal weight would be no more than 58kgs (130 pounds). Calculate your BMI and use it to determine what your target weight should be.

Also, research from America, Japan and France has confirmed that a tendency to over-eat and to store fat is largely controlled by biochemical signals emitted by a part of the brain called the hypothalamus. As well as governing many important processes such as temperature and hormone balance, the hypothalamus also controls the feeling of being satisfied. It also interprets emotional upset, stress or low blood sugar as hunger, and sends a message to the body to eat. Snacking on sugary foods gives the brain a quick energy boost for a short time, but then triggers a further drop in blood sugar levels, which causes the hypothalamus to demand more fuel. This vicious cycle can trigger numerous symptoms ranging from chronic exhaustion, mood swings and brain "fog" to black outs. The answer is to keep the hypothalamus happy by controlling blood sugar levels (see *Low Blood Sugar* and *Sugar* for more details).

Don't omit all your favourite foods at once, as this will cause you to become despondent and go on a binge. The slower you do this, the easier it will be for your body to adjust. Sugar is highly addictive and it takes a good month to educate your body to a new way of eating.

The high protein/low carbohydrate diet has attracted a lot of attention in recent years (often called the Atkins diet). The theory is that carbohydrates are bad for weight control, being turned into sugars and then fat. But it's mostly the refined "white" carbohydrates that cause the weight gain, not the unrefined ones like brown rice.

Therefore many of the "new" diets suggest lots of protein and no carbohydrates at all. But protein can be harder to digest and metabolize, releasing energy more slowly and not being stored as fat. This diet isn't a good long-term weight loss strategy. Excessive protein is very acidic in the body and therefore could contribute to osteoporosis in later life. The kidneys become stressed, metabolism is imbalanced and the saturated fat that accompanies animal protein can increase the risk of heart disease. People do experience initial weight loss on this diet, perhaps due in large part to the exclusion of wheat and sugar (most people's main carbohydrate). A better approach is to eat as great a variety of foods as possible and to make a life-long change to your diet, whilst cutting down on wheat-based foods (see *Diet – The Stay Younger Longer Diet* on page 114).

Many people find that on a trial "exclusion diet" for food allergies or intolerance they lose weight easily, while eating heartily. The common food intolerances are usually starchy or sugary in nature (wheat, corn, milk, sugar and potato) and this is not unlike the low carbohydrate diet mentioned above. But avoiding any food which is badly tolerated, whether it be "fattening" or not, usually enables rapid weight loss. Not only that, but you will feel much better and look younger.

This was the theme of the world's first ever Anti-ageing Book, *How to Live 100 Years* by Luigi Cornaro. The author was a 15th-century Italian nobleman who decided he didn't want to die in his 40s of excess food and drink. He began eliminating what he termed "rough" foods. We would say foods to which we have a sensitivity. In an age when the average life expectancy was under 40, he lived until 98!

Finally, don't be tempted to cut corners and use weight-loss pills claiming to be fat blockers or fat magnets. These products encourage you to eat a cheeseburger, then take a pill and you won't gain weight. This is definitely not the way to try to improve your health and like low-fat diets, they can stop you absorbing essential fats (the good ones) plus other fat-soluble nutrients that depend on fats to be transported into the body, such as vitamins A, D, E and K. Weight loss is best done slowly and for the long haul if you want to improve not just your weight but your health too.

Foods to Avoid

■ Cut down on the refined carbohydrates, croissants, Danish pastries, meat pies, desserts, burgers, pizzas and melted cheese-type snacks. By all means have a treat, once a week or so, but once you start losing weight and stop eating these foods all the time, your need for them will gradually disappear.

■ Artificial sweeteners found in over 3,000 foods and low-calorie drinks places a strain on the liver and can slow weight loss. The worst offender is aspartame.

■ Cut down on fried, fast foods and high-fat takeaways – Indian foods in sauces are one of the worst offenders.

■ Keep in mind that most low fat foods are high in sugar or sweeteners; check labels. Reduce foods high in sugar – sugar turns to fat inside the body if it is not used up during exercise. We all need a certain amount of fat and fat free diets are dangerous (see *Fats For Anti-ageing*).

■ Avoid salted nuts and highly preserved meats.

■ Reduce sodium-based table salt.

■ Avoid all hard margarines, full-fat milk, chocolate and full-fat cheeses.

■ Stop ordering desserts when you eat out or try the fruit salad.

■ It is the foods that you eat every day, and crave the most, that trigger the majority of your problems, keep a food diary and check what you eat the most.

Friendly Foods

■ Eat more organic foods which contain fewer pesticides – pesticides live in your fat tissue and are really hard to eliminate.

■ Eat nothing but fruit before midday – this is a great way to kick start a sluggish metabolism.

■ Instead of white flour-based foods, use wholemeal bread and experiment with various pastas made from corn, rice, lentil and potato flour.

■ Instead of wheat-based breads try amaranth crackers, rice or oatcakes, spread with a little houmous or cottage cheese – add a tomato and cucumber for a quick snack.

■ Eat more brown rice, lentils, chickpeas, barley and dried (or tinned) beans.

■ Eat plenty of fresh fruits and vegetables – the more fibre the better. Cabbage, broccoli, Brussels sprouts, cauliflower, onions, ginger, spring greens, spinach, pak choy, celery, pineapple and apples are all great foods for assisting weight loss. Radiccio, fennel, celeriac and bitter foods help to cleanse the liver, which aids weight loss (see *Liver in Ageing p189*).

■ Use organic rice milk, or skimmed milk instead of full-fat milk.

■ Eat quality protein twice daily, such as fish, eggs, chicken, as protein balances blood sugar for a longer period. Try and eat the protein at breakfast or/and lunchtime.

■ A jacket potato is fine, but fill it with low-fat yoghurt and chives instead of butter.

■ Always eat breakfast; there are dozens of organic low-sugar cereals now available and a great breakfast is organic porridge made with half water and half rice milk. Use a few raisins and a chopped apple to sweeten.

■ If you are desperate for sugar, use a little fructose which is many times sweeter than ordinary sugar, so you use far less and it has a lower glycaemic index (see *Sugar in Ageing*).

■ Drink lots of herbal teas and at least six to eight glasses of water a day. Water suppresses appetite and helps prevent fat depositing in the body, and it reduces water retention and encourages toxins to be flushed through the body.

■ Essential fats are vital if you want to lose weight (see *Fats For Anti-ageing p139*).

■ Use rice or oat bran for extra fibre.

- Ask at your health shop for a magnesium and potassium-based salt.
- Vegetarians tend to suffer less obesity, less heart disease and significantly less cancer.
- Caffeine is an appetite suppressant, though a fairly toxic one.

Useful Remedies

- Junk foods deplete many vital minerals from the body and virtually everyone who eats too many refined foods is lacking in the mineral chromium. Begin taking 200mcg daily to help reduce your chance of developing late-onset diabetes and to reduce cravings for sweet and refined foods. Take 200mcg twice daily in-between meals.
- Take a high-strength B-complex to support your nerves and aid digestion.
- Include a good-quality multivitamin/and mineral in your regimen, see page 348.
- The essential fatty acid conjugated linoleic acid (CLA) helps to burn fat while increasing muscle mass. Call BioCare for details (see page 13).
- Co-EnzymeQ10 is needed for the conversion of fat into energy within the cells. Research shows that half of all obese people are deficient in CoQ10. Take 30–150mg per day.
- Soluble fibre such as ready cracked flax/linseed seeds such as Linusit Gold or psyllium husks taken prior to meals has been shown to induce the feeling of fullness. Try having a heaped teaspoon of psyllium husks in a full glass of water 30 minutes before meals. They taste awful, but do the job!
- The amino acid, tyrosine, helps you maintain your chosen weight once you have reached it.

Helpful Hints

- Some people find it easier to lose weight by "grazing" all day on healthy snacks, to balance their blood sugar. A study published in the *New England Journal of Medicine* in 1989 proved that eating small healthy snacks every hour or so released far less of the stress hormone cortisol, which is very ageing. So constant nibbling is one of the simplest but effective ways to start losing weight. Others says that if they eat three sensible meals a day – which includes a porridge type breakfast, a good lunch (without dessert) and a light supper, with no snacks in-between, they also lose weight. Listen to your body.
- Have a look at the *Blood Type in Ageing* section page 51, as many people who have stubborn weight that won't budge – even with a sensible diet and exercise – often lose the last unwanted pounds when they "Eat Right for Their Blood Type".
- Nobel Prize winner and pioneer of optimum nutrition, Linus Pauling, advised avoiding fad diets you can't stick to. To reduce your calorie intake from all sources, eat a diet you like and can continue.
- Regular exercise increases your metabolic rate, decreases fat deposits, reduces food cravings and suppresses appetite. Regular exercise also increases muscle mass, which burns

more energy just to keep the muscles functioning properly. The most important part of regular exercise is that it needs to be regular and burning yourself out in the first week is the surest way to not continue.

- Gradually build the intensity, and vary the style of exercise. Consider joining a local dance, aerobic exercise or swimming club. It really helps if you work with people who have the same goal in mind. For this reason join Weight Watchers, call 08457 123000 to find your nearest club or log on to www.weightwatchers.co.uk

- Eat the majority of your food before 7pm if possible and try to make breakfast and lunch your larger meals of the day.

- An excess of oestrogen can cause weight gain and water retention if your body is low in progesterone (for details of natural progesterone cream see *Menopause p212*).

- One of the best books I have seen which clearly explains how to permanently control your weight is *Body Wise* by Dr John Briffa, Cima Books.

- Try the book *Grow Young and Slim* by Nick Delgado. He also has a website: at www.growyoungandslim.com

- An interesting book is *The Detox Diet* by Dr Paula Baillie-Hamilton. She argues that our natural weight regulation system is being poisoned by the toxic chemicals we encounter in our everyday lives, and that this damage makes it increasingly difficult to control our weight.

- As Dr Dean Ornish likes to point out, his complex carbohydrate diet is the only one scientifically proven to work against ageing. Try reading his book *Eat More, Weigh Less*, Quill Press.

- If you suffer from an eating disorder, get professional help. Contact The Eating Disorders Association, 1st Floor, Wensum House, 103 Prince of Wales Road, Norwich NR1 1DW or call their Helpline 0845 634 7650, open Monday to Friday, 9.00am–6.30pm, or their youth helpline 0845 634 7650, open Monday to Friday, 4.00pm–6.00pm. Their website is www.edauk.com, or email info@edauk.com to join.

WOMEN'S HORMONES IN AGEING

(See also *Menopause, Osteoporosis* and *Other Vital Hormones*)

We are all living much longer and the average life span of a woman has increased from 48 years in the year 1900, to 85 years in the year 2001. Unfortunately, our glands do tend to slow down and no longer produce the abundant hormones of youth after middle age. Women's hormones go through a complex series of changes from menses through menopause and finally into post-menopause. Many changes occur throughout each of these phases of hormonal life. The major hormones involved in the menstrual cycle are oestradiol, progesterone, luteinizing hormone (LH), and follicle stimulating hormone (FSH). However other hormones such as testosterone and DHEA have an important role in a woman's overall hormonal health.

Everything you eat, drink and do, and how you live your life will affect your hormone levels and hence the way you look and feel, as well as the state of your overall health. From your mid-20s or even younger if you are experiencing health problems you should get your hormone levels checked to ensure these are optimal. If they are sub-optimal they could be affecting your health and wellbeing.

Ideally the menstrual cycle will remain virtually unchanged until peri-menopause begins. More likely though, we see abnormal hormonal changes that can bring about PMT or failed ovulations or abnormal hormonal changes after pregnancy, or a build-up in the body of oestrogen-like chemicals from the environment, all of which contribute to the ageing effects that we see. Menopause and post-menopause is covered in another section (see *Menopause p212*).

Premenstrual Tension (PMT)
PMT is most often caused by a high oestrogen to progesterone ratio, called oestrogen dominance. This can be due to any of the following causes, high follicle stimulating hormone (FSH) levels, menstrual cycles with failed ovulation, imbalance in nutrition, impaired liver function, or a build-up of oestrogen-like chemicals from the environment. The symptoms are bloating, weight gain, headache, backache, irritability, depression, breast swelling or tenderness, loss of libido, and fatigue. These symptoms usually occur a week to 10 days before menstruation. These symptoms are most often corrected by improving the nutritional status and if needed, supplemental natural progesterone to offset the increased oestrogen activity.

Endocrine Disrupting Chemicals (EDCs)
Become informed about EDCs – *Hormone Deception* by D. Lindsey Berkson is a useful book on the subject. EDCs are abundant in our modern world, in solvents, plastics, air fresheners, packaging, animal fats, pesticides etc but can be avoided if you are aware. These oestrogen mimics can have insidious side-effects and unbalance our natural hormones. Many are not easily broken down by the body and can accumulate within our tissues. Most are stored in the body's fat and are there for many years, even decades. In a woman's body, fatty tissue is concentrated in the breast and ovaries, and in the placenta during foetal development, but is also found in other organs, including the brain, as well as throughout the body for padding, insulation, and as caloric reserves.

Pregnancy
After the birth of a child, progesterone levels drop rapidly from the level needed during pregnancy back to the normal non-pregnant levels. This often causes a drop in adrenal function, which leads to tiredness. It is even believed that the drop in progesterone level is responsible for the post-partum depression that occurs in some women, and natural progesterone has been used successfully to treat this condition. In some women, the balance between the oestrogen and progesterone activity is never fully restored and a long-term hormonal imbalance results.

Peri-menopause
Peri-menopause is the time period from 3 to 5 years before menopause when the hormonal levels are very unstable. The oestrogen levels go from low to very high day-to-day, and menstruation becomes very irregular. Characteristically there is a low progesterone level.

Foods to Avoid

- Among the foods contraindicated in PMT are heavily salted foods, junk foods, fatty foods, and tea and coffee. Consumption of dairy products and carbohydrates should be limited.

- Limit animal fats as they have a high concentration of EDCs.

- Eat fresh organic food – food grown without pesticides, herbicides, or synthetic fertilizer.

- Minimize plastic food and water containers especially when heating food in the microwave oven.

Friendly Foods

- Eat whole, fresh, preferably organic foods and avoid refined and processed foods, additives, preservatives, and colourings.

- Eat a plant-based diet, emphasizing plenty of fresh, preferably organic vegetables, wholegrains, legumes, nuts, and fruit.

- Eat modest servings of eggs, yoghurt, and deep-sea, cold-water fish ocean fish four to five times a week.

- Emphasize olive oil and avoid hydrogenated oils and most vegetable oils.

Useful Remedies

- Take Vitamin B-complex, 100mg per day. It is needed for the liver to process oestrogens.

- Take a multimineral complex to supply minerals critical to hormonal function.

- Linseed oil, 1000mg per day, helps improve the hormone balance in the body.

- Natural progesterone. If you are suffering the symptoms of oestrogen dominance, supplementation with natural progesterone helps to rebalance the hormones. Natural progesterone is made entirely from the wild yam and can be applied on the skin. It is available in the UK on prescription or through PharmWest UK, Freephone 00800-8923-8923. For more help see *Menopause, Osteoporosis* **and** *Other Vital Hormones*.

* * * * * * * * * * * * * *

Well, after eight months of interviewing specialists and typing for England, I can hardly believe I have reached the end of what I, Bob, Steve and Shane pray will be a useful and inspiring book. Meanwhile, with computer-sore eyes and a numb backside – I'm off to start practising what I have preached in this book– and then some! I apologise if a specific condition in which you have an interest is not mentioned, but if I had written about every illness associated with ageing, this book would have run to thousands of pages. Otherwise, have a look at my revised and updated book *500 of The Most Important Health Tips You'll Ever Need*, which offers advice in the same format as this book for more than 200 common conditions.

Good luck on your journey.

Hazel Courteney
www.hazelcourteney.com

USEFUL INFORMATION AND ADDRESSES

ACUPUNCTURE

Practitioners use fine, sterile needles inserted into specific points to stimulate energy and to move it more easily around the body, which encourages the body to heal itself. Acupuncture is marvellous for a whole myriad of problems for erectile dysfunction to back pain. To find your nearest practitioner contact:

British Acupuncture Council
63 Jeddo Road, London W12 9HQ
Tel: 020 8735 0400
Website: www.acupuncture.org.uk or e-mail: info@acupuncture.org.uk

ALEXANDER TECHNIQUE

A great technique for helping prevent rounded shoulders and "stooping" as you get older. Once you stand and walk properly, it gives you a greater air of self-confidence. Teaches you how to use your body more efficiently and how to have balance and poise with minimum tension in order to avoid pain, strain and injury. To find your nearest practitioner, or list of affiliated societies worldwide, contact:

Society of Teachers of the Alexander Technique
1st Floor, Linton House, 39-51 Highgate Road, London, NW5 1RS
Tel: 0845 230 7828
Website: www.stat.org.uk, or e-mail: office@stat.org.uk

AROMATHERAPY

If you are under stress, in pain or simply in need of a treat, there is nothing better than having a full body aromatherapy massage in a cosy warm room. Within 15 minutes of being applied, the oils are absorbed into the body and a relaxing/or uplifting effect is felt, depending on the oils used. Excellent theraputic grade oils are available in the UK via Susie Anthony, Tel: 01749679900, or try logging onto www.psa lifemastery.com. For a register of practitioners contact:

International Federation of Aromatherapists (IFA)
61-63 Churchfield Road, London, W3 6AY
Tel: 020 8992 9605
Website: www.ifaroma.org, or e-mail: office@ifaroma.org
or
The International Society of Professional Aromatherapists (IFPA)
82 Ashby Road, Hinckley, Leicestershire, LE10 1SN
Tel: 01455 637 987
Website:www.ifparoma.org, or e-mail admin@ifparoma.org

BACH FLOWER REMEDIES

A healing system used to treat emotional problems such as fear and hopelessness. The liquid remedies are made from the flowers of wild plants, bushes and trees. For further information contact:

The Dr. Edward Bach Centre
Mount Vernon, Bakers Lane, Brightwell-cum-Sotwell, Oxon, OX10 0PZ
Tel 01491 834 678
Website: www.bachcentre.com or e-mail: mail@bachcentre.com
Naturopath Jan De Vries has also formulated a marvellous range of flower remedies. For details log on to www.avogel.co.uk

BOOKS

If you have difficulty finding any of the recommended books, or simply want to find a book on your condition, the NutriCentre bookshop in London carry an extensive library of self-help books and are happy to order for you, or give assistance on specific subjects. Tel: 020 7323 2382.

Most of my favourite books are mentioned throughout the book under the various conditions, but I also recommend *Ultimate Health* by Dr John Briffa, Penguin Books. He is not only a good friend, but a brilliant nutritional physician. This book will help you to be well in mind, body and in spirit.

If you do not find your specific condition in this book, then have a look at my last book, *500 of The Most Important Health Tips You'll Ever Need*, Cico Books, – which covers over 200 conditions in the same format as this book.

CHIROPRACTIC

Manipulation to treat disorders of the joints and muscles and their effect on the nervous system. Chiropractors treat the entire body to bring it back into balance and restore health. I visit my chiropractor every few months, who keeps my spine and neck mobile and almost free of pain after an injury several years ago. To find a practitioner contact:

The British Chiropractic Association
Blagrave House, 17 Blagrave Street, Reading, Berkshire RG1 1QB
Tel: 0118 950 5950
Website: www.chiropractic-uk.co.uk or e-mail: enquiries@chiropractic-uk.co.uk
or
McTimoney Chiropractic Association
Wallingford, Oxon, OX10 8DJ
Tel: 01491 829211
Website: www.mctimoney-chiropractic.org
or e-mail admin@mctimoney-chiropractic.org

COLONIC HYDROTHERAPY

A method of cleansing the colon to gently flush away toxic waste, gas, accumulated faeces and mucous deposits. Check with your GP before undertaking this therapy. Colonics are very useful if you are chronically constipated or have taken antibiotics or painkillers, which can cause constipation. I have a colonic whenever I have taken antibiotics or had any kind of surgery to help remove the toxins from my system. I visit Margie Finchell who is brilliant. Tel: 020 7724 1291. You can also buy small individual boxed enemas made by Fletchers, which can be purchased from all good chemists. You simply lie on your side, insert the plastic nozzle and gently squeeze in the contents. Then stay on your back to allow the liquid to penetrate and then sit on the loo for a few minutes. It is not anything like the full colonic, but very useful for occasional constipation. To find your nearest practitioner contact:

The Guild of Colonic Hydrotherapists
16 Drummond Ride, Tring, Hertfordshire, HP23 5DE
Tel: 01442 825632
Website: www.colonic-association.com

COUNSELLING

If you, or a member of your family, are in need of professional counselling, to find your nearest practitioner contact:

British Association for Counselling and Psychotherapy
BACP House, 35-37 Albert Street, Rugby, Warwickshire, CV21 2SG
Tel: 01788 550899
Website: www.bacp.co.uk, or e-mail: bacp@bacp.co.uk

CRANIAL OSTEOPATHY

A gentle method of osteopathy concentrating on nerves and bones in the head, neck and shoulders. Many people have reported relief from ME (Chronic Fatigue Syndrome), facial pain, jaw pain and arthritis from this therapy. To find your nearest practitioner, contact:

International Bio-Cranial Academy
1 High Street Manor, Comber, County Down BT23 5TF
Tel: 028 9187 1334
Website:www.biocranial.com or e-mail: bcranial@aol.com

FOOD COMBINING

Nutritionist Kathryn Marsden, has made this subject her speciality and her books have sold by the millions worldwide. If you are interested in Food Combining there is no better book than *The Complete Book of Food Combining* by Kathryn Marsden. Piatkus Books, or *The Food Combining Diet*, HarperCollins.

INSTITUTE FOR COMPLEMENTARY MEDICINE
If you want to know more about specific alternative therapies, the Institute will be happy to give you advice and put you in touch with the practitioners and societies that now meet with their high standards of practice and therapy. Contact:

Institute for Complementary Medicine
PO Box 194, London SE16 1QZ
Tel: 020 7237 5165
Website: www.i-c-m.org.uk or e-mail:info@I-c-m.org.uk

HALE CLINIC
This clinic is the largest alternative treatment centre in Europe with over 100 practitioners, many of whom are also qualified medical doctors. Some of the best people working in alternative medicine in the UK are based at this clinic.

The Hale Clinic
7 Park Crescent, London W1N 3HE
Tel: 0870 167 6667 Website: www.haleclinic.com

HERBALISM
Using plants to treat disease. Treatment may be given in the form of fluid extracts, tinctures, tablets or teas. For further details, or a register of qualified members, contact:

The National Institute of Medical Herbalists (NIMH)
Elm House, 54 Mary Arches Street, Exeter, EX4 3BA
Tel: 01392 426022
Website: nimh.org.uk or e-mail: nimh@ukexter.freezerve.co.uk

Specialist herbal supplies
Supply organic source whole herbs. For further details contact:
Tel: 0870 774 4494. Website: www.shs100.com

HOMEOPATHY
Works in harmony with the body to stimulate the body's natural healing mechanisms. For a register of professional qualified homeopaths and general information about homeopathy contact:

The Society of Homeopaths
11 Brookfield, Duncan Close, Moulton Park, Northampton, NN3 6WL
Tel: 0845 450 6611
Website: www.homeopathy-soh.org or e-mail: info@homeopathy-soh.org

or Homeopathic Medical Association (HMA)

6 Livingstone Road, Gravesend, Kent DA12 5DZ

Tel: 01474 560336

Website: www.the-hma.org. or e-mail: info@the-hma.org

or British Homeopathic Association (BHA)
Hahneman House, 29 Park Street West, Luton, LU1 3BE
Tel : 0870 444 3950
Website: www.trusthomeopathy.org

HYPNOTHERAPY

With deep relaxation techniques you can access the subconscious mind – the computer programme which contains everything that you have ever experienced. In this way the therapist can trace back to the root cause for many problems including stress, phobias, weight problems, some medical conditions and unwanted emotional and addictive behaviours such as smoking. The therapist and client can then help reprogramme and heal the problems. To find your nearest practitioner, contact:

The General Hypnotherapy Register
PO Box 204, Lymington, Hants SO41 6WP
Tel (24hr answerphone): 01590 683770
Website: www.general-hypnotherapy-register.com. or e-mail
admin@general-hypnotherapy-register.com

Or the National Council for Hypnotherapists.
Tel: 0800 952 0545
Website www.hypnotherapists.org.uk or e-mail: admin@hypnotherapists.org.uk
Over the years I have visited Leila Hart in London – she is a brilliant and highly qualified therapist who really helps me to relax. Monday–Friday 10am–6pm. Tel: 0207 402 4311.

INSTITUTE OF OPTIMUM NUTRITION

The Institute of Optimum Nutrition prints a wonderful quarterly magazine which is packed with up-to-date health news and the latest research in alternative medicine. The Institute also holds seminars on health and have in-house nutritionists. For further information contact (or for a directory of practitioners send £5) :

Institute for Optimum Nutrition (ION)
Avalon House, 72 Lower Mortlake Rd, Richmond, Surrey, TW9 2JY
Tel: 0870 979 1122
Website: www.ion.ac.uk or e-mail: info@ion.ac.uk

KINESIOLOGY
The science of testing muscle response to discover areas of impaired energy and function in the body. Kinesiology is especially useful if you think you have an allergic reaction either to a food or an external allergen. To find your nearest practitioner contact:

Association of Systematic Kinesiology
47 Seedlescombe Road South, East Sussex, TN38 0TB
Tel: 0845 020 0383
Website: www.systematic-kinesiology.co.uk

MANUAL LYMPHATIC DRAINAGE
A very gentle pulsing massage, which helps to drain the lymph nodes, thereby reducing swelling and pain related to the lymph glands. Especially useful after breast surgery. To find your nearest practitioner, contact:

MLD UK
PO Box 14491, Glenrothes, Fife KY6 3YE
Tel: 01592 840799
Website: www.mlduk.org.uk or e-mail: admin@mlduk.org.uk

NATUROPATHY
Practitioners use diet, herbs, natural hormones and supplement therapy to treat the root cause of any illness, thereby boosting the immune system and restoring health. For details of qualified practitioners, contact:

General Council and Register of Naturopaths (GCRN)
Goswell House, 2 Goswell Road, Street, Somerset BA16 0JG
Tel: 08707 456984
Website: www.naturopathy.org.uk e-mail: admin@naturopathy.or.uk

Remember that two of my co-authors Bob Jacobs (tel: 0207 487 4334) and Steve Langley (tel: 0207 631 0156) are both highly qualified and experienced naturopaths.

The Colleges of Naturopathic Medicine (CNM) are located in London, Manchester, Belfast, Dublin, Cork and Galway. For information call 01342 410505 or visit their website www.naturopathy.com

NEURO-LINGUSTIC PROGRAMMING
This is a profound and yet simple way to re-programme any negative thoughts or habits to more positive ones. Great for phobias, panic attacks and for attaining the goals in your life. For further information on NLP contact:

ANLP
PO Box 3357, Unit 14, Barnet, EN5 9AJ
Tel: 0870 444 0790
Website: www.anlp.org, or e-mail: admin@anlp.org

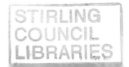

If you find any products in this book hard to find in your local health store, then either call the NutriCentre or the Sloane Health Shop. You can also speak to their in-house nutritionists free of charge – details below:

THE NUTRICENTRE

The NutriCentre, located on the lower ground floor of the Hale Clinic at 7 Park Crescent, London, is unique in being able to supply almost every alternative product currently available from any country, including specialized practitioner products. The NutriCentre offers an excellent and reliable mail order service worldwide for all its products.

> For supplements – Tel: 020 7436 5122
> For books – Tel: 020 7323 2382
> Website: www.nutricentre.com or e-mail: enq@nutricentre.com

THE SLOANE HEALTH SHOP

(If you find any supplements hard to find, the staff and nutritionists at Sloane Health are there to help you.)

> 27 King's Road, Chelsea, London SW3 4RT
> Tel: 020 7730 7046

ORGANIC FOOD AND DELIVERIES

Simply Organic is the largest supplier and home delivery service in the UK. Either log on to: www.simplyorganic.net, or call 01604 791911.

NUTRITIONAL THERAPY

To find your nearest qualified nutritionist who can help you to balance your diet and suggest the correct vitamins and minerals for your particular needs, contact:

> The British Association of Nutritional Therapists
> 27 Old Gloucester Street, London WC1N 3XX
> Tel: 0870 606 1284
> e-mail: bant.org.uk

NUTRITIONIST WHO IS ALSO A DOCTOR

You will need to be referred by your own GP who will be able to find the address of your nearest practitioner by sending a SAE to:

> British Society for Allergy Environmental and Nutritional Medicine (BSAENM)
> PO Box 7, Knighton, Powys, LD7 1WT
> Tel: 01547 550 380

ORGANIC PRODUCE

The Soil Association has published an Organic Directory, which is packed with information on where to buy organic produce throughout the country. To obtain a copy, send £7.95 plus £1 p&p to:

Soil Association
Bristol House, 40-56 Victoria Street, Bristol BS1 6BY
Tel: 0117 314 5000
Website: www.soilassociation.org e-mail: info:soilassociation.org

OSTEOPATHY

It's amazing how many people who are in skeletal pain, end up at their doctors, who then refer them for physiotherapy, which can take months. Then an X-ray may be needed which can take several more months on another waiting list. It amazes me as to why more people don't just go and see a good osteopath or chiropractor who can most probably give help on the spot, or at the very least have a better idea than a doctor as to the root cause of the problem. Practitioners use manipulation, massage and stretching techniques. To find your nearest practitioner, contact:

Osteopathic Information Service
Osteopathy House, 176 Tower Bridge Road, London SE1 3LU
Tel: 020 7357 6655 Ext 242
Website: www.osteopathy.org.uk or e-mail: info@osteopathy.org.uk

PILATES

Pilates is powerful way of exercising that is totally brilliant if you have suffered any type of injury that prevents you from working out properly. I ruptured two discs in my back a couple of years ago and after trying many treatments, Pilates has truly reduced the pain and given me the confidence to start exercising properly again. For your nearest practitioner send an SAE to:

The Pilates Foundation UK Ltd
PO Box 36052, London SW16 1XQ
Tel: 07071 781859
Website: www.pilatesfoundation.com
Anoushka Boone is my teacher and if you live near London, she has worked miracles with me. Tel: 0208 746 1199.

REFLEXOLOGY

Although it may seem that little is happening, I love reflexology. The therapist can always tell you about the problem areas in the body and by stimulating the associated points in the feet and hands, energy blockages can be removed which encourages the body to heal itself. This is a great way to boost circulation and is really relaxing. To find your nearest practitioner, contact:

Association of Reflexologists
27 Old Gloucester Street, London WC1N 3XX
Tel: 0870 567 3320 Website: www.aor.org.uk or e-mail aor@reflexology.org

or The British Reflexology Association
Monks Orchard, Whitbourne, Worcester WR6 5RB
Tel: 01886 821207 Website: www.britreflex.co.uk or e-mail:bra@britreflex.co.uk.

REIKI

Reiki (pronounced ray-key) is a Japanese word meaning Universal Life energy, an energy which is all around us. Reiki is a system of natural hands on healing, which evolved in Japan from ancient teachings. The whole person is treated, rather than specific symptoms, by a practitioner through whom the energy is channelled by the need or imbalance in the recipient. The energy goes where it is needed. A full treatment can take up to 1 hour. I have an hour of Reiki healing every week and it is magical and very relaxing; it has certainly helped me to keep going whilst I have been writing this book! For further details contact:

The Reiki Association
2 Spa Terrace, Fenay Bridge, Huddersfield, HD8 0BD
Tel: 0901 8800 009, Website: www.reikiassociation.org.uk

WEIGHT WATCHERS

As obesity is now reaching epidemic proportions – and being overweight can greatly reduce your life expectancy –– join a club where you will meet others who will give encouragement and support. Call 08457 123000 to find your nearest club, or log on to: www.weightwatchers.co.uk

WHAT DOCTORS DON'T TELL YOU

What Doctors Don't Tell You is still one of my favourite monthly newsletters packed with alternative health information, up-to-date health news and warnings about the side-effects of prescription drugs. Lynne McTaggart is famous throughout the health industry as not being afraid to tell the truth. The newsletter also has an extensive range of books on subjects ranging from cancer to the dangers of vaccinations. For details write to:

What Doctors Don't Tell You
Satellite House, 2 Salisbury Road, London SW19 4EZ
Tel: 0870 444 9887
Website: www.wddty.co.uk or e-mail: wddty@zoo.co.uk

YOGA

The ancient principles of yoga are beneficial for staying healthy and supple well into one's 80s and beyond. Yoga teaches relaxation and breathing techniques, together with gentle stretching exercises, which help keep the 'whole' self fit for life. Especially useful for keeping the organs functioning well and the spine strong. To find your nearest class, contact:

The British Wheel of Yoga
25 Jermyn Street, Sleaford, Lincolnshire NG34 7RU
Tel: 01529 306851
Website: www.bwy.org.uk or e-mail: office@bwy.org.uk

YORK LABORATORIES

I have found this laboratory extremely good for pinpointing food sensitivities and they also offer a simple pin-prick test to discover your homocysteine levels that is backed by the British Cardiac Association that can be done by post. For details call York Labs on 0800 074 6185 or log on to www.yorktest.com

KUDOS 24 Multi-Active Age Management Complex

For years I have taken up to 20 nutrients a day to help boost my immune system, nourish my skin, protect my bones, eyes, heart, circulation, brain and so on, which in turn helps slow the ageing process. It has long been my wish to help develop a multinutrient, up-to-the-minute formula, containing food state, GM-free, highly absorbable nutrients that both men and women of all ages could take once daily, and which offers 24-hour protection to help slow ageing at every level. After months of research, here it is...

Available from health and department stores.
For more Information, or to order, call 0800 389 5476.
For overseas orders call: (44) (0) 208 392 6524
Fax: (44) (0)208 392 6540
E-mail: info@kudosvitamins.com
Website: www.kudosvitamins.com

This formula is suitable for vegetarians, pregnant women (under supervision of a health professional) and for men and women of all ages. It contains:

Organic Artichoke – to help cleanse and support the liver, packed with anti-ageing phytonutrients.

Organic Aloe Vera Extract – contains the essential sugar, mannose, which boosts immune function.

Antioxidants – a full spectrum of high-strength antioxidants from grape seed extract, organic broccoli and pine bark extract.

B Vitamins – a full spectrum of all the B group, including folic acid, B1, B3, B6, B12 and biotin – all needed to support your nervous system, your hair, skin and nails and helps in the control of cholesterol.

Vitamin C – a vital antioxidant crucial for collagen production, the immune system and for more than 50 processes in the body.

Boron – an essential mineral for healthy bones and vital for people with inflammatory conditions such as arthritis.

Calcium – for healthy bones and teeth. A natural tranquilliser, also involved in nerve and muscle control.

Broccoli Extract – packed with antioxidants and helps re-alkalize the body.

Bromelain – extracted from pineapples, is highly anti-inflammatory, reduces bruising, aids digestion and absorption of nutrients from your diet.

Natural Source Carotenes – vital for a healthy immune system, for healthy eyes and skin which convert to vitamin A in the body.

Co-EnzymeQ10 – which helps your heart and gives you energy.

Carnosine – regenerates ageing cells and skin, improves muscle tone, reduces arterial plaque and is an important antioxidant.

Chromium – a mineral greatly lacking in our diets that helps reduce the cravings for sugar and reduces the likelihood of developing late-onset diabetes.

Copper – which helps in the manufacture of neurotransmitters in the brain.

Vitamin D – to promote healthy bones.

Essential Fats – extracted from hemp seed – a fantastic source of omega-3 and 6 essential fats. Vital for hydrated, younger looking skin, for the brain, for hormone production and weight loss.

Vitamin E – full spectrum vitamin E, vital for healthy skin, an antioxidant which also helps keep your blood and circulation healthy.

Glutiathione – a star brain anti-ageing nutrient, which aids brain function and detoxifies the liver.

Iron – traces of iron from organic asparagus, very safe and will not accumulate in the body.

Manganese – needed for reproduction processes and sex hormone formation.

Magnesium – equally as important as calcium for healthy bones, for lung health, for reducing stress and for keeping the body more alkaline.

Molybdenum – an anti-ageing enzyme that helps maintain DNA.

PhosphatidylSerine – a vital "good mood" brain nutrient that aids memory and learning.

Selenium – an antioxidant that helps protect against cancers and degenerative disease.

Soya Isoflavones – they help protect against hormone disrupting chemicals found in pesticides and herbicides. Regulates hormones in both sexes and helps protect against cancer. Helps keep calcium in the bones.

Soya Isolate - a complete protein that helps slow ageing.

Stomach Acid (Betain HCl) – to aid digestion and increase absorption of nutrients from your diet.

Turmeric – is anti-cancerous, anti-inflammatory and helps keep Alzheimer's disease at bay.

Zinc – essential for healthy skin, wound healing, fertility and a healthy sex life.

All these nutrients provide an excellent base for anti-ageing at every level.

INDEX